STRUCTURE AND FUNCTION
OF CEREBRAL COMMISSURES

STRUCTURE AND FUNCTION OF CEREBRAL COMMISSURES

Edited by
I. STEELE RUSSELL
MRC Unit on Neural Mechanisms of Behaviour

M. W. VAN HOF
Department of Physiology 1, Erasmus University, Rotterdam

G. BERLUCCHI
Institute of Physiology, University of Pisa

UNIVERSITY PARK PRESS
Baltimore

First published 1979 by
The Macmillan Press Ltd
London and Basingstoke

Published in North America by
UNIVERSITY PARK PRESS
233 East Redwood Street
Baltimore, Maryland 21202

Printed in Great Britain

Library of Congress Cataloging in Publication Data

Workshop on the Structure and Function of the Cerebral Commissures, Erasmus University Medical School, 1977.
   Structure and function of cerebral commissures.

   "A collection of papers culled from the European Brain Behaviour Society's Workshop on the Structure and Function of the Cerebral Commissures, which was held at the Erasmus University Medical School from March 30 to April 2, 1977."
   Bibliography: p.
   Includes index.
   1. Neuropsychology—Congresses. 2. Corpus callosum—Congresses.
I. Russell, I. Steele. II. Hof, Marius Wilhelm van, 1927– III. European Brain Behaviour Society. IV. Title. V. Title: Cerebral commissures.
QP360.W67 1977   599'.01'88   78-27587
ISBN 0-8391-1391-9

CONTENTS

LIST OF CONTRIBUTORS AND PARTICIPANTS AT THE EBBS WORKSHOP 1977

Amore, R., Center for Cerebral Neuro-
physiology, National Research Council
Institute of Neurophysiopathology,
University of Genoa, Italy

Antonini, A., Istituto di Fisiologia,
Universita di Pisa, 56100 Pisa, Via S.
Zeno 29–31, Pisa, Italy

Atal Russell, G., Wellcome Institute
for the History of Medicine,
183 Euston Road, London
NW1 2BP

Bateson, P. P. G., Department of Zoology
University of Cambridge, Cambridge

Beaubaton, D., Institut de Neurophysio-
logie et de Psychophysiologie, Departe-
ment de Psychophysiologie Generale,
C.N.R.S.–INP 4–31, chemin Joseph-
Aiguier, 13274 Marseille Cedex 2,
France

Beauvois, M. F., Laboratoire de Neuropsychologie INSERM U. 84, Hôpital de
la Salpetrière, 47 Boulevard de l'Hôpital,
75634 Paris Cedex 13, France

Berlucchi, G., Istituto di Fisiologia,
Universita di Pisa, 56100 Pisa, Via S.
Zeno 29–31, Pisa, Italy

Bertelson, P., Laboratoire de Psychologie
experimentale, Université Libre de
Bruxelles, Avenue Adolphe Buyl 117,
1050 Bruxelles, Belgium

Bookman, J., MRC Unit on Neural Mechanisms of Behaviour, 3 Malet Place,
London WC1E 7JG

Burkhalter, A., Institute for Brain Research,
University of Zurich, August-Forel
Strasse 1, CH-8029 Zurich, Switzerland

Butler, S., The University of Birmingham,
Department of Anatomy, Medical School,
Vincent Drive, Birmingham B15 2TJ

Caminiti, R., Istituto di Fisiologia Umana,
via Grotte di Posatora, 60100, Ancona,
Italy

Corvaja, N., Istituto di Fisiologia Umana, Via
S. Zeno 31, 56100 Pisa, Italy

Cuénod, M., Institute for Brain Research,
University of Zurich, August-Forel
Strasse 1, CH-8029 Zurich, Switzerland

Cupello, A., Center for Cerebral Neuro-
physiology, National Research Council
Institute of Neurophysiopathology,
University of Genoa, Italy

Doty, R. B., Center for Brain Research, Box
605, University of Rochester, Rochester,
New York 14642, U.S.A.

Downer, J. L. deC., Department of Physiology, King Faisal University Colleges of
Medicine and Medical Sciences, P.O. Box
2114 Damman, Saudi Arabia

Ettlinger, G., Institute of Psychiatry, De
Crespigny Park, Denmark Hill, London
SE5 8AF

Ferrilo, F., Center for Cerebral Neuro-
physiology, National Research Council
Institute of Neurophysiopathology,
University of Genoa, Italy

Garey, L. J., Institut d'Anatomie, Université
de Lausanne, Rue du Bugnon 9, CH-
1011 Lausanne, Switzerland

Giurgea, C. E., UCB, Division Pharmaceutique, 68 rue Berkendael, B-1060,
Bruxelles, Belgium

Goodale, M. A., Department of Psychology,
University of Western Ontario, London,
Ontario, Canada

Gordon, H. W., The Aba Khoushy School of
Medicine in Haifa, Department of
Behavioral Biology, Gutwirth Building,
Technion City, Haifa, Israel

Graf, M., Swiss Federal Institute for
Technology Zurich, Department of
Behavioral Science, Turnerstrasse 1,
CH-8006 Zurich, Switzerland

Grangetto, A., Institut de Neurophysiologie
et de Psychophysiologie, Département de
Psychophysiologie Generale, C.N.R.S.-
INP 4–31, chemin Joseph-Aiguier,
13274 Marseille Cedex 2, France

Graves, J. A., Psychological Laboratory, University of St Andrews, St Andrews, Fife, Scotland

Guiard, Y., Département de Psychobiologie Experimentale, Institut de Neurophysiologie et de Psychophysiologie, C.N.R.S.-INP 3-31, chemin Joseph-Aiguier, 13274 Marseille Cedex 2, France

Hoogland, P. V., Department of Anatomy, Free University, P.O. Box 7161, Amsterdam, The Netherlands

Horn, G., Department of Zoology, University of Cambridge, Cambridge

Innocenti, G. M., Institut d'Anatomie, Université de Lausanne, Rue du Bugnon 9, CH 1011 Lausanne, Switzerland

Kemali, M., Laboratorio di Cibernetica CNR, 80072 Arco Felice, Naples, Italy

Kuypers, H.G.J.M., Department of Anatomy Erasmus University, P.O. Box 1738, Rotterdam, The Netherlands

Lazzarini, G., Center for Cerebral Neurophysiology, National Research Council Institute of Neurophysiopathology University of Genoa, Italy

Lhermitte, F., Laboratoire de Neuropsychologie INSERM U.84, Hôpital de la Salpetrière, 47 Boulevard de l'Hôpital, 75634 Paris Cedex 13, France

Lohman, A.H.M., Department of Anatomy, Free University, P.O. Box 7161, Amsterdam, The Netherlands

Maier, V., Institut für Hirnforschung der Universität, August-Forel Strasse 1, CH-8008 Zurich, Switzerland

Manzoni, T., Istituto di Fisiologia Umana, via Grotte di Posatora, 60100, Ancona, Italy

Marzi, C. A., Istituto di Fisiologia, Universita di Pisa, 56100 Pisa, Via S. Zeno 29-31, Pisa, Italy

Meinardi, H., Instituut voor Epilepsiebestreiding, "Meer en Bosch", Achterweg 5, Heemstede, The Netherlands

Meininger, V., Laboratoire de Neuropsychologie INSERM U.84, Hôpital de la Salpetrière, 47 Boulevard de l'Hôpital, 75634 Paris Cedex 13, France

Mergner, T., Istituto di Fisiologia Umana, Via S. Zeno 31, 56100 Pisa, Italy

Mohn, G., MRC Unit on Neural Mechanisms of Behaviour, 3 Malet Place, London WC1E 7JG

Moore, J. W., Department of Psychology, Middlesex House, University of Massachusetts, Amherst, Massachusetts 01002 U.S.A.

Morais, J., Laboratoire de Psychologie experimentale, Université Libre de Bruxelles, Avenue Adolphe Buyl 117, 1050 Bruxelles, Belgium

Morgan, S. C., MRC Unit on Neural Mechanisms of Behaviour, 3 Malet Place, London WC1E 7JG

Mosidze, V. M., Institute of Physiology, Academy of Sciences of the Georgian SSR, Gotua st. N 14, Tbilisi, U.S.S.R.

Moyersoons, F., UCB, Division Pharmaceutique, 68 rue Berkendael, B-1060, Bruxelles Belgium

McQueen, J. K., MRC Brain Metabolism Unit, University Department of Pharmacology, 1 George Square, Edinburgh EH8 9JZ, Scotland

Negrão, N., Laboratorio de Neurofisiologia, Departmento de Fisiologia, Instituto de Ciencias Biomedicas, Universidade de São Paulo, C.P. 4368, São Paulo, S.P. 01000, Brasil

Overman, W. H., Center for Brain Research, Box 605, University of Rochester, Rochester, New York 14642, U.S.A.

Paillard, J., Institut de Neurophysiologie et de Psychophysiologie, Département de Psychophysiologie Generale, C.N.R.S.-INP 4-31, chemin Joseph-Aiguier, 13274 Marseille Cedex 2, France

Pompeiano, O., Istituto di Fisiologia Umana, Via S. Zeno 31, 56100 Pisa, Italy

Poppel, E., Max-Planck-Institut für Psychiatrie, Deutsche Forschungsanstalt für Psychiatrie, 8 Munchen 40, Kraepelinstrasse 2, Postfach 401240, Germany

Preilowski, B., Universität Konstanz, Fachgruppe Psychologie, Postfach 7733, D-7750 Konstanz, B.R.D.

Rizzolatti, G., Istituto di Fisiologia Umana, Universita di Parma, Via Gramsci 14, Parma, Italy

Rosadini, G., Center for Cerebral Neurophysiology, National Research Council Institute of Neurophysiopathology, University of Genoa, Italy

Rose, S.P.R., Brain Research Group, The Open University, Walton Hall, Milton Keynes

Russell, I. Steele, MRC Unit on Neural Mechanisms of Behaviour, 3 Malet Place, London WC1E 7JG

Saillant, B., Laboratoire de Neuropsychologie INSERM U.84, Hôpital de la Salpetrière, 47 Boulevard de l'Hôpital, 75634 Paris Cedex 13, France

Sanides, D., Max-Planck-Institut für Biophysikalische Chemie, Postfach 968, D-3400 Gottingen-Nikolausberg, B.R.D.

Savage, G. E., Department of Zoology and Comparative Physiology, Queen Mary College, Mile End Road, London E1 4NS

Schenk, V. W. D., Departments of Neuropathology and Neuroanatomy, Erasmus University, Rotterdam, The Netherlands

Simoni, A., Istituto di Fisiologia Umana, Via San Zeno 29–31, 56100 Pisa, Italy

Singer, W., Max-Planck-Institut für Psychiatrie, Deutsche Forschungsanstalt für Psychiatrie, 8 Munchen 40, Kraepelinstrasse 2, Postfach 401240, B.R.D.

Spidalieri, G., Istituto di Fisiologia Umana, via Fosato di Mortara 64/b, 44100, Ferrara, Italy

Sprague, J. M., Department of Anatomy, University of Pennsylvania, Philadelphia, Pennsylvania, U.S.A.

Starr, B., Psychology Academic Group, School of Natural Sciences, The Hatfield Polytechnic, P.O. Box 109, College Lane, Hatfield, Herts AL10 9AB

Stefanko, S. Z., Departments of Neuropathology and Neuroanatomy, Erasmus University, Rotterdam, The Netherlands

Stefano, M. Di, Istituto di Fisiologia Umana, via San Zeno 29–31, 56100 Pisa, Italy

Stock, G., Department of Physiology, University of Heidelberg, Im Neuenheimer Feld 326, D-6900 Heidelberg, B.R.D.

Sturm, V., Department of Physiology, University of Heidelberg, Im Neuenheimer Feld 326, D-6900 Heidelberg, B.R.D.

Swadlow, H. A., Department of Psychology, University of Connecticut, Storrs, Connecticut 06268, and Department of Neurology, Harvard Medical School, Beth Israel Hospital Boston, Massachusetts 02215, U.S.A.

Van Haelen, H., Laboratoire de Psychologie experimentale, Université Libre de Bruxelles, Avenue Adolphe Buyl 117, 1050 Bruxelles, Belgium

Van Hof, M. W., Department of Physiology 1, Erasmus University, P.O. Box 1738, Rotterdam, The Netherlands

Waxman, S. G., Department of Neurology, Stanford University School of Medicine, Veterans Administration Medical Center, Palo Alto, California 94394, U.S.A.

Weiskrantz, L., Department of Experimental Psychology, University of Oxford, South Parks Road, Oxford OX1 3UD

Whitteridge, D., Department of Physiology, University of Oxford, South Parks Road, Oxford OX1 3PT

Wolff, J. R., Max-Planck-Institut für Biophysikalische Chemie, Department Neurobiology, Postfach 968, D-3400 Gottingen-Nickolausberg, B.R.D.

Yeo, C. H., MRC Unit on Neural Mechanisms of Behaviour, 3 Malet Place, London WC1E 7JG

Záborszky, L., 1st Department of Anatomy, Semmelweis University Medical School, Budapest, Hungary

Zeier, H., Swiss Federal Institute of Technology Zurich, Department of Behavioral Science, Turnerstrasse 1, CH-8006 Zurich, Switzerland

Zielinski, K., Nencki Institute of Experimental Biology, 3 Pasteur Street, 02-093 Warsaw, Poland

Zihl, J., Max-Planck-Institut für Psychiatrie, Deutsche Forschungsanstalt für Psychiatrie, 8 Munchen 40, Kraepelinstrasse 2, Postfach 401240, B.R.D.

PREFACE

The present book contains a collection of papers culled from the European Brain Behaviour Society's Workshop on *The Structure and Function of the Cerebral Commissures*, which was held at the Erasmus University Medical School from March 30 to April 2, 1977. The meeting was supported by the Gerrit Jan Mulder Stichting, Rotterdam. Funds were also generously donated by: the European Brain Behaviour Society; the Erasmus University; the Fonds Medische Faculteit Rotterdam; Blydorp Zoo, Rotterdam; Ciba-Geigy; Heineken Breweries; Nefarma; Organon; Unilever and Union Chemique Belge. Both the editors and the contributors wish to express their appreciation to these organisations for making the Workshop possible.

The editors are also grateful to the staff of the Department of Physiology at Rotterdam, especially to Dr Jackie van Hof-van Duin, for dealing with the local arrangements and accommodation so efficiently and pleasantly. We should also like to express our appreciation to Mary James and Hannie Kouer who assisted so ably with the many secretarial problems associated with the preparation of this edition. Finally we are grateful to Mediha Atal for her assistance in the preparation of the cover for the book.

I. Steele Russell
M. W. van Hof
G. Berlucchi

INTRODUCTION TO THE BEGINNINGS
OF COMMISSURE RESEARCH

G. ATAL RUSSELL and I. STEELE RUSSELL

The origins of the work on interhemispheric relations arise from partly philosophical and partly medical concerns with the explanation of the unity of perception or consciousness. As such the various theories and speculations have essentially focused on two principal structures in the brain. In the periphery the optic chiasma was early considered as a mechanism of visual integration. The unity of consciousness was believed to be a product of central integration which was originally thought to occur in the ventricular system; and much later this function was assigned to the commissures.

The earliest written description of the optic chiasma and its connections with the brain in fish was provided by Aristotle (384-322 B.C.). Believing that the brain was little more than an accessory to the heart, he attached no particular significance to the chiasma. Herophilus (fl. c. 300 B.C.) and Erasistratus (fl. c. 260 B.C.), the pioneers of the Alexandrian school of anatomy and medicine, correctly identified the visual role of the optic chiasma. The optic nerves, believed to be hollow tubes were described in Rufus of Ephesus (fl. c. A.D. 98-117) as emerging from the base of the brain and meeting in the chiasma, and then bifurcating laterally to enter both eyes. Aretaeus, the Cappadocian (c. A.D. 81-138 or c. 131-200) described them, however, as completely decussated in the form of the letter χ.

The influence of Galen (A.D. 129-199) in physiology and anatomy, and in particular concerning brain function was a watershed in science. His treatment and interpretation of the visual system were the first attempt to provide a coherent mechanistic explanation of visual perception in anatomical terms. Morphologically he regarded each optic tract not as nerves but as tubular extensions of the brain itself, originating from the lateral ventricles which he termed *thalami* or cavities. The optic nerves were considered to extend from the brain separately, to come together without any decussation, and to end inside the eyes. There each nerve thins out to form the retina (*arachnoeides hitôn*) which extends as far as the lens (*krystalloeides hitôn*).

The function of this system was to provide a hydraulic exchange circuit in the eye to permit the transfer of information from the environment to the brain. Galen believed the ventricles contained a *luminous air* (*pneuma horatikon*) which circulated via the channels of the optic nerves to the eye, and from there to the outside where, in the presence of light, it altered or 'stressed' the surrounding air.

The impression of the object to be perceived was then transmitted to the eye by this 'stressed' air in the form of the Euclidian cone with its base on the object and its apex at the pupil. The two were connected by 'visual rays' which were to be thought of as straight lines analogous to a multitude of fine gossamer threads. Galen regarded the lens as the principal organ of vision or the structure where photoreception occurred. Its alleged function was to act as an exchange membrane where the pneuma could be 'charged' with the images located there by the visual rays (*opseis*). Visual perception was completed only when the pneuma conveyed these images back to the brain, which was the ultimate site of consciousness. Without the transfer of information by the lens, vision would not be possible.

Galen's views on the optic chiasma were also obscure. Its principal function was to ensure a proper distribution of pneuma from the brain to both eyes. During monocular vision it acted to redeploy all of the available pneuma to the open eye, thus to compensate for the loss of one receptor by doubling the power of the other. At the same time the chiasma served to prevent diplopia.

Further developments in our understanding of the function of the optic chiasma had to wait until the early beginnings of modern physiology and the rise of experimental scientific enquiry. This began with the recognition of the eye as an optic instrument in Islamic science. A significant feature of Arabic treatises and books on medicine and physics is their detailed description of the structure and function of the eye. What is perhaps more important is the fact that for the first time in history they use detailed illustrations of the eye, optic nerves, and the brain. For example, Hunain ibn Isḥāq (Johannitius, A.D. 809–877) produced a diagram of the eye (see figure I.1) that was not only remarkable for its detail and clarity, but represents a genre that powerfully influenced all early European diagrams of the eye by Roger Bacon, Pecham, Witello, and even da Vinci and Vesalius. Such early Arab physicians as ibn Isḥāq were, however, adherents of the emanation doctrines as well as being assiduous practitioners of Galenic principles.

The most comprehensive and systematic alternative to classical optical theories was formulated by the mathematician–physicist Ibn al-Haytham (Alhazen, A.D. 965–1039) who had a profound influence on Western science. His principal work on optics (*Kitab al-Manāzir*) was already translated into Latin by the thirteenth century and together with Risner's printed edition, *Opticae thesaurus* (1572) dominated European thought until the seventeenth century. It is for this reason that he is known as the father of ophthalmology.

The essential feature of Ibn al-Haytham's system is his theory of direct vision and his uncompromising rejection of emanation theory. His statement that 'the act of vision is accomplished by means of light rays coming from external objects and entering the eye . . . and the belief of those who think that something comes out of the eye is false' is both trenchant and clear. Of paramount importance was his belief that an unqualified reliance on naive sensory observation was inherently undesirable. He gives as an example of this the illusion of seeing the moon move when it is observed in the wake of morning clouds. True scientific knowledge, Ibn al-Haytham insisted, could only come from anchoring all observations to

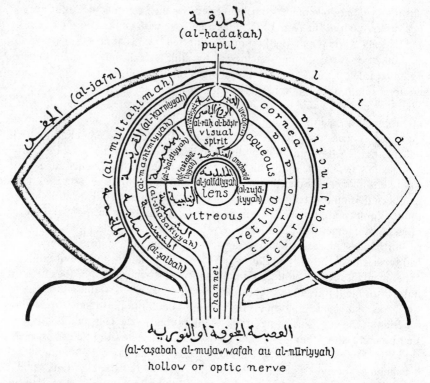

الْحَدَقَة
(al-ḥadaḳah)
pupil

(al-ʿaṣabah al-mujawwafah au al-nūriyyah)
hollow or optic nerve

Figure I.1 Adapted from a diagram of the eye contained in a manuscript written by Hunain ibn Ishāq entitled *Ten Treatises on the Structure of the Eye, its Diseases and their Treatment*. The approximate date of the original manuscript is A.D. 860. The manuscript in which the figure was found was dated at A.D. 1196. The text was preserved in Europe in pseudonymous Latin translations of such great plagiarists as Constantine, The African

quantitative measurement or by finding systematic agreement among several unrelated observations.

Nowhere is this better illustrated than with his investigations of the linear transmission of light. He used a dark chamber with a small aperture in one wall to provide a narrow point source of light. Filling the room with dust allowed the beam of light to be both visualised and tested for linearity against a rule. Similarly, stretching a thread along the path of a light beam in a dust-free chamber was shown to give the same results. Finally using an angled light from the wall to the floor he measured the height of the beam at various distances from the wall. By this method it was shown that the path taken by the light was the hypoteneuse of a triangle where the remaining sides were the wall and floor respectively.

Considering the nature of light, Ibn al-Haytham concluded that it was a form of energy related to heat because the sun's rays are both luminous and warm, as is light from fire. Furthermore he demonstrated that when light rays are reflected by a concave mirror they will burn objects placed at the focus, dependent on the intensity of the light. The effect of such intense lights on the eye is both to blur vision and to induce pain, which indicated to Ibn al-Haytham that vision could only result from light rays entering the eye from the outside world. The emission of the eye's own rays could not be responsible for the experience of pain. Similarly he argued that the phenomenon of visual after-images was due to the external bright light producing a temporary injury to the eye.

In optics he made significant contributions to both catoptrics and dioptrics. Not only did he experimentally confirm the first law of reflection, but he was responsible for the second law that the incident, normal and reflected rays always lie in the same plane. His major contribution was, however, his experimental studies of light refraction. He was the formulator of the first law of refraction and part-discoverer of the second law. By careful and systematic observation he established the fact that the angle of incidence is always greater than the angle of refraction. Further, he noted that when the angle of incidence is less than $20°$ the ratio of the two angles is constant. For angles of incidence greater than this the ratio was variable. Despite his familiarity with trigonometric tables he did not compare the sines of the angles, and thus left the complete formulation of the second law of refraction to Snell to complete in 1621. Ibn al-Haytham was mainly limited in studies of dioptrics to considering the refraction of light from air to water. However, preliminary observations on the refraction of light by water-filled glass bottles led him to explore the mathematical properties of magnifying lenses, which due to the inadequacies of the technology of his day were not taken further. Finally he performed numerous experiments with the pin-hole camera, where he first demonstrated how the image of an external candle was inverted on the screen inside the chamber.

In his treatment of the eye Ibn al-Haytham for the first time gave us the modern synthesis of anatomy and physical optics. His description of the structure and mechanisms of the eye is a model of clarity and attention to detail, suggesting that his knowledge of the anatomy of the eye came from dissection and detailed observation. In particular his exact description of the lens illustrates this point. To Ibn al-Haytham the round shape of the lens with its biconvex lateral appearance resembled a lentil grain. He further noted that the anterior surface of the lens was relatively flat compared with the posterior surface which has a much shorter radius of curvature. The Arabic word *adasa* (lentil) was translated into Latin as *lenticula* which is the origin of the English word lens. Another example of the early diffusion of Arabic influences to the West is seen with the word cornea. The transparent anterior surface of the eye was called *al-qarniyya* in Arabic to refer to a protrusion or horn. This was conveyed directly into Latin as cornea with no attempt being made to translate it.

Ibn al-Haytham likened the eye to a modified 'dark chamber' or pin-hole camera, where the pupil acts as an aperture to project an upright image on the back of the posterior chamber of the eye. Despite his pioneering investigations into refraction he totally failed to appreciate the true function of the lens. Instead he believed it was that part of the eye where visual sensations are first experienced as is the case when intense light induces pain. Light rays were refracted by the vitreous humour in such a way as to form an upright image. This image was created by the perpendicular light rays from the object to the eye so that each point of the object has a corresponding spatially organised point on the retinal image. This image or pattern of stimulation was thought to be preserved as it travelled in the hollow optic nerve to the brain where conscious perception of the object occurred. These ideas of Ibn al-Haytham clearly represent one of the earliest formulations of the concept of topographic retinal projection to the cerebrum.

Furthermore this notion of retinal information having a punctate organisation in the optic nerve was a cardinal assumption in his explanation of both the unity of perception and the function of the optic chiasma (see figure I.2). He believed the chiasma to be an association nerve (al-asaba al-jawfa al-mushtarika) where the contents of the two optic nerves came together and were mixed. This enabled the separate images from the two eyes to be superimposed and establish an exact match to generate a single fused image which in turn was conveyed to the brain resulting in a single visual experience.

An alternative view of the chiasma was provided by ibn Sina (Avicenna, A.D.

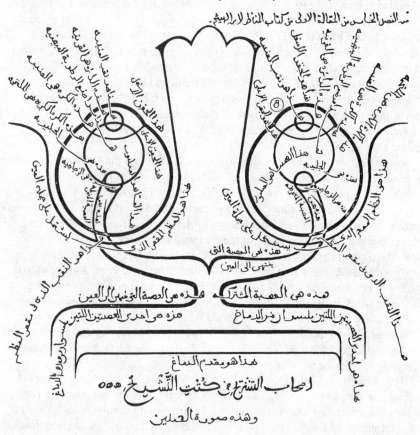

Figure I.2. Drawing adapted from a diagram of the visual system from the oldest copy of the *Kitab al-manazir* by Ibn al-Haytham. Manuscript dated A.D. 1083 in the possession of the Fatih Library, Istanbul. For identification of parts represented see Figure 8, p. 41 in S. Polyak, *The Retina*

980-1037) the great savant from Bukhara in Turkistan. In contrast to Ibn al-
Haytham he believed the optic nerves in the chiasma to be completely crossed
(see figure I.3) such that the separate images from the eyes are conveyed to
opposite lateral ventricles. He provided the answer to the problem of the unity
of consciousness by having the third and fourth ventricles act as association
chambers to unite the separate images.

Thus by the end of the eleventh century both a peripheral and a central theory
of the unity of consciousness had been promulgated in terms that were to remain

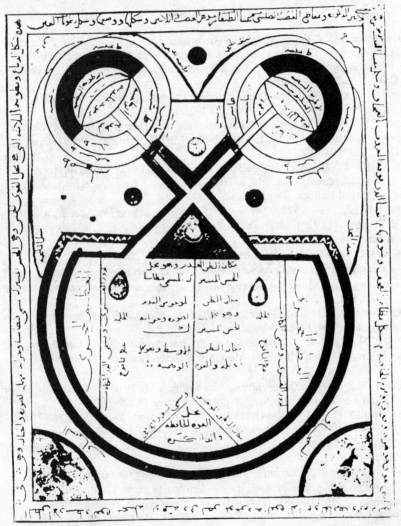

Figure I.3. Diagram of the visual system from a manuscript by Khalifa *c* A.D. 1266. The upper
part shows the two lateral ventricles, with the third and fourth ventricles of the brain in the
midline. The complete crossing of the optic nerves in the chiasma is shown. See S. Polyak, *The
Vertebrate Visual System*

essentially unchanged for the next 600 years. It was not until Descartes published his *Traité de l'Homme* in 1686 that a neural alternative was proposed to the ventricular hydraulic model. With the advantages of the new knowledge in optics and mathematics Descartes was able to reformulate Ibn al-Haytham's ideas of projection in modern form. The pineal gland then became the neural site where binocular integration occurred during vision. It was not until 1903 that the central integrating role of the corpus callosum was discovered (Immamura, 1903).

REFERENCES

Clarke, E. and O'Malley, C. D. (1968). Aretaeus, the Cappadocian, p. 282; Aristotle, p. 9, *The Human Brain and Spinal Cord: A Historical Study Illustrated by Writings from Antiquity to the Twentieth Century*. University of California Press, Berkeley

Crombie, A. C. (1967). The mechanistic hypothesis and the scientific study of vision. *Proc. R. Microsc. Soc.*, **2**(1), 12–22

Galen (129–199). The Eyes, *On the usefulness of the parts of the body. De usu partium*, translated by M. T. May (1968). Cornell University Press, Ithaca; **II, X**, 463–504

    Siegel, R. E. (1970). *Galen on Sense Perception*: His doctrines, observations, and experiments on vision, hearing, smell, taste, touch, and pain, and their historical sources. Karger, Basel

Hunayn b. Ishaq (809–877). *The Book of Ten Treatises on the Eye*, ed. and trans. M. Meyerhof (1928). Government Press, Cairo

Ibn al-Haytham (965–1039).

    Grant, E. (ed.) (1974). *A Source Book in Medieval Science.* Harvard University Press, Cambridge Massachusetts, 376–432.

    Lindberg, D. C. (1967). Alhazen's theory of vision and its reception in the West. *ISIS*, **581**, 327–41.

    Lindberg, D. C. (1976). *Theories of Vision from al-Kindi to Kepler.* University of Chicago Press, Chicago

    Nazif, M. (1942–43), *Al-Hasan ibn al-Haytham buhuthuhu wa-kushūfuhu al-basariyya* (Ibn al-Haytham: His Optical Researches and Discoveries) 2 vols, Cairo

    Omar, S. B. (1977). *Ibn al-Haytham's Optics*: A Study of the Origins of Experimental Science. Bibliotheca Islamica, Chicago, **iii**, 59–100

    Sabra, I. A. (1972). 'Ibn al-Haytham', *Dict. of Scient. Biogr.*, **VI**, 189–210.

Ibn Sina (980–1037). *Psychologie d'Ibn Sina (Avicenne) d'apres son oeuvre as-Sifa*, ed. Jan Bakoš. (French trans. and Arabic text) (1956) 2 vols, Prague, Book 6, Part 4

    Rahman, F. (1952). *Avicenna's Psychology: An English translation of the Kitab al-Najāt*. Book III, vi. Oxford University Press, London

Immamura, A. (1903). Über die kortikalen Storungen des Sehaktes und die Bedeutung des Balkens. *Pflügers Arch.*, **100**, 495–531

Polyak, S. (1941). *The Retina*, University of Chicago Press, Chicago Part II, vii–ix

Polyak, S. (1957). *The Vertebrate Visual System*. University of Chicago Press, Chicago Part I, i, 1–4; ii, 1–6

1

ANATOMY OF CEREBRAL COMMISSURES IN REPTILES

A. H. M. LOHMAN and P. V. HOOGLAND

INTRODUCTION

It is the purpose of this chapter to present a brief survey of the commissures in the forebrain of reptiles. Before discussing this particular topic, an overview of the normal anatomy of the reptilian cerebral hemispheres will be given. Secondly, reference will be made to the experimental anatomical studies which during the last decade have been carried out on the afferent relationships of the forebrain of reptiles. It is perhaps superfluous to state that a detailed knowledge of the input to the forebrain is an essential prerequisite for an understanding of the functional significance of the commissures that connect the right and left cerebral hemispheres.

NORMAL ANATOMY OF THE CEREBRAL HEMISPHERES

The cerebral hemispheres can be divided into a roof or pallium and a basis or subpallium. The subpallium consists of three zones: a medial zone or septal area, a lateral zone or strio-amygdaloid complex and a ventral zone which encompasses the nucleus accumbens and the olfactory tubercle (figures 1.1–1.3). (See table 1.1 for an explanation of abbreviations used in figures 1.1–1.4.)

In the pallium, three longitudinal cellular strips can be distinguished. By the end of the last century these zones had already been described in detail by Edinger (1896) and had been labelled by him according to their position: mediodorsal cortex, dorsal cortex and lateral cortex. In many reptiles the mediodorsal cortex can be further subdivided into a medial or small-celled part and a dorsal or large-celled part. Most recent descriptions of the reptilian brain follow the nomenclature of Edinger, although minor modifications are in use. For instance, the mediodorsal cortex is designated by Senn and Northcutt (1973) medial cortex, whereas in snakes Ulinski (1974) calls the small-celled part of this cortical field medial cortex and the large-celled part dorsomedial cortex. An exception to the wide usage of Edinger's terminology is made by Hall and Ebner (1970a, 1970b), who for the cortical fields in the turtle forebrain use the nomenclature introduced by Johnston

Table 1.1

Abbreviations used in figures 1.1–1.4

Acc	nucleus accumbens
Alh	lateral hypothalamic area
Amc	central amygdaloid nucleus
Ame	external amygdaloid nucleus
Ami	internal amygdaloid nucleus
Amm	marginal amygdaloid nucleus
ca	anterior commissure
Ce	cerebellum
cfd	commissura fornicis dorsalis
cfv	commissura fornicis ventralis
ch	habenular commissure
cho	optic chiasm
cp	posterior commissure
cpa	anterior pallial commissure
cpp	posterior pallial commissure
Cx dors	dorsal cortex
Cx lat	lateral cortex
Cx mediodors	mediodorsal cortex
Hyp	hypothalamus
Inst	nucleus interstitialis
Iped	nucleus intrapeduncularis
lfb	lateral forebrain bundle
Nca	nucleus of the anterior commissure
Ns	nucleus sphaericus
n III	nervus oculomotorius
Peh	nucleus periventricularis hypothalami
Pepo	nucleus periventricularis preopticus
postcfx	postcommissural fornix
precfx	precommissural fornix
Sd	dorsal striatum
Sel	nucleus septi lateralis
Seli	nucleus septi lateralis, pars inferior
Sels	nucleus septi lateralis, pars superior
Sept	septal area
sm	stria medullaris
Sv	ventral striatum
Subc layer	subcortical layer
Svl	ventral striatum, large-celled part
Svs	ventral striatum, small-celled part
Tec	optic tectum
tol	lateral olfactory tract
Thal	thalamus

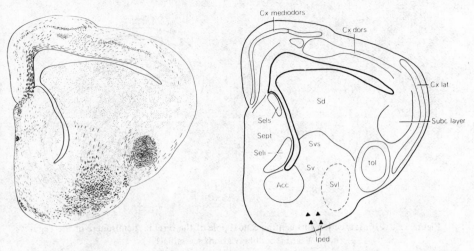

Figure 1.1. Frontal section through the rostral pole of the cerebral hemisphere of the Tegu lizard (for abbreviations see table 1.1)

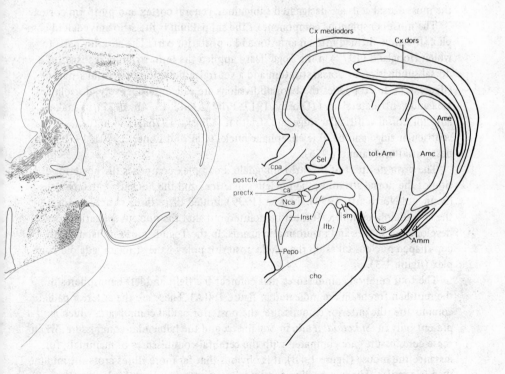

Figure 1.2. Frontal section through the middle of the cerebral hemisphere of the Tegu lizard (for abbreviations see table 1.1)

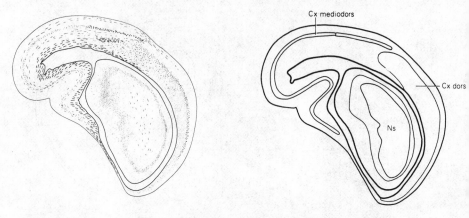

Figure 1.3.   Frontal section through the caudal pole of the cerebral hemisphere of the Tegu
lizard (for abbreviations see table 1.1)

(1915). From medial to lateral they call the three fields: hippocampus, of which
the most dorsal cells are designated subiculum, general cortex and pyriform cortex.

The most conspicuous component of the subpallium is the strio-amygdaloid complex. It can be divided into an anterior and a posterior part. The anterior part, to
which Hoogland (1977) in the Tegu lizard applied the term striatum, consists of a
dorsal subdivision or dorsal striatum and a ventral subdivision or ventral striatum
(figure 1.1). In crocodiles the two subdivisions are called, respectively, dorsolateral
area and ventrolateral area (Crosby, 1917; Pritz, 1974a, 1974b, 1975), in snakes
anterior dorsal ventricular ridge and striatum (Ulinski, 1976a), and in turtles dorsal
ventricular ridge and basal telencephalic nuclei (Hall and Ebner, 1970a, 1970b) or
basal striatum (Parent, 1976).

The posterior part of the strio-amygdaloid complex comprises the posterior division of the dorsal striatum, the nucleus sphaericus and the nucleus ventromedialis
(Senn and Northcutt, 1973). Curwen (1939) termed these three structures together
the amygdaloid complex. It must be pointed out that the nucleus sphaericus is well
developed in snakes and macrosmatic lizards. In the Tegu lizard, for instance, the
cup-shaped nucleus takes up the whole posterior pole of the strio-amygdaloid complex (figure 1.3).

The four cerebral commissures that connect the right and left hemispheres of
the reptilian forebrain are indicated in figure 1.4(A). These are the anterior pallial
commissure, the anterior commissure, the posterior pallial commissure which is
present only in *Sphenodon* and in Squamata, and the habenular commissure. When
these commissures are compared with the cerebral commissures of mammals, for
instance the mouse (figure 1.4B), it is obvious that far more fibres cross the midline
than in reptiles. The mammalian corpus callosum and the dorsal and ventral com-
missurae fornicis are represented in reptiles only by the far smaller commissura
pallii anterior.

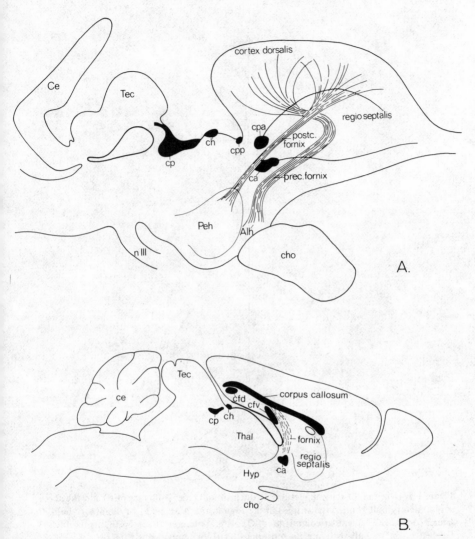

Figure 1.4. Sagittal sections through the brain of a Tegu lizard (A) and a mouse (B) showing the cerebral commissures (for abbreviations see table 1.1)

THE HABENULAR COMMISSURE

The commissure that at present is best known in reptiles is the habenular commissure. From the experimental studies of Gamble (1952, 1956), Heimer (1969) and Halpern (1976) we know that this commissure is made up of fibres that take their origin from the main olfactory bulb. As can be seen in figure 1.5, in the Tegu lizard these fibres travel caudally in the medial olfactory tract, cross the midline in the

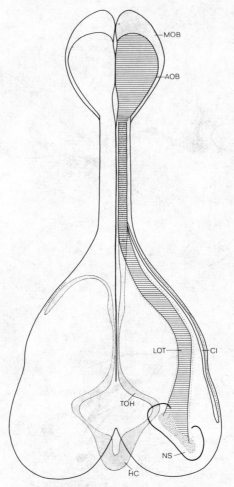

Figure 1.5. Diagram of the connections of the main olfactory bulb (stippled) and the accessory olfactory bulb (horizontal stripes) in the Tegu lizard. AOB, accessory olfactory bulb; Cl, lateral cortex; HC, habenular commissure; LOT, lateral olfactory tract; MOB, main olfactory bulb; NS, nucleus sphaericus; TOH, olfactohabenular tract

habenular commissure, and then course, again in the medial wall of the hemisphere, in a rostral direction. They reach the anterior part of the contralateral lateral cortex where they terminate superficially in the molecular layer. No fibres have been found that cross the midline in the anterior commissure.

Figure 1.5 also shows that a second contingent of fibres from the main olfactory bulb distributes to the ipsilateral cortex. Their mode of termination is the same as at the contralateral side. From our own experimental work in the Tegu lizard (Lohman and Mentink, 1972) it appeared that the lateral cortex, in turn, has a direct projection to the mediodorsal cortex. Following lesions destroying the cell layer of the lateral cortex, degenerated fibres could be traced in a medial direction under the surface of the forebrain to the small-celled part of the mediodorsal cortex. Here, the degenerated terminals are found in the superficial part of the molecular layer where, apparently, they synapse on the distal segments of the apical dendrites emanating from the more deeply situated cell bodies.

ASCENDING CONNECTIONS TO THE FOREBRAIN

As regards the ascending fibres that reach the reptilian forebrain from the diencephalon and more caudal levels, it must be pointed out that an analysis of these connections has so far been attempted only in a few species, and that even in these animals the analysis has not been completely worked out. Hall and Ebner (1970a, 1970b) could demonstrate that in the turtle the dorsal thalamus as well as the mid-

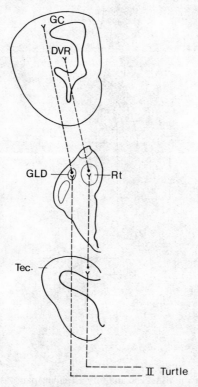

Figure 1.6. Diagram of the two visual pathways in the turtle. II, nervus opticus. One pathway projects to general cortex (GC) after a relay in the dorsal lateral geniculate nucleus (GLD); the other projects to the dorsal ventricular ridge (DVR) after relaying first in the optic tectum (Tec) and then in nucleus rotundus (Rt)

brain projects to the forebrain. The fibres from the midbrain which, according to Parent (1976), have their cell bodies in the lateral portion of the tegmentum distribute mainly to the basal telecephalic nuclei, whereas the thalamic fibres terminate in the basal telencephalic nuclei, the core of the dorsal ventricular ridge and superficially in the general cortex. The authors could further make the point that there are two visual relay nuclei in the dorsal thalamus of the turtle: one is the nucleus rotundus which is reached by fibres from the optic tectum and projects to the dorsal ventricular ridge; the other, the dorsal lateral geniculate nucleus, receives a direct input from the retina and projects to the general cortex where the axons terminate in the molecular layer just beneath the pial surface (figure 1.6).

Very recently, the pathway from the dorsal lateral geniculate nucleus to the

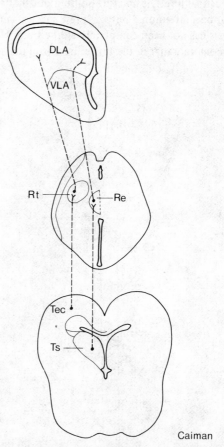

Figure 1.7. Diagram of the visual and auditory ascending pathways to the forebrain in caiman. The visual pathway originates from the optic tectum (Tec) and projects to the lateral portion of the dorsolateral area (DLA) above the ventrolateral area (VLA) after a relay in nucleus rotundus (Rt). The auditory pathway originates from the torus semicircularis (Ts) and projects to the medial portion of the dorsolateral area after relaying in nucleus reuniens (Re)

general cortex in the turtle brain has been confirmed by Hall *et al.* (1977). Further-more, it has been shown by these authors that the general cortex receives additional afflux from two other dorsal thalamic nuclei: nucleus ventralis and nucleus dorso-lateralis anterior. As stated by Hall *et al.*, the demonstration that the nucleus ven-tralis projects to general cortex may be of special interest, since there are several findings suggesting that this nucleus serves as a relay in an ascending sensory path-way. At present it is unknown which afferent fibres reach the nucleus dorsolateralis anterior, and therefore the functional significance of its connections to the general cortex still remains unknown.

Experiments in reptiles other than the turtle have confirmed the projection from nucleus rotundus to the anterior dorsal ventricular ridge (Distel and Ebbesson, 1975; Pritz, 1975). In addition, it has been shown that auditory impulses also can reach the forebrain by way of the dorsal thalamus (figure 1.7). This conduction route has been worked out by Pritz (1974a, 1974b) who found in caiman that the nucleus reuniens of the thalamus receives a projection from the torus semicircularis and, in turn, projects to the anterior dorsal ventricular ridge (i.e. dorsolateral area). On the other hand, evidence is accumulating that the direct projection from the dorsal lateral geniculate nucleus to the cortex of the forebrain might well be a unique feature of the turtle brain. Wang and Halpern (1977) found that in garter snakes the dorsal lateral geniculate nucleus projects to the dorsal ventricular ridge. Moreover, the findings of Distel and Ebbesson (1975) and of ourselves (Lohman and van Woerden-Verkley, 1976b) suggest that in lizards the exclusive site of origin of the thalamocortical projection is the nucleus dorsolateralis anterior. In the Tegu lizard it has been found by us that the major portion of the fibres arising from this nucleus distributes ipsilaterally to a distinct zone in the middle of the molecular layer of the small-celled part of the mediodorsal cortex. The rest of the fibres ter-minate bilaterally beneath the pial surface above the medial part of the dorsal cortex.

THE ANTERIOR AND POSTERIOR PALLIAL COMMISSURES

In view of the fact that in the Tegu lizard the small-celled part of the mediodorsal cortex is not only the main target of the fibres originating in the dorsal thalamus but also receives olfactory input from the lateral cortex, it could be thought that for the sake of a rapid transfer of sensory information from one hemisphere to the other it is just this cortical field that is the main origin of the fibres constituting the anterior pallial commissure. However, it was found by us that not the small-celled part of the mediodorsal cortex but the large-celled part, which receives no extrinsic afferent fibres, emits the commissural fibres (Lohman and Mentink, 1972). It is of interest to point out that this condition to some extent parallels the interhemisphe-ric neocortical connections in mammals. Yorke and Caviness (1975) demonstrated in the mouse that of the cortical areas receiving thalamic input those that represent highly lateralised sensory functions do not give rise to callosal fibres. Instead, the cells of origin of these fibres are located in immediately adjoining zones of the neocortex.

The fibres which cross the midline in the anterior pallial commissure of the Tegu lizard terminate in the contralateral hemisphere in two layers just superficial and deep to the cell layer of the small-celled part of the mediodorsal cortex. Furthermore, there is a projection to the outer part of the molecular layer above the large-celled part of this cortical field (Lohman and Mentink, 1972). Identical origin and termination of the fibres of the anterior pallial commissure have recently been reported by Ulinski (1976b) in water and garter snakes. In addition, it was found by Ulinski that, at least in snakes, the commissure also contains fibres that originate in the small-celled part of the mediodorsal cortex of one hemisphere and terminate dorsally in the septal area of the contralateral hemisphere (Ulinski, 1975).

As has already been said before, the large-celled part of the mediodorsal cortex is not known to receive any extrinsic afferent input. It receives, however, a projection from the small-celled part (Ulinski, 1975; Lohman and Mentink, 1972), and via this projection sensory information that reaches the small-celled part might be relayed to the cells of origin of the anterior pallial commissure.

From the observations of Butler (1976) in the gecko it might be inferred that, apart from the organisation in other reptilian groups, the pattern of origin and distribution of the interhemispheric connections mediated via the anterior pallial commissure (i.e. hippocampal commissure) is not identical in all lizards and snakes. She concludes that the origin of the commissural fibres is not the mediodorsal cortex but the dorsal cortex. She further found that the termination area of the fibres in the contralateral hemisphere is not confined to the mediodorsal cortex, but also includes the dorsal cortex and the lateral edge of the dorsal ventricular ridge.

The posterior pallial commissure or commissura aberrans (Elliot Smith, 1903) has so far been investigated only in the Tegu lizard (Voneida and Ebbesson, 1969; Lohman and van Woerden-Verkley, 1976a). Although these studies did not reveal the exact origin of the commissural fibres, it is very likely that they originate from the small-celled part of the mediodorsal cortex ventrally and caudally in the forebrain. The fibres pass in the contralateral hemisphere beneath the nucleus sphaericus in a ventral direction and terminate in an area that has been termed by Ebbesson and Voneida (1969) ventral cortex.

THE ANTERIOR COMMISSURE

From the experiments of Hoogland (1977), who studied the connections of the striatum in the Tegu lizard, it has become clear that the dorsal striatum and the amygdaloid complex are the major sites of origin of the fibres of the anterior commissure. As is shown in figure 1.8, there is a projection from the caudal part of the dorsal striatum to the contralateral caudal portion of the ventral striatum, and a

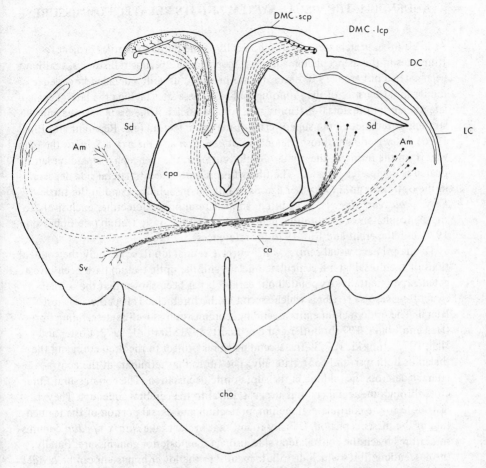

Figure 1.8. Diagram of the commissural connections via the anterior commissure, ca, in the Tegu lizard. Am, amygdala; cho, optic chiasm; cpa, anterior pallial commissure; DC, dorsal cortex; DMC-sep, dorsomedial cortex, small-celled part; DMC-lep, dorsomedial cortex, large-celled part; LC, lateral cortex; Sd, dorsal striatum; Sv, ventral striatum

projection from the amygdaloid complex to the contralateral amygdala and an area just beneath the lateral cortex. There are contradictory reports as to whether or not the lateral cortex is also a source of origin of the fibres of the anterior commissure. From her experiments in the gecko, Butler (1976) concluded that the lateral cortex does contribute fibres to the anterior commissure, whereas in the Tegu lizard (Lohman and van Woerden-Verkley, 1976a) it was found that the subcortical distribution area of the lateral cortex is wholly confined to the underlying dorsal striatum.

ADDENDUM: THE VISUAL SYSTEM AND ITS RELATED COMMISSURES

As in all other vertebrates, the ganglion cells of the retina in reptiles project to structures in the diencephalon and mesencephalon. Experimental studies, that have been carried out from 1950 onward, have provided us with a detailed knowledge of the termination sites of the retinofugal fibres. These sites include the lateral geniculate nucleus in the dorsal thalamus, most of the nuclei of the pretectal area and the stratum griseum et album superificiale of the optic tectum (e.g. Repérant and Rio, 1976). In crocodilians, most chelonians, *Sphenodon* and the lizard *Scincus* the pathway from the retina to the primary optic centres in the diencephalon and mesencephalon is completely crossed. The fibres that reach the contralateral side decussate in the optic chiasm. In all other lizards examined, in ophidians and in the turtle *Emys orbicularis* there is, in addition, an ipsilateral projection either exclusively to the diencephalon or to both the diencephalon and the optic tectum (see Ebbesson, 1970 and Repérant and Rio, 1976 for references).

Of the primary visual centres which receive retinal input, so far only the connections of the dorsal lateral geniculate nucleus and the optic tectum have been investigated experimentally. As pointed out earlier, it has been shown that the former structure gives rise to fibres which ascend to the forebrain. This pathway is ipsilateral. The optic tectum emits ascending, commissural as well as descending fibres (Hall and Ebner, 1970b; Butler and Northcutt, 1971; Braford, 1972; Foster and Hall, 1975; Ulinski, 1977). The ascending fibres project to the pretectum and the thalamus both ipsi- and contralaterally. The fibres that terminate at the contralateral side cross the midline in the supra-optic decussation. The commissural fibres cross through the tectal commissure just dorsal to the cerebral aqueduct. They distribute to the contralateral tectum, pretectum and dorsal portion of the tegmentum of the mesencephalon. Ulinsky found that in the snake *Natrix sipedon* commissural fibres reach the contralateral side also via the posterior commissure. Finally, the descending fibres which distribute mainly to the lower brainstem can be divided into an ipsilateral and a contraleteral pathway. The latter crosses in the midbrain beneath the medial longitudinal fasciculus and then descends through the brainstem as the predorsal bundle. It seems of importance to point out that Foster and Hall found in iguana that the descending pathways originate only from the deepest layers of the optic tectum. These layers are known to receive no input from the retina.

REFERENCES

Braford, M. R. Jr (1972). Ascending efferent tectal projections in the South American spectacled caiman. *Anat. Rec.*, **172**, 275–76

Butler, A. B. (1976). Telencephalon of the lizard *Gekko gekko* (Linnaeus): some connections of the cortex and dorsal ventricular ridge. *Brain, Behav. Evol.*, **13**, 396–417

Butler, A. B. and Northcutt, R. G. (1971). Ascending tectal efferent projections in the lizard *Iguana iguana*. *Brain Res.*, **35**, 597-601

Crosby, E. C. (1917). The forebrain of *Alligator mississippiensis*. *J. comp. Neurol.*, **27**, 325-402

Curwen, A. O. (1939). The telencephalon of *Tupinambis nigropunctatus*. *III. Amygdala. J. comp. Neurol.*, **71**, 613-36

Distel, H. and Ebbesson, S. O. E. (1975). Connections of the thalamus in the monitor lizard. *Neurosci. Abstr.*, **1**, 559

Ebbesson, S. O. E. (1970). On the organization of central visual pathways in vertebrates. *Brain, Behav. Evol.*, **3**, 178-94

Ebbesson, S. O. E. and Voneida, T. J. (1969). The cytoarchitecture of the pallium in the Tegu lizard (*Tupinambis nigropunctatus*). *Brain, Behav. Evol.*, **2**, 431-66

Edinger, L. (1896). Untersuchungen über die vergleichende Anatomie des Gehirns. III. Neue Studien über das Vorhirn der Reptilien. *Abh. Senckenb. Naturforsch. Gesch.*, **19**, 313-88

Elliot Smith, G. (1903). On the morphology of the cerebral commissures in the Vertebrata, with special reference to an aberrant commissure found in the forebrain of certain reptiles. *Trans. Linn. Soc. Lond. (Zool.)*, **8**, 455-500

Foster, R. E. and Hall, W. C. (1975). The connections and laminar organization of optic tectum in a reptile (*Iguana iguana*). *J. comp. Neurol.*, **163**, 397-426

Gamble, H. J. (1952). An experimental study of the secondary olfactory connexions in *Lacerta viridis. J. Anat.*, **86**, 180-96

Gamble, H. J. (1956). An experimental study of the secondary olfactory connexions in *Testudo graeca. J. Anat.*, **90**, 15-29

Hall, J. A., Foster, R. E., Ebner, F. F. and Hall, W. C. (1977). Visual cortex in a reptile, the turtle (*Pseudomys scripta* and *Chrysemys picta*). *Brain Res.*, **130**, 197-216

Hall, W. C. and Ebner, F. F. (1970a). Thalamotelencephalic projections in the turtle (*Pseudemys scripta*). *J. comp. Neurol.*, **140**, 101-22

Hall, W. C. and Ebner, F. F. (1970b). Parallels in the visual afferent projections of the thalamus in the hedgehog (*Paraechinus hypomelas*) and the turtle (*Pseudemys scripta*). *Brain, Behav. Evol.*, **3**, 135-54

Halpern, M. (1976). The efferent connections of the olfactory bulb and accessory olfactory bulb in the snakes, *Thamnophis sirtalis* and *Thamnophis radix. J. Morphol.*, **150**, 553-78

Heimer, L. (1969). The secondary olfactory connections in mammals, reptiles and shark. *Ann. N. Y. Acad. Sci.*, **167**, 129-46

Hoogland, P. V. (1977). The efferent connections of the striatum in *Tupinambis nigropunctatus. J. Morphol.*, **152**, 229-46

Johnston, J. B. (1915). Cell masses in the forebrain of the turtle, *Cistudo carolina. J. comp. Neurol.*, **25**, 393-468

Lohman, A. H. M. and Mentink, G. M. (1972). Some cortical connections of the Tegu lizard (*Tupinambis teguixin*). *Brain Res.*, **45**, 325-44

Lohman, A. H. M. and van Woerden-Verkley, I. (1976a). Further studies on the cortical connections of the Tegu lizard. *Brain Res.*, **103**, 9-28

Lohman, A. H. M. and van Woerden-Verkley, I. (1976b). The reptilian cortex and some of its connections in the Tegu lizard. In 'Afferent and Intrinsic Organization of Laminated Structures in the Brain' (O. Creutzfeld, ed), *Expl Brain Res.*, Suppl. 1, 166–70

Parent, A. (1976). Striatal afferent connections in the turtle (*Chrysemys picta*) as revealed by retrograde axonal transport of horseradish peroxidase. *Brain Res.*, **108**, 25–36

Pritz, M. B. (1974a). Ascending connections of a midbrain auditory area in a crocodile, *Caiman crocodilus. J. comp. Neurol.*, **153**, 179–98

Pritz, M. B. (1974b). Ascending connections of a thalamic auditory area in a crocodile, *Caiman crocodilus. J. comp. Neurol.*, **153**, 199–214

Pritz, M. B. (1975). Anatomical identification of a telencephalic visual area in crocodiles: ascending connections of nucleus rotundus in *Caiman crocodilus. J. comp. Neurol.*, **164**, 323–38

Repérant, J. and Rio, J. -P. (1976). Retinal projections in *Vipera aspis*. A reinvestigation using light radioautographic electron microscopic degeneration techniques. *Brain Res.*, **107**, 603–609

Senn, D. G. and Northcutt, R. G. (1973). The forebrain and midbrain of some Squamates and their bearing on the origin of snakes. *J. Morphol.*, **140**, 135–52

Ulinski, P. S. (1974). Cytoarchitecture of cerebral cortex in snakes. *J. comp. Neurol.*, **158**, 243–66

Ulinski, P. S. (1975). Corticoseptal projections in the snakes, *Natrix sipedon* and *Thamnophis sirtalis. J. comp. Neurol.*, **164**, 375–88

Ulinski, P. S. (1976a). Structure of anterior dorsal ventricular ridge in snakes. *J. comp. Neurol.*, **148**, 1–22

Ulinski, P. S. (1976b). Intracortical connections in the snakes *Natrix sipedon* and *Thamnophis sirtalis. J. Morphol.*, **150**, 463–80

Ulinski, P. S. (1977). Tectal efferents in the banded water snake, *Natrix sipedon. J. comp. Neurol.*, **173**, 251–74

Voneida, T. J. and Ebbesson, S. O. E. (1969). On the origin and distribution of axons in the pallial commissures in the Tegu lizard (*Tupinambis nigropunctatus*). *Brain, Behav. Evol.*, **2**, 467–81

Wang, R. T. and Halpern, M. (1977). Afferent and efferent connections of thalamic nuclei of the visual system of garter snakes. *Anat. Rec.*, **187**, 741

Yorke, C. H. Jr. and Caviness, V. S. (1975). Interhemispheric neocortical connections of the corpus callosum in the normal mouse: a study based on anterograde and retrograde methods. *J. comp. Neurol.*, **164**, 233–46

2
MORPHOLOGICAL RELATIONSHIP ESTABLISHED THROUGH THE HABENULO-INTERPEDUNCULAR SYSTEM BETWEEN THE RIGHT AND LEFT PORTIONS OF THE FROG BRAIN

MILENA KEMALI

INTRODUCTION

It is known that the left and right cerebral hemispheres of man are not functionally equivalent. The classification of verbal versus perceptual functions has produced the distinction of the left 'dominant' hemisphere and the right 'minor' hemisphere in man. On these grounds, we might consider the commissures, or at least some of them, as fibre bundles which connect non-homologous structures that topologically occupy the same zone in the two halves of the brain. This concept is strengthened by the observation that the different functional specialisation of the two hemispheres is probably related to their morphological asymmetry. In man the area behind the auditory cortex in the temporal lobe is larger in the left hemisphere than in the right (Geschwind and Levitzky, 1968). On the other hand, the mass of periventricular brain tissue in the posterior part of the hemisphere is greater on the right than on the left, the occipital horn of the lateral ventricle being longer on the left than on the right (McRea *et al.*, 1968).

If we search for the phylogenetic point of the appearance of a dual asymmetry in the bilaterally symmetric vertebrate brain then the answer could be found in the morphological asymmetry of the habenular nuclei in lower vertebrates. A clear instance of functional asymmetry is offered by the song pattern of birds which is greatly impaired when the descending nerve to the syrinx is destroyed on the left and less affected when the destruction occurs on the right (Nottebohm, 1970).

The habenular nuclei are part of the habenulo-interpeduncular system which exists substantially unmodified in all vertebrates and which forms the inner ring—the phylogenetically oldest portion—of the limbic circuit (Isaacson, 1974).

The function of the habenulo-interpeduncular system is still rather obscure. Through the connections established with other cerebral structures, it has been considered an extrahypothalamic feeding system that follows an epithalamic route

15

which lies parallel to the well-established lateral hypothalamic connection (Booth, 1967; Grossman, 1968) and may be crosslinked to it by transthalamic fibres (Morgane, 1961a, 1961b). This 'duplicate' feeding system is situated between the limbic forebrain and the tegmental motor system where it can mediate feeding reflexes independently of the hypothalamus (Woods, 1964). The habenulo-interpeduncular system is also involved in several other somatic and autonomic functions (Cragg, 1959; Granit and Kaada, 1953; Kaada, 1951).

The habenulo-interpeduncular system is a structurally unique complex of the vertebrate central nervous system with regard to its anatomical composition. In fact it is formed by: (1) two paired nuclei, although asymmetric in some species, which are the habenular nuclei situated on the right and left epithalamus separated by the third ventricle and united by the habenular commissure; (2) one single nucleus, the interpeduncular nucleus (ITP), situated on the midline of the mesencephalic tegmentum; (3) two bundles of fibres, one on the right and one on the left side of the epithalamus which converge in the midline of the tegmentum mesencephali and which interconnect the habenular nuclei and the ITP (fasciculus retroflexus, FR). These bundles of fibres end only partly in the ITP; the majority of them proceed caudally, decussating within the nucleus in such a zigzag fashion that the habenular nuclei of one side are contralaterally connected to the dorsal and deep tegmental nuclei of the other side through the ITP.

In the present chapter we shall consider the habenulo-interpeduncular system of the frog *Rana esculenta* from the morphological point of view and try to give an answer to the following questions: does lateral specialisation exist in the brain of a frog and how does the habenulo-interpeduncular system affect the relationship between the right and the left portions of the brain? An attempt will also be made to provide a functional explanation of this particular morphological configuration.

We have made our observations by studying normal and degeneration material both with the light and the electron microscopes, but the main contribution comes from observations of material impregnated by a modified rapid Golgi method (Kemali, 1976a).

THE HABENULAR COMPLEX

The habenulae have many connections with various telencephalic, diencephalic and mesencephalic zones which were revealed by degeneration techniques and electrophysiological experiments (Cragg, 1961; David and Herbert, 1973; Halpern, 1972; Kappers, 1971; Mitchell, 1963; Mok and Mogenson, 1972a, 1972b; Nauta, 1958; Powell, 1968; Raisman, 1966; Smaha and Kaelber, 1973).

The most interesting connection is that established with the ITP through the FR. Some of these fibres are reciprocal (Smaha and Kaelber, 1973), some end in the ITP (Lenn, 1976; Mizuno and Nakamura, 1974) and some continue caudally to end in the dorsal and deep tegmental nuclei (Akagi and Powell, 1968; Way and

Kaelber, 1969). The connection with the dorsal tegmental nucleus provides an information flow to the dorsal longitudinal fasciculus which sends terminal fibres to the motor nuclei of the trigeminal, the facial and the hypoglossal nerves, which allow the co-operative action of the striated muscles in feeding (Crosby *et al.*, 1962).

The numerous connections established by the habenular nuclei are probably mediated by different substances and in fact numerous putative neurotransmitters found in the habenular nuclei (Bjorklund *et al.*, 1972; Braak, 1970; Hokfelt *et al.*, 1975; Jacobowitz and Palkovits, 1974; Kataoka *et al.*, 1973; Kuhar *et al.*, 1975;

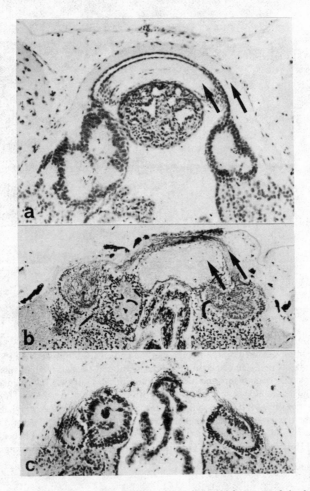

Figure 2.1 Three differently stained transverese sections of the epithalamus of the frog showing the asymmetry of the dorsal habenular nuclei and the habenular commissure. The medial portion of the left habenula is visible in the three pictures. The arrows show that the habunular commissure consists of two portions. The staining methods are: (a) Nissl; (b) Bodian; (c) Kluver–Barrera. 150×

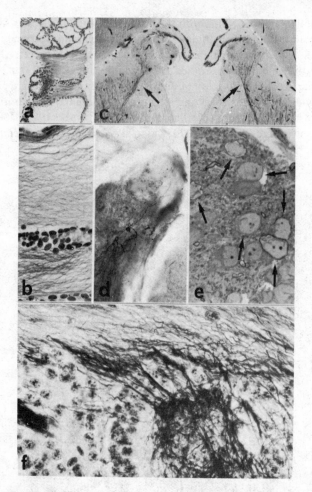

Figure 2.2   (a), (b) Unmyelinated fibres forming the two portions of the habenular commissure cut horizontally, stained by the Bodian method and enlarged, respectively 85× and 350×. (c) A horizontal section stained according to the method of Landau. The myelinated fibres are seen in the habenular commissure and in the FR of both sides (arrows). The medial portion of the left habenula does not seem to be involved with the fasciculus retroflexus. 60×. (d) Golgi method—transverse section showing cells of the lateral border of a ventral habenular nucleus sending their axons upwards to the habenular commissure. 110×. (e) Semi-thin section, 1 μm thick, showing a group of myelinated cells (arrows) in the right ventral habenular nucleus. 900×. (f) Horizontal section of a portion of the dorsal habenula showing bundles of fibres of the stria medullaris. Cajal staining. 580×

Trueman and Herbert, 1970) explain the variety of synaptic vesicles found in these nuclei (Kemali, 1976b; 1977b).

In the frog we distinguish a dorsal and a ventral habenular nucleus in both sides of the epithalamus corresponding respectively to the medial and lateral habenular

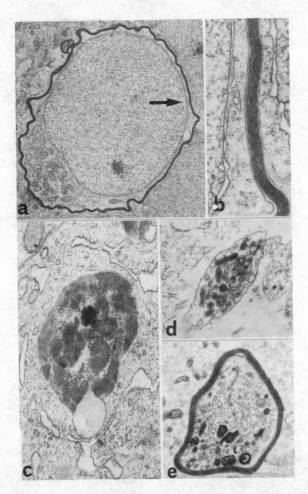

Figure 2.3.   (a) Cell of the ventral right habenula wrapped in myelin. 6600X. The arrow points
to the region enlarged in (b) (40 320X). Aldehyde fixation. (c) Intracytoplasmic polymorphic
crystal-like inclusion confined to the cells of the medial portion of the left habenula. A large
'drop' is contiguous to a cistern of the rough endoplasmic reticulum. 37 800X. Aldehyde fixation. (d), (e) Portions of degenerated fibres of the right habenula following ablation of the left
habenula. 25 200X and 15 360X, respectively. Osmium fixation

nuclei of mammals. The cells of the dorsal habenular nuclei are arranged in a ring
encircling a neuropil. Those of the ventral habenular nuclei are distributed within
the nucleus.

The dorsal habenular nuclei of frogs are asymmetric in the sense that the left
one has a more lobate structure than its right counterpart. Frontera (1952) demonstrated this in various species of frogs and Kemali and Braitenberg (1969) demonstrated it in *Rana esculenta*.

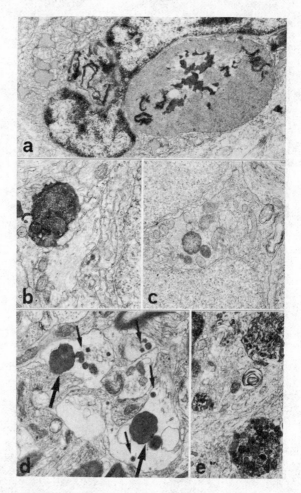

Figure 2.4. (a) Degenerated cell of the right habenula following ablation of the left habenula. 11 200X. Osmium fixation. (b) Degenerated terminal in the right habenula after ablation of the telencephalon. 24 000X. Aldehyde fixation. (c) Degeneration signs in the cytoplasm of cells of the right habenula after ablation of the telencephalon. 11 800X. Aldehyde fixation. (d) Huge dark bodies (large arrows) which appear within the large processes of the ITP cells (which contain large granules—small arrows) after ablation of the telencephalon. Compare the size of the large granules to that of conventional synaptic vesicles. 14 000X. Aldehyde fixation. (e) Degenerated elements in the cytoplasm of cells of the right habenula after ablation of the left habenula. 11 190X. Osmium fixation

When referring to the left-side habenula we can distinguish a lateral portion and a medial portion close to the third ventricle. This can be seen in figure 2.1 which shows the epithalamus of the frog in transverse section and stained by three different methods, demonstrating the cell masses (a), the unmyelinated fibres (b) and the myelinated fibres (c).

Habenular Commissure

The habenular commissure is a ribbon of fibres which stands like a bridge on the third ventricle, between the right and the left habenular nuclei. As is clearly visible in figure 2.1 and in figure 2.2(a) and 2.2(b), it consists of two portions (arrows) of different size which, according to the plane of cutting and to its rotation during histological manipulations, may be dislocated in a dorsoventral or an anteroposterior orientation because it lies above the third ventricle cavity. Some of the fibres forming the commissure are myelinated and these are confined to the external borders of the bundle as clearly illustrated in figure 2.1(c) and figure 2.2(c). It seems that the habenular commissure does not involve the medial portion of the left habenula which appears to stand apart from the entire neuronal system.

Although the habenular nuclei have been considered a crucial junction in the discharge of olfactory impulses to motor centres (Rausch and Long, 1971), there is experimental evidence (Scalia, 1976) that, in the frog, olfactory bulb efferents do not terminate in the habenular nuclei and that the lateral olfactory tract crosses to the contralateral hemisphere through the habenular commissure.

It seems to us that the habenular commissure is in part formed by axons arising in cells of the ventral habenula (figure 2.2d). These axons have been followed, using Golgi preparations, beyond the commissure to the lateral border of the contralateral habenula. On the other hand, ablation of the habenula of one side results in degeneration, seen by the electron microscope, of some fibre and cellular elements in the contralateral habenula (figure 2.3d and 2.3e; figure 2.4a and 2.4e). Ablation of the entire telencephalon resulted in degeneration, also visible with the electron microscope, of synapses in the habenular nuclei as well as degeneration in the cytoplasm of some cell populations (figure 2.4b and 2.4c).

Consequently, our observations suggest the existence of real commissural fibres which occupy a small portion of the habenular commissure, where decussating fibres of the stria medullaris also occur, and which permit a reciprocal influence between the symmetric habenulae of the two sides. They also indicate the presence of some elements of the habenular nuclei that project to the telencephalon as well as some fibres of the telecephalon that end in the habenular nuclei, suggesting that the stria medullaris establishes, at least in part, reciprocal connections. The fibres of the stria medullaris are grouped in small bundles where they traverse the cellular border of the habenular nuclei (as shown in figure 2.2f).

Asymmetry

Although cases of morphological predominance of the right habenula are reported in the literature (Jansen, 1930; Johnston, 1902) we can affirm that in the frog this predominance is always on the left side (Kemali, 1970), and quantitative studies carried out on the two sides of the epithalamus of the frog (Braitenberg and Kemali, 1970) and the eel and the newt (Kemali et al., 1971) have demonstrated that the cells of the medial portion of the left dorsal habenula are larger than those of the lateral portion and those of the right habenula. Also, in one of the reptiles, the lizard, an 'extra' nucleus has been demonstrated in the left habenula and not in the right (Kemali and Agrelli, 1972).

By means of electron microscopy we have demonstrated that the ventral habenular nuclei of the frog are asymmetric also, but in this case the asymmetry is reversed. In fact, cells which have the peculiarity of presenting their perikaryon wrapped in myelin (Kemali and Sada, 1973)—figure 2.3a and 2.3b—and whose physiological meaning is obscure, have been found grouped in a nucleus only on the right side (Kemali, 1974)—figure 2.2e.

We have seen in man that brain asymmetry does not mean dominance of one side over the other but rather a different specialisation of the two sides. May we consider, even in the brain of the frog, a different specialisation of the right and left epithalamus on the basis of their morphologic differences?

In the interpretation of our morphologic data we have confined ourselves to the dorsal habenular nuclei only, disregarding the ventral habenular nuclei where the unusual myelin is more pertinent to an electrophysiological study. By means of the electron microscope we have investigated separately the right habenula and the two portions of the left habenula (Kemali and Guglielmotti, 1977).

It was possible to demonstrate a particular type of synaptic terminal only in the left habenula and not in the right. Further, it was possible to show a particular type of inclusion confined to the medial portion of the left habenula and present in each of its cells and sometimes in their processes. Such inclusions show a polymorphic crystal-like pattern whose morphologic characteristics exclude their possible lysosomal nature. They are probably formed by the aggregation of several bodies of one type which, depending on the cutting plane, show diverse ultrastructural patterns. Dark granules—probably pigment—and light droplets—probably lipid droplets—may occur within such inclusions which are frequently close to the cisternae of the rough endoplasmic reticulum (figure 2.3c). Only in some instances is there any suggestion that fragments of a membrane seem to belong to portions of the crystal-like bodies; more usually they are devoid of a limiting membrane.

On a morphological basis we interpret these crystal-like inclusions as photosensitive organelles. In fact they are similar to photoreceptive elements seen in the frog's retina (Moody and Robertson, 1960; Porter and Yamada, 1960), to photoreceptors described in the neural tissues of the sixth abdominal ganglion of the crayfish (Uchizono, 1962) and to photoreceptors of the pineal body (Eakin et al., 1963).

Extraretinal photoreceptors may have a functional entrainment role conditioned by light cycles. In the sixth abdominal ganglion of the crayfish they are considered responsible for the locomotor activity of this invertebrate through a photochemical reaction (Uchizono, 1962); the photoreceptors of the pineal body are considered to be involved in the circadian activity rhythm of vertebrates (Wurtman et al., 1968). The habenular nuclei have been reported as being in connection with the pineal body (David and Herbert, 1973) and, due to the presence of the crystal-like inclusions confined to the medial portion of the left habenula, we suppose that only this side of the epithalamus is linked to the pineal. On the other hand, as long ago as 1930, Johnston wrote of the Petromyzon brain: 'The pineal apparatus probably functions as a light percipient organ; it is in relation with the left ganglion habenulae only' (Johnston, 1930, p. 79).

The fact that the pineal body and the medial portion of the left habenula share photoreceptive elements may indicate that they also share a functional mediation of some kind between environmental light and the organism's activity rhythm, probably through a hormonal mechanism.

In mammals circadian photoreceptors seem to be confined to the eyes. The anatomical routes through which they are coupled to regions of the brain, in order to utilise the diurnal pattern of environmental light for the generation of the organism's rhythms, are different from those involved in pattern vision. In fact the information concerning the external light that affects biochemical rhythms in the pineal apparently arrives at this organ by way of the accessory optic tract (Moore, 1974), while direct retinohypothalamic fibres may be involved in the entrainment of eating, drinking and locomotor rhythms (Stephan and Zucker, 1972).

As we have reported previously, it seems that the habenulae and the interconnected ITP are considered part of a feeding system. The parallel between the two feeding systems—the epithalamic and the hypothalamic—is further strengthened by the recent data in favour of a neurosecretory activity in the ITP (Kemali, 1977a) and the dorsal habenular nuclei of the frog (Kemali 1977b).

In our opinion there are grounds to consider the photoreceptors confined to the left side of the epithalamus as the phylogenetically oldest structures essential to the mediation between the light–dark cycle of environmental illumination and the behavioural rhythms of the animal. The hormonal nature of the mechanism cannot be excluded.

If our interpretation is correct, the morphological asymmetry of the dorsal habenular nucleus could have a functional explanation.

THE ITP

The ITP attracted the attention of early neuro-anatomists (Cajal, 1911) for its unique structure, and although many studies have been conducted since then its function has not yet been established.

A puzzling behaviour following lesion of the ITP is described by Bailey and Davis (1942). They obtained a locomotor automatism in the cat which continued without remission until the death of the animal and which they described as the 'syndrome of obstinate progression'. Herrick (1948) hypothesised the inhibitory function of the ITP which, when lost, could explain this syndrome.

The ITP establishes anatomical connections with the habenular nuclei through the FR (Smaha and Kaelber, 1973), with the dorsal and deep tegmental nuclei (Briggs and Kaelber, 1971; Morest, 1961), and it has been demonstrated (Lazar, 1969; Rubinson, 1968) that it receives bilateral projections from the optic tectum in which the ipsilateral component is the strongest.

The connection established by the FR is particularly interesting from the structural point of view. First, because it forms a connection between a pair of nuclei, one on the right and one on the left side of the brain, and one single nucleus situated on the midline of the tegmentum mesencephali. Secondly, it is interesting for the neuro-anatomically unique architectural pattern established by the fibres of the FR and the cell population of the ITP. Some of the fibres of the FR end in the nucleus (Lenn, 1976; Mizuno and Nakamura, 1974), while some traverse the nucleus and continue caudally to end in the dorsal and deep tegmental nuclei (Akagi and Powell, 1968; Way and Kaelber, 1969). In this way one short pathway connects the habenulae and the ITP while a long pathway after having traversed the ITP, connects the habenulae and the dorsal tegmental nuclei.

Short Pathway

By means of immunohistochemical techniques the habenulae and the ITP have been found to be rich in substance 'P' (Brownstein *et al.*, 1976; Leranth *et al.*, 1975). Hokfelt *et al.* (1975) demonstrated it within neurons of the habenular nuclei and electron microscopy has revealed large granules, with a sub-unit structure, probably the storage sites of this peptide, in the habenular nuclei (Kemali, 1977b) and in large processes of cells of the ITP (Kemali, 1977a) whose perikaryons lie distant from the ependymal lining of the sylvian aqueduct. The processes of such cells cross the ITP in a dorsoventral direction, perpendicular to the fibres which traverse the nucleus in the frontal plane and which belong to the long pathway. They end in foot-like expansions on the subpial ventral surface of the ITP which is above the interpeduncular cistern, where a pool of cerebrospinal fluid and large blood vessels occur, and where these cells could presumably release their content.

The ablation of the telencephalon resulted in the degeneration of these large processes (Figure 2.4d) in the ITP, thus suggesting the existence of a link between structures in the telencephalon and these particular cells in the ITP, but the anatomical route is unknown.

There is a correlation between the degeneration of the habenular nuclei and the content of substance 'P' in the ITP (Hong *et al.*, 1976). On the other hand there is evidence that the fibre tract which interconnects the habenulae and the ITP is cholinergic (Kataoka *et al.*, 1973; Kuhar *et al.*, 1975). It is possible that the portions of the FR which ends in the ITP—the short pathway—may be part of a circuit in which the neurons which use a peptide as probable neurotransmitters (habenula) or neurohormones (ITP) are of the Golgi type II and are regulated by cholinergic neurons of the Golgi type I which form part of the FR which interconnects reciprocally the habenulae and the ITP.

This portion of the habenulo-interpeduncular system, because of its topological position and the type of chemical substances within its structures, could represent a crucial circuit within the mesolimbic path in the production of the abnormal behaviour associated with schizophrenia.

Long Pathway

From the anatomical point of view the long path of the FR deserves attention. The anatomical structure of the ITP is shown in figure 2.5, where the components of the

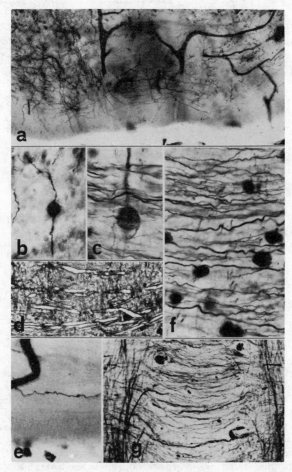

Figure 2.5. (a) The ITP seen in transverse section and impregnated according to the Golgi method. On the left the fibres of the FR entering the nucleus are shown. Two large blood vessels mark the lateral margins of the nucleus. 160×. (b), (c) Two neurons of the ITP, Golgi and Bodian preparations, respectively, showing their axons directed in opposed directions. Transverse section, 800×. (d) Semi-thin transverse section of the ITP showing myelinated axons traversing it. 340×. (e) Transverse section showing one beaded fibre traversing the ITP. Golgi preparation. 500×. (f) Transverse section of the ITP. Unmyelinated fibres of various diameters traverse the nucleus. Cajal method. 900×. (g) Horizontal section of the ITP stained according to Landau method. The fibres entering the ITP at its border are shown; the holes are blood vessels cut transversely. 140×

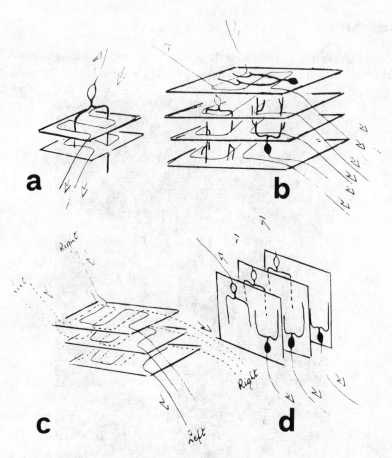

Figure 2.6.   Tridimensional sketches of the ITP of the frog in which, for simplicity, only a few elements are shown. The fibres of the FR confine their peculiar wiring to horizontal planes (a, b, c) as well as the cells with their dendrites spread horizontally (b). The fibres of the FR enter in the rostral portion and exit from the caudal portion of the ITP. In (a) and (b) only one fibre of the FR of one side is illustrated, while in (c) fibres of the FR from both sides are shown in order to demonstrate their peculiar decussations within the ITP. The cells with their dendrites spread in the sagittal direction are confined to sagittal planes within the ITP (d), but contact the fibres of the FR of several horizontal planes (a). The neurons having their axons directed caudally have black soma, while those directed rostrally have white soma. This configuration is described in detail in the text.

nucleus are illustrated in Golgi preparations and in material stained for unmyelinated and myelinated fibres. Ablation of the habenular nuclei (one at a time) and the application of a modification of the degenerative technique of Nauta (Eager, 1970) has shown that in the frog there is no difference between the projections of the habenular nuclei of the two sides to the ITP (Kemali and Guglielmotti, 1973) and this observation could be in favour of the hypothesis that the medial portion of the left habenular nucleus could be considered a metabolically different zone within the habenulo-interpeduncular system. The degenerative methods have also shown that some fibres proceed caudally, flanking the ITP, while others enter the nucleus where they form the well-known peculiar wiring.

The Golgi method has shown that the fibres of each FR enter the ITP from one side, traverse it to reach the opposite side, then loop over and cross the nucleus again to reach the first side where they loop over to traverse it again and then continue caudally, establishing contralateral connections with the more caudal nuclei.

The loops described are confined to the horizontal plane and cross within the nucleus the loops formed by the fibres of the FR entering the nucleus from the other side. Thus the fibres of the FR which enter the ITP may be considered to be decussating fibres, as they connect the habenula of one side with the contralateral dorsal and deep tegmental nuclei through the wiring of the fibres within the nucleus, where they establish contact 'en passant' with the cell population.

By means of this long path the fibres of the right and left FR have the opportunity of contacting the entire cell population of the ITP. The fibres of the FR of both sides enter the nucleus at different levels in the frontal plane. Thus we shall see a stack of several such loops in this plane of section, the stack being separated into discrete levels, each level containing its decussations (figure 2.6).

The cells of the ITP are bipolar with a dendritic trunk which arborises widely and an axon which projects outside the nucleus. Some of the cells are oriented with the dendritic arborisation on the horizontal plane and with the axon directed caudally. Some have the dendritic arborisation directed vertically and widely spread in the sagittal plane at right angles to the fibres of the FR which traverse the nucleus in the horizontal plane (Cajal likened this arrangement to that of the parallel fibres with the Purkinje cells of the cerebellar cortex). This latter type of neuron can have its axons in opposite directions. In fact some of them send their axons upwards to join the FR and are probably responsible for the feedback path from the ITP to the habenular nuclei. Another portion sends the axons caudally to join the fibres of the FR which do not end in the ITP but proceed caudally. The dendrites of both types of neuron are, of course, oriented in opposite directions with regard to their axons.

The result of this schematised geometric arrangement (figure 2.6) is that the neurons with the dendrites spread in the horizontal plane contact the loops of the FR which are confined to this plane and are formed by one fibre from the right FR and one from the left. Those directed vertically contact all the loops of the different horizontal planes at the various levels and are in connection with the whole output of the FR from both sides.

In this way, depending on the spreading of the dendritic arborisation, the fibres of the FR can deliver several impulses displaced in time to the same neuron, so that there is a temporal control of the sequence of the axonal firing. If these impulses, although separated by small delays, are below the threshold firing level but arrive within the excitation time of the neuron, their signal can be summated and cause the firing of the neuron. This may apply to all the cells having this particular type of construction and could produce a general firing with a consequent massive output.

Due to the geometric arrangement of the cell population of the ITP with the fibres of the FR traversing the nucleus, it is sufficient to have a stimulus arriving from only one FR (i.e. from the right or left side of the brain) to influence all the ITP efferents (i.e. caudal motor structures of both sides) as well as the habenular nuclei of both sides via feedback connections.

This simplification is suggested by the observation of the Golgi impregnated material. The neuropil of the ITP is very complex when examined by the electron microscope and shows a variety of synaptic vesicles. Furthermore, as already noted, there are cells whose secretory nature is assumed and from which it appears that the habenulo-interpeduncular system of the frog offers an example of interrelationship between functions mediated by neurotransmitters and by neurohormones.

However, the most important feature of the habenulo-interpeduncular system, from the anatomical point of view, seems to be its neuronal circuitry which suggests a device for modulating the correct timing and sequencing for selected patterns of movement of an articulate motor organ, as for instance the tongue.

It is known that the prey-catching behaviour of a frog is put in motion by a mechanism of visually guided behaviour in which the thalamus and the telencephalon might be involved (Ingle, 1976) and which ends in the 'firing' of the tongue on the prey with great precision and at exactly the right moment. The optic tectum has fibres projecting to the ITP (Lazar, 1969; Rubinson, 1968) and neurons able to modify snapping and tongue movement (Grusser and Grusser-Cornehls, 1976). The visual input, in general, is a sort of predictive input, as it can locate a target position prior to the initiation of the motor response and guide the movement towards the source of stimulation.

To accomplish the prey-catching behaviour the frog needs a precisely timed monitoring and controlling mechanism for its tongue. The ITP provides, through the long thin fibres which traverse it, a delay line to allow this appropriate timing. With the various sizes and the different degrees of myelination of its fibres and with the particular geometric arrangement of its cells, it provides the possibility of discharging its entire cell population simultaneously to a caudal motor pool, regardless of whether the stimulus impinges on the right or left side structures of the brain. In other words, a stimulus from only one side is sufficient to produce a massive output of the entire ITP which will influence simultaneously and bilaterally the caudal motor structures. Furthermore, a feedback circuit to the habenular nuclei supplies a monitoring and control action on its massive output. In addition, a feedback control from the periphery cannot be excluded, as we have demonstrated in the tongue of the frog, by means of the Ruffini method, the presence of spiral nerve endings which could represent a specialised form of proprioceptor (Kemali, 1973).

In conclusion we suggest that a portion of the habenulo-interpeduncular complex represents a neural system which controls the lingual motor activity of the frog.

This is an hypothesis which needs the demonstration of a direct anatomical link between the ITP and the hypoglossal nuclei.

ACKNOWLEDGEMENT

We wish to thank Professor E. Caianiello for his encouragement in this research and E. Casale, D. Gioffré, V. Guglielmotti and E. Sada of Laboratorio di Cibernetica and G. Dafnis of Stazione Zoologica of Naples for their valuable technical assistance.

SUMMARY

By means of the functional interpretation of the neuro-anatomy of the habenulo-interpeduncular system of the frog, we wish to call attention to the important role that this circuit might have within the vertebrate central nervous system. The habenulo-interpeduncular system is of particular interest for its position in the limbic circuit and for being the site rich in substance 'P' which might be stored in structures which we have identified with the electron microscope. Furthermore the ultrastructure of the habenulo-interpeduncular system favours the hypothesis that it is the site of a relationship between neural and hormonal functions.

The results of the examination of traditional histological and electron microscope preparations and the observation made on degeneration material suggest that the medial portion of the left habenula stands alone among the other structures of the system and may share with the pineal body a functional mediation of some kind between environmental light and the organism's activity rhythms which would be in favour of a functional specialisation of the left side of the brain. Commissural fibres in the habenular commissure indicate a mutual interaction between the symmetric habenulae.

The interpeduncular nucleus (ITP) through the peculiar decussation of the fibres of the fasciculus retroflexus (FR) may influence simultaneously the bilateral structures of the brainstem as a consequence of homolateral stimulation.

The neuro-anatomically unique architectural pattern between the cells and the fibres of the ITP suggests that the stimulation of the afferences from either side to the ITP results in a massive simultaneous output. We hypothesise that a portion of the habenulo-interpeduncular system represents in the frog the anatomical circuit responsible for the projection of the tongue towards an edible target.

Note added in proof

Since submitting this manuscript several papers concerning the habenular connections of the rat have been published. Afferents to the lateral habenula of striatal origin (Herkenham and Nauta, 1977) and lateral habenula afferents to midbrain raphe (Aghajanian and Wang, 1977) have been reported by means of the horse-radish peroxidase retrograde transport method. Cuello *et al*. (1978) have also reported an interaction between the substance P containing neurons of the medial habenula and the A-10 group of catecholaminergic neurons which are located around the ITP and which are the origin of the dopaminergic mesocortical and mesolimbic systems. A probable projection from the mesocortical system to the habenula has also been reported (Bjorklund, 1978). The habenulae then, as stressed also by the above literature, seem to be, in addition, prominent structures, where inputs of both striatal and limbic origin converge, which are interposed in those dopaminergic circuits that are believed to be involved in some psychiatric disorders.

REFERENCES

Aghajanian, G. K. and Wang, R. Y. (1977). Habenular and other midbrain raphe afferents demonstrated by a modified retrograde tracing technique. *Brain Res.*, **122**, 229-42

Akagi, K. and Powell, E. W. (1968). Differential projections of the habenular nuclei. *J. comp. Neurol.*, **132**, 263-73

Bailey, P. and Davis, E. W. (1942). The syndrome of obstinate progression in the cat. *Proc. Soc. exp. Biol. Med.*, **51**, 307

Bjorklund, A. (1978). Dopaminergic pathways in the rat CNS. *Neurosci. Lett.* Suppl. 1, S418

Bjorklund, A., Owman, Ch. and West, K. A. (1972). Peripheral sympathetic innervation and serotonin cells in the habenular region of the rat brain. *Z. Zellforsch.*, **127**, 570-79

Booth, D. A. (1967). Localization of the adrenergic feeding system in the rat diencephalon. *Science*, **158**, 515-17

Bowman, J. P. (1971). *The Muscle Spindle and Neural Control of Tongue*, C. C. Thomas, Springfield, Illinois

Braak, H. (1970). Biogene Amine im Gehirn von Frosch (*Rana esculenta*). *Z. Zellforsch.*, **106**, 269-308

Braitenberg, V. and Kemali, M. (1970). Exceptions to bilateral symmetry in the epithalamus of lower vertebrates. *J. comp. Neurol.*, **138**, 137-46

Briggs, T. L. and Kaelber, W. W. (1971). Efferent fiber connections of the dorsal and deep tegmental nuclei of Gudden. An experimental study in the cat. *Brain Res.*, **29**, 17-29

Brownstein, M. J., Mroz, E. A., Kizer, J. S., Palkovits, M. and Leeman, S. E. (1976). Regional distribution of substance P in the brain of the rat. *Brain Res.*, **116**, 299-305

Cajal, R. Y. S. (1911). *Histologie du Système Nerveux de l'Homme et des Vertébrés*, vols I and II, Madrid (traduit par le L. Azoulay, Paris, A. Maloine, 1909-1911)

Cragg, B. G. (1959). A heat-loss mechanism involving the habenular, interpeduncular and dorsal tegmental nuclei. *Nature*, **184**, 1724

Cragg, B. G. (1961). The connections of the habenula in the rabbit. *Expl. Neurol.*, **3**, 388-409

Crosby, E. C., Humphrey, T. and Lauer, E. W. (1962). *Correlative Anatomy of the Nervous System*. McMillan, New York

Cuello, A. C., Emson, P. C., Paxinos, G. and Jessell, T. (1978). Substance P containing and cholinergic projections from the habenula. *Brain Res.*, **149**, 413-29

David, C. F. X. and Herbert, J. (1973). Experimental evidence for a synaptic connection between habenula and pineal ganglion in the ferret. *Brain Res.*, **64**, 327-43

Eager, R. P. (1970). Selective staining and degenerative axons in the central nervous system by a simplified silver method: spinal cord projections to external cuneate and inferior olivary nuclei in the cat. *Brain Res.*, **22**, 137-41

Eakin, R. M., Quay, W. B. and Westfall, J. A. (1963). Cytological and cytochemical studies on the frontal pineal organs of the treefrog '*Hyla regilla*'. *Z. Zeitforsch.*, **59**, 663-83

Frontera, J. G. (1952). A study of the anuran diencephalon. *J. comp. Neurol.*, **96**, 1-69

Geschwind, N. and Levitzky, W. (1968). Human brain: left-right asymmetries in temporal speech region. *Science*, **161**, 186-89

Granit, R. and Kaada, B. R. (1953). Influence of stimulation of central nervous system structures of muscle spindles in cat. *Acta physiol. scand.*, **27**, 130-60

Grossman, S. P. (1968). Hypothalamic and limbic influences on food intake. *Fedn Proc.*, **27**, 1349-60

Grusser, O. -J. and Grusser-Cornehls, U. (1976). Neurophysiology of the anuran visual system. In *Frog Neurobiology*, Springer-Verlag, Heidelberg, pp. 297-385

Halpern, M. (1972). Some connections of the telencephalon of the frog *Rana pipiens*. *Brain, Behav. Evol.*, **6**, 42-68

Herkenham, M. and Nauta, W. H. (1977). Afferent connections of the habenular nuclei in the rat. A Horseradish Peroxidase study, with a note on the fiber-of-passage problem. *J. comp. Neurol.* **173**, 123-46

Herrick, C. J. (1948). *The Brain of the Tiger Salamander*, University of Chicago Press

Hokfelt, T., Keller, J. O., Nilsson, G. and Pernow, B. (1975). Substance P localization in the central nervous system and in some primary sensory neurons. *Science*, **190**, 889-90

Hong, J. S., Costa, E. and Yang, H. -Y. T. (1976). Effects of habenular lesions on the substance P content of various brain regions. *Brain Res.*, **118**, 523-25

Ingle, D. (1976). Behaviour correlates of central visual function in anurans. In *Frog Neurobiology*, Springer-Verlag Heidelberg, pp. 435-51

Isaacson, R. L. (1974). *The Limbic System*, Plenum Press, New York

Jacobowitz, D. M. and Palkovits, M. (1974). Topographic atlas of catecholamine and acetylcholinesterase-containing neurons in the rat brain. 1. Forebrain (telencephalon, diencephalon). *J. comp. Neurol.*, **157**, 13-28

Jansen, J. (1930). The brain of *Myxine glutinosa*. *J. comp. Neurol.*, **49**, 359-507

Johnston, J. B. (1902). The brain of Petromyzon. *J. comp. Neurol.*, **12**, 1-86

Kaada, B. R. (1951). Somato-motor, autonomic and electrocorticographic responses to electrical stimulation of 'rhinencephalic' and other structures in primates, cat and dog. *Acta physiol. scand.*, **24**, Suppl. 83, 1-285

Kappers, J. A. (1971). The pineal organ: an introduction. In *The Pineal Gland* (J. Knight, ed.), Ciba Foundation Symposium, Churchill, London, pp. 3-25

Kataoka, K., Nakamura, Y. and Hassler, R. (1973). Habenulo-interpeduncular tract: a possible cholinergic neuron system in rat brain. *Brain Res.*, **62**, 264-67

Kemali, D., Bartholini, G. and Richter, D., eds. (1976). *Schizophrenia Today*, Pergamon Press, Oxford

Kemali, M. (1970). Asimmetria: regola o eccezione? *Acta Neurol.*, **XXV**, 476-88
Kemali, M. (1973). Lingual nerve-endings in the frog. *A. Mikrosk-Anat. Forsch.*, 87, 544-48
Kemali, M. (1974). Ultrastructural asymmetry of the habenular nuclei of the frog. *J. Hirnforsch.*, **15**, 419-26
Kemali, M. (1976a). A modification of the rapid Golgi method. *Stain Technol.*, **51**, 169-72
Kemali, M. (1976b). The electron microscopy of the synaptic vesicles of the frog habenular nuclei. *Brain Res.*, **112**, 156-61
Kemali, M. (1977a). The interpeduncular nucleus (ITP). Ultrastructure data indicative of a possible neurosecretory activity. *Cell Tissue Res.*, **178**, 83-96
Kemali, M. (1977b). The ultrastructure of the large granular vesicles of the frog's habenula. *Neurosci. Lett.*, 5, 21-4
Kemali, M. and Agrelli, I. (1972). The habenulo-interpeduncular nuclear system of a reptilian representative *Lacerta sicula. Z. Mikrosk.-Anat. Forsch.*, 85, 325-33
Kemali, M. and Braitenberg, V. (1969). *Atlas of the Frog's Brain*, Springer-Verlag, Heidelberg.
Kemali, M. and Guglielmotti, V. (1973). Studio preliminare sulle fibre efferenti degenerate dei nuclei abenulari di *Rana esculenta. Acta Neurol.*, **XXVIII**, 225-30
Kemali, M. and Guglielmotti, V. (1977). An electron microscope observation of the right and the two left portions of the habenular nuclei of the frog. *J. comp. Neurol.*, **176**(2). 133-48
Kemali, M. and Sada, E. (1973). Myelinated cell bodies in the habenular nuclei of the frog. *Brain Res.*, **54**, 355-59
Kemali, M., Casale, E., Guglielmotti, V. and Sada, E. (1971). Indagine quantitativa su una zona epitalamica asimmetrica nel tritone e nell'anguilla. *Boll. Soc. It. Biol. Sper.*, **XLVII**, 472-75
Kuhar, M. J., De Haven, R. N., Yamamura, H. I., Rommelspacher, R. and Simon, J. R. (1975). Further evidence for cholinergic habenulo-interpeduncular neurons: pharmacologic and functional characteristics. *Brain Res.*, **97**, 265-75
Lazar, G. (1969). Efferent pathways of the optic tectum in the frog. *Acta Biol. Acad. Sci. Hung.*, **20**, 171-83
Lenn, N. J. (1976). Synapses in the interpeduncular nucleus: electron microscopy of normal and habenular lesioned rat. *J. comp. Neurol.*, **166**, 73-100
Leranth, Cs., Brownstein, M., Zaborszky, L., Jaranyi, Zs. and Palkovits, M. (1975). Morphological and biochemical changes in the rat interpeduncular nucleus following the transection of the habenulo-interpeduncular tract. *Brain Res.*, **99**, 124-28
McRea, D. L., Branch, C. L. and Milner, B. (1969). The occipital horns and cerebral dominance. *Neurology.*, **18**, 95-98
Mitchell, R. (1963). Connections of the habenula and of the interpeduncular nucleus in the cat. *J. comp. Neurol.*, **121**, 441-53
Mizuno, N. and Nakamura, Y. (1974). An electron microscope study of terminal degeneration of the fasciculus retroflexus Meynerti within the interpeduncular nucleus of the rabbit. *Brain Res.*, **65**, 165-69
Mok, A. C. S. and Mogenson, G. J. (1972a). An evoked potential study of the projections to the lateral habenular nucleus from the septum and the lateral preoptic area in the rat. *Brain Res.*, **43**, 343-60
Mok, A. C. S. and Mogenson, G. J. (1972b). Effect of electrical stimulation of the septum and the lateral preoptic area on unit activity of the lateral habenular nucleus in the rat. *Brain Res.*, **43**, 361-72

Moody, M. F. and Robertson, J. D. (1960). The fine structure of some retinal photoreceptors. *J. biophys. biochem. Cytol.*, **7**, 87–92

Moore, R. Y. (1974). Visual pathways and the central neural control of diurnal rhythms. In *The Neurosciences*, 3rd Study Program, MIT Press, Cambridge, Massachusetts, 537–42

Morest, D. K. (1961). Connexions of the dorsal tegmental nucleus in rat and rabbit *J. Anat.*, **95**, 229–46

Morgane, P. J. (1961a). Medial forebrain bundle and 'feeding centers' of the hypothalamus. *J. comp. Neurol.*, **117**, 1–25

Morgane, P. J. (1961b). Alterations in feeding and drinking behavior in rats with lesions in globi pallidi. *Am. J. Physiol.*, **201**, 420–28

Mulder, A. H. and Snyder, S. H. (1976). Putative central neurotransmitters. In *Molecular and Functional Neurobiology* (W. H. Gispen, ed.), Elsevier, Amsterdam, pp. 161–220

Nauta, W. J. H. (1958). Hippocampal projections and related neural pathways to the midbrain in the cat. *Brain*, **81**, 319–40

Nottebohm, F. (1970). Ontogeny of bird song: different strategies in vocal development are reflected in learning stages, critical periods, and neural lateralization. *Science*, **167**, 950–56

Porter, K. R. and Yamada, F. (1960). Studies on the endoplasmic reticulum. I. Its form and differentiation in pigment epithelial cells of the frog retina. *J. biophys. biochem. Cvt.*, **8**, 181–204

Powell, E. W. (1968). Septohabenular connections in the rat, cat and monkey. *J. comp. Neurol.*, **134**, 145–150

Raisman, G. (1966). The connexions of the septum. *Brain*, **89**, 317–48

Rausch, L. J. and Long, C. J. (1971). Habenular nuclei: a crucial link between olfactory and motor system. *Brain Res.*, **29**, 146–50

Rubinson, K. (1968). Projections of the tectum opticum of the frog. *Brain, Behav. Evol.*, **1**, 529–61

Scalia, F. (1976). Structure of the olfactory and accessory olfactory system. In *Frog Neurobiology*, Springer-Verlag, Heidelberg, pp. 213–33

Smaha, L. A. and Kaelber, W. W. (1973). Efferent fiber projections of the habenula and the interpeduncular nucleus. An experimental study in the opossum and cat. *Expl Brain Res.*, **16**, 291–308

Snyder, S. H. (1972). Catecholamines in the brain as mediators of amphetamine psychosis. *Archs gen. Psych.*, **27**, 169–79

Stephan, F. K. and Zucker, I. (1972). Circadian rhythms in drinking behaviour and locomotor activity of rats are eliminated by hypothalamic lesions. *Proc. natn Acad. Sci. U.S.A.*, **69**, 1583–86

Trueman, J. and Herbert, J. (1970). Monoamines and acetylcholinesterase in the pineal gland and habenula of the ferret. *Brain Res.*, **109**, 83–100

Uchizono, K. (1962). Structure of possible photoreceptive elements in the 6th abdominal ganglion of crayfish. *J. Cell Biol.*, **15**, 151–54

Way, J. S. and Kaelber, W. W. (1969). A degeneration study of efferent connections of the habenular complex in the opossum. *Am. J. Anat.*, **124**, 31–46

Woods, J. W. (1964). Behavior of chronic decerebrate rats. *J. Neurophysiol.*, **26**, 635–44

Wurtman, R. J., Akelrod, J. and Kelly, D. E. (1968). *The Pineal*, Academic Press, New York

3
INTEROCULAR TRANSFER AND COMMISSURE FUNCTION IN LOWER VERTEBRATES, WITH SPECIAL REFERENCE TO FISH

GEORGE E. SAVAGE

INTRODUCTION

The vast majority of studies on interhemispheric relations in lower vertebrates have utilised the interocular transfer of various types of visual discrimination. Fish in particular have proved to be ideal animals for such investigations, because their visual system is capable of discriminating fine colour and shape differences, and their behaviour is sufficiently variable to allow them to be trained with a wide variety of regimes (see, for example, Behrend and Bitterman, 1964; Bitterman *et al.,* 1958).

Lower vertebrates in general have two distinct advantages as subjects for interocular transfer experiments. First, the entire optic input from one eye projects to the contralateral optic tectum; hence, sectioning of the optic chiasm, and the attendant visual deficits, can be avoided. Fish have the added advantage of simplicity in visual system structure, for in the teleost fish at least, there is no evidence for a visual projection to the telencephalon (Karamian *et al.,* 1966).

Schroeder and Ebbesson (1974) have demonstrated thalamic projection to the telencephalon in sharks, and have suggested that this is partially visual, on the basis of evoked-potential evidence (Cohen *et al.,* 1973). However, it is necessary to show caution in such an interpretation, for Karamian has demonstrated how easily visual evoked potentials can spread from the tectum to other areas of the brain. The interpretation of the behavioural evidence for lack of vision following telencephalic ablation in sharks (Graeber *et al.,* 1972) has been questioned elsewhere (Savage, 1978) as being due to the delayed reward technique used. The matter of a telencephalic visual projection in elasmobranchs is thus uncertain

Secondly, the majority of lower vertebrates possess little binocular overlap, and hence it is often quite simple to present stimuli to one eye without the need to cover the other eye. Quite apart from the procedural simplifications permitted by these anatomical peculiarities, the fact that the two visual fields hardly overlap, and that the visual projections are exclusively contralateral, means that there must normally

be continual and effective correlation of two separate visual worlds in lower vertebrates. This must occur at a high level in the central nervous system, and leads to
the expectation of efficient interocular transfer of learned information in these
animals. Thus the study of lower forms of vertebrate neural organisation may help
us to understand the origin and significance of commissural systems, by examining
such systems in their simplest manifestation. In particular, the absence of any true
cerebral organisation focuses our attention on subcortical mechanisms of learning
and cross-brain transfer.

THE MAJOR COMMISSURES OF THE PROSENCEPHALON AND MESENCEPHALON OF FISH

The Telencephalon

The telencephalic hemispheres of fish are characterised by a lack of neocortical
development. Homologies with the brains of higher vertebrates are difficult, for
the telencephalon shows an eversion during development, which makes topological
relations difficult to ascertain (see, for example, Bannister, 1973; Herrick, 1922;
Nieuwenhuys, 1959). However, such homologies as are possible suggest that the
fish telencephalon represents the early stages of development of the basal ganglia
and limbic system. (The dorsomedial areas have been characterised as hippocampal,
the anterior dorsolateral areas as pyriform, the posterior dorsolateral areas as
amygdaloid, and the dorsocentral areas as striatal (Schnitzlein, 1964; Sheldon,
1912).

The two sides of the telencephalon are linked by the anterior commissure,
which in fact consists partly of large numbers of decussating fibres of the olfactory
tracts and forebrain bundles. Despite this, there are true commissures linking the
ventral telencephalic areas, which Nieuwenhuys (1959) has characterised as primarily
olfactory, and the dorsal telencephalic areas, which receive little direct olfactory
input, and which have been implicated in the organisation of some innate (de Bruin,
1978) and learned (Savage, 1978) behaviours. The dorsolateral, medial and central
areas, whose possible homologies were discussed above, are all linked with the
equivalent area of the contralateral side by way of the anterior commissure
(Nieuwenhuys, 1959).

The Diencephalon

There are three major diencephalic commissures. These lie close together immediately behind the optic chiasm, and are often known collectively as the postoptic commissures. Closest to the chiasm, and often appearing to be part of it, is the transverse
commissure. This links areas of the dorsal thalamus, and probably contains tectal
fibres. Behind this are two commissures lying one above the other—the dorsal minor

and the ventral horizontal commissures. The minor commissure links pretectal areas and also parts of the posterior hypothalamus. The horizontal commissure links areas of the anterior thalamus and of the posterior hypothalamus (Ariëns Kappers *et al.*, 1935).

Although all three commissures link areas which have considerable probable visual projection, no definite statements can be made as to the terminations of commissural fibres, for as yet there have been no degeneration or dye studies on the projections of these systems.

The Mesencephalon

The mesencephalon contains two commissures—the posterior and the tectal. The former lies in the anterior dorsal tegmentum, and projects to the pretectal area, the dorsal thalamus and the tectum (Ariëns Kappers *et al.*, 1935; Hocke Hoogenboom, 1929; Schnitzlein, 1962). The tectal commissure forms a ladder-like link between the two optic tecta. Fibres have been shown to run into a deep white zone, then ascend through the grey layers to terminate in the superficial fibrous marginal layer (Marlotte and Mark, 1975).

BEHAVIOURAL TECHNIQUES FOR DEMONSTRATING TRANSFER

Two paradigms in particular have lent themselves to studies of interocular transfer in fish; these are classical conditioning of the bradycardiac response to shock (figure 3.1), and instrumental avoidance of shock (figure 3.2). Both types of task may be used with single or differential stimulus presentations, and their great advantage lies in the fact that fish are confined in a narrow chamber, so that a stimulus can be presented to one eye alone, without the contralateral eye needing to be covered. Hence, one eye only can learn a discrimination, while both eyes learn any movements necessary to perform the response. The importance of this will be shown below. The disadvantage of these methods stems from a peculiarity of fish, namely that they cannot be trained to respond to stationary shapes when the animals themselves are stationary, although they are immediately able to identify the same stationary shapes in an identical situation when they themselves are free to move. Thus, shape stimuli must be moved when presented to fish, although higher vertebrates can learn when presented with stationary shapes. Such a difference may be an expression of a movement-scanning mode of shape analysis in fish, or of an inbuilt mechanism to select attention only for objects moving against a background. There have been several attempts to identify shape-sensitive neurons in the optic tectum of goldfish, but without success. However, Guthrie (personal communication) has found such units in the tectum of the perch, and it may be that different species of fish analyse shapes in different ways, as suggested by Trevarthen (1968).

Moving shapes and their attendant extraneous cues can be avoided if fish are trained to swim to stationary shapes to obtain food, for instance in the simultaneous choice chamber designed by Meesters (1940) and used extensively for visual studies by Sutherland (1969). Such experimental situations necessitate the fitting of eye occluders if monocular presentation is desired, and the use of occluders causes problems of interpretation in transfer studies in fish.

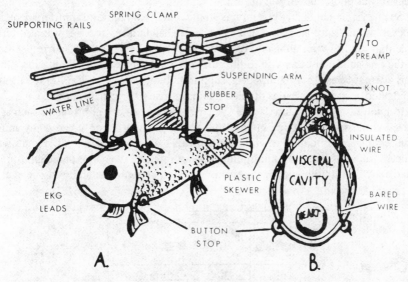

Figure 3.1. (A) Technique used for restraining fish during cardiac conditioning and tests for transfer of the conditioned cardiac response. (B) Schematic cross-section of fish at level of heart showing buried EKG electrodes in place (McCleary, 1960)

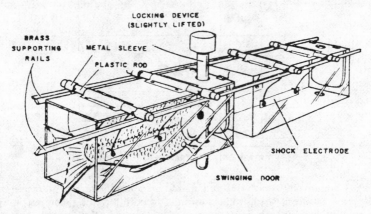

Figure 3.2. Double-box apparatus for avoidance training of fish. (The subjects are trained to swim forward to the anterior box when positive stimulus is presented and to remain in place when the neutral stimulus is presented) (McCleary, 1960)

The earliest study on fish interocular transfer, that of Sperry and Clark (1949), encountered this problem. Gobies (*Bathygobius soporator*) were trained to swim to small high white lures, and not to large low red lures, to obtain food. Although the animals acquired the task rapidly, occlusion of the trained eye caused a disruption of discriminative responses, although these returned immediately when the trained eye was uncovered, and the naive eye patched. It was concluded that interocular transfer was poorly developed in fish.

Such a finding in higher vertebrates would indicate a failure to transfer adequately an engram, but since animals failed to respond at all in many cases, it was also possible that the fish were unable to organise the actual operant response, irrespective of the availability or otherwise to the naive eye of the relevant discrimination engram. This alternative explanation has been supported by work by McCleary (1960), who conducted an extensive series of experiments on fish interocular transfer. Early tests involved training fish with one eye covered, on a variety of problems such as mazes, visual discriminations and multiple-choice learning. In no case did any animal manifest signs of retention when tested using its naive eye. However, if animals were trained using the classical conditioning of heart rate and avoidance paradigms outlined above, with both eyes open, but with stimuli presented laterally to one eye,

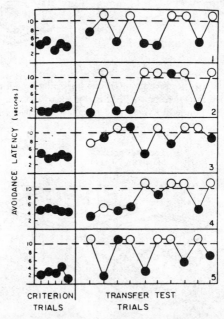

Figure 3.3. Results on five individual fish, trained and tested for interocular transfer in the double-box avoidance apparatus without use of blinders. (Filled circles show response latencies to the positive stimulus; open circles show latencies in response to the neutral stimulus. Since transfer trials were terminated after 10 s, points above the dashed line indicate that no avoidance response was made) (McCleary, 1960)

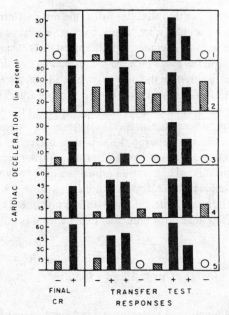

Figure 3.4. Individual data for five fish, showing, on the left, size of final cardiac CR after conditioning the 'training' eye. (Transfer-test responses show the differential cardiac responses resulting when the stimuli are presented to the contralateral, 'naive' eye. The naive eye was covered during conditioning, and the training eye was covered during the tests for transfer (McCleary, 1960)

perfect transfer was observed (figure 3.3). Further, when fish were trained on these problems, but with monocular occlusion, the cardiac response transferred (figure 3.4), whereas the avoidance response did not. It appears that the information relating to the reinforcement associated with shapes can transfer if occluders are used, as seen in the cardiac conditioning experiments, but that transfer of the information relating to the response is inhibited by the use of patching. This distinction is upheld by the results obtained by McCleary using several instrumental paradigms, where he observed that while fish being tested to the naive eye might not show skilled responses, they nevertheless gave greater or lesser arousal responses to the positive or neutral shapes, indicating that some discriminative information was available to the naive side of the brain. This peculiarity of interocular transfer in fish may possibly extend to other lower vertebrates, but there are as yet no observations on it.

In view of this experiential factor in fish visual transfer, it is important to demonstrate adequate response transfer before levels of discriminative transfer can be assessed. An elegant study by Shapiro (1965) is an example of such an approach. Goldfish were trained to press a paddle to obtain food, when a light came on, and were then trained with a red/green problem. Once they reached criterion, they received training with occluders fitted, and the eye being patched was alternated daily. Thus there was no question that the fish could not perform the response using either eye. Finally, animals were trained using a vertical versus horizontal bar problem, and the side with an occluder was alternated daily. One group of fish always saw the same shape as positive, a second group saw one shape positive in one eye, the other shape as positive in the other eye, and a third group was presented with random shape reinforcements. Only the first group learned, showing that transfer occurred, for the second group, receiving opposite information on the two sides of the brain, showed no acquisition. This suggests that there is an efficient system of information transfer between the two brain halves.

As McCleary has pointed out, interocular transfer in lower vertebrates is all the more impressive in that it is often between retinal sectors having no binocular overlap. He specifically examined this (McCleary and Longfellow, 1961) by training in the far lateral (temporal) field, where no overlap was possible. The levels of transfer were high, demonstrating that prior binocular experience was not necessary for transfer to occur.

LEVELS OF TRANSFER

The only detailed examination of conventional transfer levels in fish is that of Schulte (1957) using carp (*Carassius carassius*) fitted with occluders, and trained in an approach situation, using simultaneous shape presentations. His initial tests measured acquisition rates for monocularly and binocularly learned problems. Fish consistently took greater numbers of trials to reach criterion when using just one eye, than when using both eyes. This may possibly indicate that the side of the brain without optic input does not participate in acquisition, hence a 'mass action' deficit is seen, but in the absence of motor controls for unilateral visual deprivation such a conclusion is extremely tentative.

When fish received transfer trials there was no relation between the difficulty of learning the task and the degree of interocular transfer manifested. For instance, fish trained with ⌋ versus ∴ took an average of 475 trials to reach criterion, whereas the problem ||||| versus ▌▌▌▌ took 825 trials, but transfer levels of 80-90% were obtained for both problems.

Other types of visual problem have been shown to transfer. For example, Bernstein (1962) has demonstrated transfer of a colour discrimination, and this and a flash frequency discrimination have been shown to transfer during experiments carried out in the author's laboratory. (Cardiac conditioning was used in all three experiments.)

THE LIMITS OF TRANSFER

The type of transfer failure phenomenon outlined previously, namely an inability to transfer response information under certain conditions, suggests that interocular transfer in lower vertebrates may not be the apparently automatic and inevitable process it appears to be in the higher forms. Such considerations have led to a search for the limits of transfer, limits which may provide important clues to the functioning of the system.

Schulte (1957) examined transfer limits by presenting his fish with generalisation problems to both trained and naive eyes. In general, the greater the difference of the generalisation shapes from the original discrimination, the greater differences in performance were obtained between the two eyes; the naive eye appeared unable to cope with large generalisation shifts, and Schulte concluded that the memory established on the trained side was stronger than that on the untrained side. Such an assumption of bilateral engrams, rather than of access failure by the naive side, was of course speculative, although it has recently received direct proof (see chapter 4).

A considerable contribution to our knowledge of transfer limits has come from the work of Ingle, using the differential avoidance paradigm, in which response transfer appears to be automatic; hence, transfer failure may be assumed to relate to the discrimination. An early experiment (Ingle, 1965) showed that engrams involving colour appeared to transfer more easily than those involving shape, for if fish were trained with stimuli differing in colour and shape, and then both eyes were tested with the cues confounded, the trained eye responded to shape, the untrained eye to colour. With regard to shape, 'easy' tasks appeared to transfer more easily than 'difficult' ones (Ingle, 1968a). Thus responses to a $52°$ orientation difference in stripe patterns transferred, whereas responses to a $23°$ difference did not. When the $23°$-trained animals were tested with an easier ($38°$) pair to the naive eye, they did not respond, but $52°$-trained animals did. Ingle concluded that the failure to transfer was not failure to gain access to a contralateral engram, but a failure to lay down an ipsilateral engram. ($52°$-trained animals showed responses to $38°$, whereas the same transferable task did not give results in the $23°$-trained animals.)

Such evidence for a limit to the transfer of information led Ingle to attempt simultaneously to train opposing discriminations to the two eyes. Since fish could learn such a problem, he assumed that they were capable of independent action in the two halves of the brain, but it is possible that they could learn by *using* transfer, and hence learn HL/VR versus HR/VL as compound stimuli. However, other evidence makes the former explanation more likely. Fish could learn a discrimination trained to one eye, even if an irrelevant stimulus were presented to the other eye during training. When they were tested to the naive eye, no transfer occurred, but if there were as few as three trials without the irrelevant stimulus present, transfer occurred. It appears that a direct input to one tectum dominates its attention, and prevents the transfer of memory, but that very few undistracted trials are needed for such memory transfer to occur. A very similar phenomenon has been reported by Bureš and his co-workers, using spreading depression (Bureš and Burešová, 1971).

There is an apparent inconsistency between these results and those of Shapiro (1965) cited above, where Shapiro failed to train goldfish to learn opposing discriminations in opposite eyes. However, Shapiro's animals received training to one eye only each day, hence there was no stimulus in the opposite eye, and thus no inhibition of transfer to the naive side. Hence, each day there would be transfer of an opposing discrimination, totally irreconcilable with that established the previous day. In Ingle's paradigm, each tectum was dominated by its own direct input, and inhibited transfer of the reverse problem.

TRANSFER OF MIRROR IMAGE INFORMATION

Since the report of paradoxical interocular transfer of mirror images in pigeons (Mello, 1965), and reports of similar results in primates (Hamilton *et al.,* 1973; Noble, 1968; see also chapter 28), there has been considerable disagreement as to the interpretation of the phenomenon. Ingle (1968b) has suggested that the transfer of such shapes is dependent on their interpretation by the animal, and that this is in turn dependent on the size of shape used. Since fish eyes are situated laterally, a > shape presented to the left eye will point forwards, but if presented to the right eye, will point backwards (figure 3.5). The use of the term 'veridical' to describe such transfer is thus confusing, and Ingle has suggested the term 'L/R equivalence'. If a fish responds to > to the left eye by choosing < using the right eye, i.e. by choosing two nasally-directed arrowheads, it is said to show 'front/back equivalence'; this is synonymous with paradoxical transfer in higher vertebrates. Ingle found that small (subtending < 8°) objects showed L/R equivalence on transfer, whereas large (subtending > 22°) objects showed front/back equivalence. Small objects are con-

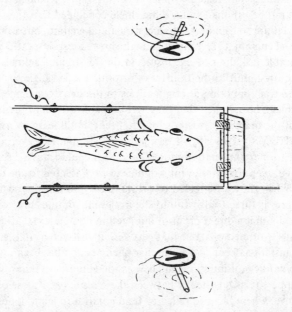

Figure 3.5. An 'equivalent' pair of shapes, as judged by interocular transfer tests following monocular training on 'forward' versus 'backward' arrowheads. This kind of transfer equivalence is called L/R. During a conditioned avoidance response, the subject swims forward through the door into the identical goal box (Ingle, 1968b)

sidered to be seen as units, and are therefore expected to retain the relation between their two ends, hence the veridical transfer, whereas large objects are seen as two or more separate 'bits', one of which is in front of the other in the visual field, hence the paradoxical transfer. Campbell (1971) has shown that if fish are presented with $\sim 16°$ shapes, they appear to have difficulty in recognising shapes as one class or the other, and hence transfer is neither veridical nor paradoxical.

AREAS OF THE LOWER VERTEBRATE BRAIN INVOLVED IN LEARNING

Only the telencephalon and the optic tectum have been the subject of any memory localisation studies, primarily in fish, and of the two areas the telencephalon has received by far the greater amount of attention.

Delay and trace classical conditioning (Farr and Savage, 1978; Overmier and Curnow, 1969; Overmier and Savage, 1974) and positively reinforced visual discriminations (Janzen, 1933; Savage, 1969b) are learned equally well by normal and telencephalon-ablated fish (figure 3.6). However, simple and differential avoidance, and some instrumental delay tasks, are poorly learned, and their retention is abolished, following telencephalic ablation (Aronson and Kaplan, 1968; Hainsworth *et al.,* 1967; Savage, 1969a). It is currently suggested that the telencephalon causes an arousal, which allows the utilisation of secondary reinforcement (see, for example,

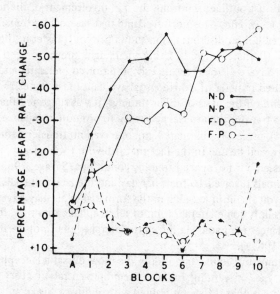

Figure 3.6. Mean percentage heart rate change during the CS–US interval for the normal delay-conditioning group (N–D), forebrain-ablated delay-conditioning group (F–D), normal pseudo-conditioning group (N–P), and the forebrain-ablated pseudo-conditioning group (F–P). Each point represents the mean of five trials for each of four fish (Overmier and Savage, 1974)

Farr and Savage, 1978; Flood *et al.*, 1976; Savage, 1978). Thus, for instance, fish which have been classically conditioned to light and shock will change their side preference in a T maze if 'rewarded' with light for turns to the preferred side; telencephalon-ablated fish, unable to use reinforcement derived from the light, show no preference change (Farr and Savage, 1978). With regard to other lower vertebrates, Bianki (1972) has shown deficits in classical conditioning in amphibia following telencephalic damage, so that it is possible that the telencephalic involvement in learning is greater in amphibians and reptiles than it is in fish.

Evidence for tectal involvement in learning in lower vertebrates is extremely tenuous. Tectal damage causes visual and motor deficits (Healey, 1957) which make interpretation of any learning deficits extremely difficult. For instance, Sears (1934) showed that a simple conditioned reflex was not abolished by tectal ablation, whereas Sanders (1940) found that retention of a maze paradigm was poor. Unpublished observations by the present author suggest that the learning and retention of avoidance problems are affected only to the extent that motor disorders are caused by the ablation.

COMMISSURES AND TRANSFER

The Anterior Commissure

In view of the results just outlined, showing the non-involvement of the telencephalon in classical conditioning, it is not surprising that interocular transfer of a classically conditioned colour discrimination shows perfect transfer in the absence of the telencephalon (Bernstein, 1962). Using a paradigm known to need telencephalic participation, Savage (1969a) severed the anterior commissure, and observed that there was impaired transfer of a differential avoidance task. Since the savings were considerable, and on the basis of other findings, it was suggested that there had been a failure to transfer the arousal necessary to promote avoidances. Ingle and Campbell (1974), using a similar paradigm, observed no transfer deficits, but this discrepancy may well be due to the fact that fish with total telencephalic ablation learn under massed but not spaced training conditions (Savage, 1968); hence, since the former animals received 10 trials per day and the latter all trials in one day, the telencephalic involvement in learning in the former animals may have been far greater. There is certainly some lateralisation of telencephalic function, for unilateral lesions impair avoidances mediated via the contralateral eye but not via the ipsilateral eye (Savage, 1969a).

The anterior commissure connects not only the more dorsal telencephalic regions implicated in some types of learning, but also the more ventral olfactory regions. Bianki (1972) has shown that if fish are trained with auditory, visual and olfactory discriminations, section of the anterior commissure has no effect on performance of the first two tasks but causes deficits in the third. In amphibia trained with auditory and visual tasks, section of the commissure causes decreases in the magnitude and accuracy of conditioned responses. While these studies support a greater telencephalic involvement in learning in amphibia than in fish, as suggested above, the lack of available detail makes interpretation difficult. Possibly commissure section has its effect by reducing the amount of nervous tissue which can act in synchrony to promote a response—a type of mass action effect.

The Tectal Commissure

In view of the importance of the tectum in lower vertebrates, as the primary visual area, there has been interest in the obvious link between the two tecta, the superficially situated tectal commissure.

Mark (1966) trained specimens of *Astronotus ocellatus* to swim to one of two shapes floating on the surface, to obtain food. Animals were pretrained to the response, then fitted with occluders and trained to discriminate the shapes. On training via the naive eye, high levels of transfer were demonstrated. Animals which underwent prior section of the tectal commissure showed normal rates of learning, but poor transfer, with much increased reaction times (figure 3.7). In a second series of experiments (Mark *et al.*, 1973), goldfish and carp (*Carassius carassius*) were trained in a differential avoidance situation. Xylocaine was injected into one eye to anaesthetise it. Animals were pretrained binocularly with a simple light avoidance problem, then trained monocularly with a red/green discrimination. Animals with section of the tectal commissure showed transfer failures (figure 3.8). However, despite such results, the reacquisition on the naive side was shorter than the original learning, suggesting some degree of transfer.

Despite the pretraining received by fish in these experiments, there is a possibility that transfer failures were due more to a failure to organise a movement than to

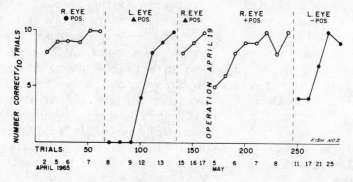

Figure 3.7. Learning curves and the results of interocular transfer tests in fish No. 2. Note how the fish persisted in striking at the filled circle when eye use was changed from right to left even though reward pairing was reversed at the same time. After the reverse habit had been learned it transferred back to the right eye. A similar test performed 16 days after section of the tectal commissure showed that changing eye use and reversing reward pairing had no significant effect on the learning through the second eye (Mark, 1966)

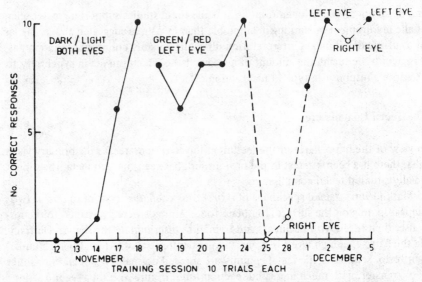

Figure 3.8. Learning curves from a fish in which the posterior commissure was intact but in which the tectal commissure had been cut. The dark–light discrimination was learned through both eyes, the green–red discrimination through the left eye alone. On the first trial with the right eye there was no behavioural evidence of the colour discrimination achieved through the left eye and little improvement on the second day's training. The left eye had retained the discrimination, and, on retesting with the right eye two days later, the score was as good as with the left. This shows that initial learning through the left eye was not immediately available to the right eye but that learning through the right eye was possible (Mark *et al.*, 1973)

recognise the significance of the stimuli. The movement to swim up to the shapes is very skilled, and since the avoidance box used was large compared to the fish used, the movements involved are more complex than are usual in the more conventional narrow fish avoidance box. If learning in such a situation is viewed as classical, with an added instrumental component, it is possible that the former but not the latter transferred. Such difficulties can be avoided by the use of a differential classical conditioning paradigm (Yeo and Savage, 1975; see also chapter 4), where no transfer deficits are seen in fish with section of the tectal commissure. Alternatively, extensive binocular and monocular pretraining of the sort used by Shapiro (1965) can remove this objection. Using such techniques, Ingle and Campbell (1977) have shown good transfer of a differential avoidance paradigm in operated fish. Thus the tectal commissure may be involved in motor, but not discrimination, transfer.

Johnstone and Mark (1969) have demonstrated the existence of units in the tectal commissure, which fire just before an eye movement, and they have suggested that such firing represents the efference copy generated before a movement, to preserve perceptual stability. If section of the commissure disrupts eye movement stabilisation, the two tecta may fall out of perceptual synchrony, and hence there

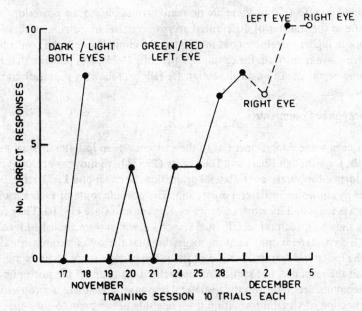

Figure 3.9. Learning curves from a fish in which the posterior commissure had been cut but the tecta commissure was intact. The dark–light discrimination was learned through both eyes, the green–red discrimination through the left eye alone as the right eye was blinded by local anaesthetic before each training session. On the first and second trial, with the right eye working and the left eye blinded, the score was not significantly below that recorded the day before, indicating that learning through the left eye was available to sensory messages arriving from the right eye (Mark *et al.*, 1973)

may be failure to show accurate movements when the naive side is being used. Some measure of such visuomotor failure might be gained from operated fish extensively trained monocularly on both sides with a differential cardiac response, then trained monocularly on differential avoidance using the same discrimination, and tested on the naive eye, with the sure knowledge of a high level of transfer of the classical basis of the task, and of experience of the response by the naive eye. The only report that section of the commissure may have a profound effect on retention comes from Bianki (1972), who reported that fish showed failures in a binocular visual discrimination task following operation, possibly as a result of failures to reconcile their two visuomotor co-ordinations.

The Posterior Commissure

Mark *et al.* (1973) and Ingle and Campbell (1977) sectioned this commissure in fish trained with differential avoidance problems. There were no suggestions of any interference with transfer. Yeo and Savage (1976; see also chapter 4) examined the effects of the operation on transfer of a differential classical conditioning paradigm and obtained no effect. Thus there are no reasons to implicate the posterior commissure in the transfer of differential aversive classical or instrumental tasks. Since work in higher vertebrates has implicated the commissure in the control of vertical eye movements (see, for example, Christoff, 1974), it is possible that tasks emphasising height/depth might show transfer failures following posterior commissure section.

The Diencephalic Commissures

There has been some disagreement as to the existence of an ipsilateral visual projection in fish, for although Buser and Dussardier (1953) have shown electrophysiological evidence for purely contralateral projection, Springer and Landreth (1977) have recently shown an ipsilateral projection. The possible route of such a projection in fish is suggested by work on frogs by Keating and Gaze (1970). They found that frogs showed ipsilateral tectal visual responses, which were abolished by ablation of the contralateral optic tectum, suggesting that there was a commissural relay back to the ipsilateral tectum. Section of the tectal and posterior commissures did not abolish the response, but section of unspecified members of the postoptic group of commissures removed the ipsilateral response. Thus there is a route for direct projection of visual information from one side of the brain to the other. Meier (1971) has shown the importance of these commissures for interocular transfer in pigeons.

Using a stereotaxic atlas for goldfish, devised by Roberts (1973), Yeo and Savage (1976; see also chapter 4) showed that section of the minor and horizontal commissures caused transfer failure in differentially classically trained goldfish. (Section of the transverse commissure has not been attempted, on account of its extreme proximity to the optic chiasm.) Section of the minor and horizontal commissures after training caused fish to show discriminated responses with both eyes; thus it appears that engrams are laid down bilaterally during monocular learning. The effect of postoptic commissure section on transfer of postoperatively trained tasks has also been demonstrated by Ingle and Campbell (1977), using differential avoidance training.

CONCLUSIONS

There are vast gaps in our knowledge of interhemispheric phenomena in lower vertebrates. In particular we know nothing of the time course of transfer. If it is possible accurately to apply spreading depression to the midbrain, it may prove possible to train simple paradigms unilaterally, then to examine the rates of transmission and consolidation of such information, as seen in rats (Bureš and Burešová, 1971). It may also prove possible to see whether transfer failure is really due to lack of a bilateral memory, or of access to memory on the contralateral side.

On the positive side, there is evidence for a route of transfer of both instrumentally and classically trained information, and the simple structure of lower vertebrate brains makes attractive the experiment of combining unilateral lesions and commissure sections. In addition, the simple vertebrate system may prove a useful neurophysiological model for studies of neural information transfer.

Secondly, although the postoptic commissures attract attention for learning studies, the other commissures are easily accessible and may prove useful for the study of vertebrate cross-brain relations in general.

REFERENCES

Ariëns Kappers, C. U., Huber, G. C. and Crosby, E. C. (1935). *Comparative Anatomy of the Nervous Systems of Vertebrates, including Man,* Macmillan, London

Aronson, L. R. and Kaplan, H. (1968). Function of the teleostean forebrain. In *The Central Nervous System and Fish Behavior* (D. J. Ingle, ed.), University of Chicago Press, pp. 107-25

Bannister, L. H. (1973). Forebrain structure in *Phoxinus phoxinus,* a member of the Cyprinid family. *J. Hirnforsch.,* **14**, 413-33

Behrend, E. R. and Bitterman, M. E. (1964). Avoidance conditioning in the fish: further studies of the CS-US interval. *Am. J. Psychol.,* **77**, 15-28

Bernstein, J. J. (1962). Role of the telencephalon in color vision of fish. *Expl Neurol.,* **6**, 173-85

Bianki, V. L. (1972). The hypothesis on the origin factors of the forebrain paired structures in the phylogenesis of the vertebrates. In *Cerebral Interhemispheric Relations* (J. Černaček and F. Podivinsky, eds.), Vydavatelstvo Slovenskej Akademie Vied, Bratislava, pp. 29-42

Bitterman, M. E., Wodinsky, J. and Candland, D. K. (1958). Some comparative psychology. *Am. J. Psychol.,* **71**, 94-110

Bureš, J. and Burešová, O. (1971). The reunified split brain. In *The Neural Control of Behavior* (R. E. Whalen, R. F. Thompson, M. Verzeano, and N. M. Weinbergen, eds.), Academic Press, New York, pp. 211-38

Buser, P. and Dussardier, M. (1953). Organisation des projections de la rétine sur le lobe optique, étudiée chez quelques Téléostéens. *J. Physiol. (Paris),* **45**, 57-60

Campbell, A. (1971). Interocular transfer of mirror-images by goldfish. *Brain Res.,* **33**, 486-90

Christoff, N. (1974). A clinopathologic study of vertical eye movements. *Archs Neurol.,* **31**, 1-8

Cohen, D. H., Duff, T. A. and Ebbesson, S. O. E. (1973). Electrophysiological identification of a visual area in shark telencephalon. *Science,* **182**, 492-94

de Bruin, J. P. C. (1978). Telencephalon and behavior in teleost fish: a neuroethological approach. In *Comparative Neurology: The Telencephalon* (S. O. E. Ebbesson, ed.), Academic Press, New York, in press

Farr, E. J. and Savage, G. E. (1978). First- and second-order conditioning in the goldfish, and their relation to the telencephalon. *Behav. Biol.,* **22**, 50-59

Flood, N. B., Overmier, J. B. and Savage, G. E. (1976). Teleost telencephalon and learning: an interpretive review of data and hypotheses. *Physiol. Behav.,* **16**, 783-98

Graeber, C. G., Schroeder, D. M., Jane, J. A. and Ebbesson, S. O. E. (1972). The importance of telencephalic structures in visual discrimination learning in nurse sharks. Paper presented at 2nd Annual Meeting of Society for Neuroscience, Houston, Texas

Hainsworth, F. R., Overmier, J. B. and Snowdon, C. T. (1967). Specific and permanent deficits in instrumental avoidance responding following forebrain ablation in the goldfish. *J. comp. physiol. Psychol.* **63**, 111-16

Hamilton, C. R., Tieman, S. B. and Brody, B. A. (1973). Interhemispheric comparison of mirror image stimuli by chiasm-sectioned monkeys. *Brain Res.*, **58**, 415-25

Healey, E. G. (1957). The nervous system. In *The Physiology of Fishes* (M. E. Brown, ed.), vol. 2, Academic Press, New York, pp. 1-119

Herrick, C. J. (1922). Functional factors in the forebrain of fishes. In *Libro en Honor de S. Ramon y Cajal*, vol. 1, Madrid, pp. 143-202

Hocke Hoogenboom, K. J. (1929). Das Gehirn von *Polyodon folium* Lacép. *Jahrb. Morphol. Anat. Zeit Forsch.*, **18**, 311

Ingle, D. J. (1965). Interocular transfer in goldfish: color easier than pattern. *Science*, **149**, 1000-1002

Ingle, D. J. (1968a). Interocular integration of visual learning in the goldfish. *Brain, Behav. Evol.*, **1**, 58-85

Ingle, D. J. (1968b). Spatial dimensions of vision in fish. In *The Central Nervous System and Fish Behavior* (D. J. Ingle, ed.), University of Chicago Press, pp. 51-59

Ingle, D. J. and Campbell, A. (1977). Interocular transfer of visual discriminations by goldfish with selective commissure lesions, *J. comp. physiol. Psychol.*, **91**, 327-35

Janzen, W. (1933). Untersuchungen über Grosshirnfunktion des Goldfisches (*Carassius auratus*). *Zool. Jahrb. Zool. Physiol.*, **52**, 591-628

Johnstone, J. R. and Mark, R. F. (1969). Evidence for efference copy for eye movements in fish. *Comp. Biochem. Physiol.*, **30**, 931-39

Karamian, A. I., Vesselkin, N. P., Belekhova, M. G. and Zagorulko, T. M. (1966). Electrophysiological characteristics of tectal and thalamocortical divisions of the visual system in lower vertebrates. *J. comp. Neurol.*, **127**, 559-76

Keating, M. J. and Gaze, R. M. (1970). The ipsilateral retinotectal pathway in the frog. *Q. Jl exp. Physiol.*, **55**, 284-92

Mark, R. F. (1966). The tectal commissure and interocular transfer of pattern discrimination in cichlid fish. *Expl Neurol.*, **16**, 215-25

Mark, R. F., Peer, O. and Steiner, J. (1973). Integrative functions in the midbrain commissures of fish. *Expl Neurol.*, **39**, 140-56

Marlotte, L. R. and Mark, R. F. (1975). Ultrastructural localization of synaptic input to the optic lobe of carp (*Carassius carassius*). *Expl Neurol.*, **49**, 772-89

McCleary, R. A. (1960). Type of response as a factor in interocular transfer in the fish. *J. comp. physiol. Psychol.*, **53**, 311-21

McCleary, R. A. and Longfellow, L. A. (1961). Interocular transfer of pattern discrimination without prior binocular experience. *Science*, **134**, 1418-19

Meesters, A. (1940). Über die Organisation des Gesichtsfeldes der Fische. *Z. Tierpsychol.*, **4**, 84-149

Meier, R. E. (1971). Interhemisphärischer transfer visueller Zweifachwahlen bei kommissurotomierten tauben. *Psychol. Forsch.*, **34**, 220–45

Mello, N. K. (1965). Interhemispheric reversal of mirror-image oblique lines following monocular training in pigeons. *Science*, **148**, 252–54

Nieuwenhuys, R. (1959). The structure of the telencephalon of the teleost *Gasterosteus aculeatus. Kon. Ned. Akad. Wetensch. Amsterdam*, **C62**, 341–62

Noble, J. (1968). Paradoxical interocular transfer of mirror-image discrimination in the optic chiasm sectioned monkey. *Brain Res.*, **10**, 127–51

Overmier, J. B. and Curnow, P. F. (1969). Classical conditioning, pseudoconditioning and sensitization in 'normal' and forebrainless goldfish. *J. comp. physiol. Psychol.*, **68**, 193–98

Overmier, J. B. and Savage, G. E. (1974). Effects of telencephalic ablation on trace classical conditioning of heart rate in goldfish. *Expl Neurol.*, **42**, 339–46

Roberts, M. G. (1973). Experimental studies on the hypothalamus and related brain regions of the goldfish. *Ph.D. thesis*, University of London

Sanders, F. K. (1940). Second-order olfactory and visual learning in the optic tectum of the goldfish. *J. exp. Biol.*, **17**, 416–34

Savage, G. E. (1968). Temporal factors in avoidance learning in normal and forebrainless goldfish (*Carassius auratus*). *Nature (Lond.)*, **218**, 1168–69

Savage, G. E. (1969a). Telencephalic lesions and avoidance behaviour in the goldfish (*Carassius auratus*). *Anim. Behav.*, **17**, 362–73

Savage, G. E. (1969b). Some preliminary observations on the role of the telencephalon in food-reinforced behaviour in the goldfish, *Carassius auratus. Anim. Behav.*, **17**, 760–72

Savage, G. E. (1978). The fish telencephalon and its relation to learning. In *Comparative Neurology: The Telencephalon* (S. O. E. Ebbesson, ed.), Academic Press, New York, in press.

Schnitzlein, H. N. (1962). The habenula and the dorsal thalamus of some teleosts. *J. comp. Neurol.*, **118**, 225–68

Schnitzlein, H. N. (1964). Correlation of structure and habit in the fish brain. *Am. Zool.*, **4**, 21–32

Schroeder, D. M. and Ebbesson, S. O. E. (1974). Nonolfactory telencephalic afferents in the nurse shark (*Ginglymostoma cirratum*). *Brain, Behav. Evol.*, **9**, 121–55

Schulte, A. (1957). Transfer- und Transpositionsversuche mit monokular dressierten Fischen. *Zeit. vergl. Physiol.*, **39**, 432–76

Sears, R. R. (1934). Effect of optic lobe ablation on the visuo-motor behaviour of goldfish. *J. comp. Psychol.*, **17**, 233–65

Shapiro, S. M. (1965). Interocular transfer of pattern discrimination in the goldfish. *Am. J. Psychol.*, **78**, 21–38

Sheldon, R. E. (1912). The olfactory tracts and centers in teleosts. *J. comp. Neurol.*, **22**, 177–338

Sperry, R. W. and Clark, E. (1949). Interocular transfer of visual discrimination habits in a teleost fish. *Physiol. Zool.*, **22**, 372–78

Springer, A. D. and Landreth, G. E. (1977). Direct ipsilateral retinal projections in goldfish (*Carassius auratus*). *Brain Res.*, **124**, 533–37

Sutherland, N. S. (1969). Shape discrimination in the rat, octopus and goldfish: a comparative study. *J. comp. physiol. Psychol.*, **67**, 160–76

Trevarthen, C. (1968). Vision in fish: the origins of the visual frame for action in vertebrates. In *The Central Nervous System and Fish Behavior* (D. J. Ingle, ed.), University of Chicago Press, pp. 61-94

Yeo, C. H. and Savage, G. E. (1975). The tectal commissure and interocular transfer of a shape discrimination in the goldfish. *Expl Neurol.,* **49**, 291-98

Yeo, C. H. and Savage, G. E. (1976). Mesencephalic and diencephalic commissures and interocular transfer in the goldfish. *Expl Neurol.,* **53**, 51-63

4
INTEROCULAR TRANSFER IN THE GOLDFISH

CHRISTOPHER H. YEO

Bykov and Speransky (1924) demonstrated that salivary conditioning to unilateral tactile stimulation of the flank of a dog could be lateralised by surgical transection of the corpus callosum. After commissurotomy, a response conditioned to stimulation of the left side could not be elicited by stimulation of the right side. Apart from this early study, there have been no reports of the successful lateralisation of classical conditioning, but it would seem that 'split brain' studies might be powerful methods for an analysis of the mechanisms of such learning.

The interocular transfer of a classically conditioned visual discrimination in the fish was first demonstrated by McCleary (1960), and it would seem that commissurotomy studies of this system offer several unique advantages. The fish cardiac conditioning preparation allows the rapid, monocular training of pattern and colour discriminations, and the ability to restrain the fish during conditioning allows precise control over spatial aspects of stimulus presentation. In addition, it has been shown that complete telencephalic ablation causes no disruption of trace or delay classical conditioning in the fish (Bernstein, 1962; Overmier and Curnow, 1969; Overmier and Savage, 1974) and so it is reasonable to direct attention towards diencephalic and mesencephalic commissures in the investigation of the interocular transfer of classical conditioning.

Commissurotomy studies have already implicated the tectal commissure in the interocular transfer of instrumental learning; Mark (1966) demonstrated deficits in the interocular transfer of food-reinforced approach learning in tectal commissure-sectioned oscar fish, and Mark *et al.* (1973) found poor interocular transfer of shock-avoidance learning in tectal commissure-sectioned goldfish and carp. This latter study reported unimpaired interocular transfer in posterior commissure-sectioned fish. The postoptic commissure of the diencephalon has not been studied with lesion methods.

This chapter describes a series of experiments designed to define the commissure involved in the interocular transfer of a classically conditioned shape discrimination, and to obtain information about the lateralisation of monocular conditioning in the goldfish *Carassius auratus*.

METHODS

The fish were anaesthetised in MS 222 solution and were implanted with ECG electrodes using the method of Roberts *et al.* (1973) and immediately afterwards a brain operation was performed. The skull was opened and a rectangle of bone above the optic tecta was removed in one piece. Control animals were given a 'sham operation' in which the fat overlying the surface of the brain was removed by gentle aspiration. A second group of animals sustained section of the tectal commissure, accomplished under direct vision using an electrolytically-sharpened, tungsten wire hook. A third group underwent combined transection of the habenular and posterior commissures, which lie just ventral to the anterior extent of the tectal commissure. The lobes of the telencephalon and the optic tecta were gently separated, and the wire hook was passed between them to cut the commissures from below. The final group underwent transection of the postoptic commissure complex, which was located stereotaxically, using the atlas of Roberts (1973), and was cut using a very fine knife inserted vertically down the ventricle. The small piece of skull bone was then replaced in all animals, and was sealed into place using a cyanoacrylate adhesive and acrylic dental cement. The fish were then allowed a 24-hour postoperative recovery period, which in all cases was sufficient for the resumption of normal feeding and swimming activities.

The fish were conditioned in black Perspex restraining chambers, 12.5 cm long, 6.5 cm high and 3 cm wide. They were able to see out through vertical slots in the side walls of the chambers into the right and left lateral visual fields. These areas were illuminated from above, and the discriminanda were presented here, at a distance of 9.5 cm from the eye, against the matt-black walls of the aquaria surrounding the restraining chambers. The discriminanda were horizontal and vertical white plastic rectangles, 0.4 cm × 2.0 cm in size. The conditional stimulus (CS) duration was 10 s, during which period the stimulus was 'bobbed' vertically at a frequency of 1 Hz and with an amplitude of approximately 1 cm. This is found to be necessary to ensure reliable conditioning. The unconditional stimulus (US) was a 0.1 s, 4 V a.c. electric shock of 1.4 mA current, coterminous with the CS. It was delivered to the tail of the fish via two copper plate electrodes attached to the side of the restraining chamber.

Before differential conditioning, the fish were given between 8 and 24 unreinforced habituation presentations of the CS to the right eye, until any cardiac decelerations (CD) judged to be present were habituated. Horizontal and vertical stimuli were alternated in a semi-random sequence. Training trials were then given to the right eye, with the animals trained against any preference which they may have demonstrated during the habituation presentations. In most fish, there was no evidence of such preferences. The intertrial interval (ITI) in habituation and training sessions was 105 ± 15 s.

The tectal commissure-sectioned fish were trained to a criterion of 75% bradycardia (see below for calculation). Because of the difficulty in measuring this criterion during the conditioning, the other groups were trained with the number of trials fixed at 68, which gave final bradycardiac responses of approximately 75%. The method chosen to quantify the interocular transfer, however, allows valid comparison of these groups.

The last eight training trials were given in the sequence: 0++0+00+ (where 0 represents the unreinforced stimulus and + represents the reinforced stimulus). Immediately after training, a block of eight unreinforced interocular transfer test trials was delivered to the left, naive side, using the same 0++0+00+ sequence. Since there was an initial 'novelty' response by the untrained side to the first presentation of a stimulus, the first trial of the test block was always the neutral stimulus, so avoiding bias in favour of transfer. After training and testing, the brains of the fish were examined histologically for completeness of commissure transection.

Cardiac decelerations (CD) were calculated from the formula:

$$CD = \frac{\text{No. of beats in 10 s period pre CS} - \text{No. of beats during CS}}{\text{No. of beats in 10 s period pre CS}}$$

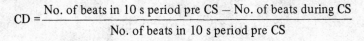

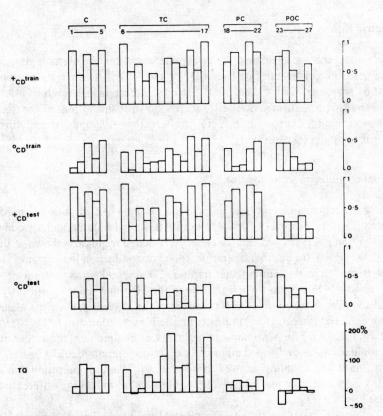

Figure 4.1. | Cardiac decelerations (CD) and transfer quotients (TQ) of control (C), tectal commissure-sectioned (TC), posterior commissure-sectioned (PC) and postoptic commissure-sectioned (POC) goldfish

CDs for the last four reinforced stimulus presentations of the training session were averaged to give $^+\text{CD}^{\text{train}}$. CDs for the last four unreinforced stimulus presentations of the training session were averaged to give $^\circ\text{CD}^{\text{train}}$. Similarly, $^+\text{CD}^{\text{test}}$ and $^\circ\text{CD}^{\text{test}}$ values for the interocular transfer test were calculated.

An expression of interocular transfer, calculated as the discrimination performance by the untrained side, is given by the transfer quotient (TQ):

$$TQ = \frac{(^+\text{CD}^{\text{test}} \div \, ^\circ\text{CD}^{\text{test}}) - 1}{(^+\text{CD}^{\text{train}} \div \, ^\circ\text{CD}^{\text{train}}) - 1} \times 100$$

Figure 4.1 shows the CD scores and the TQ measures of all control (C), tectal commissure-sectioned (TC), posterior and habenular commissures-sectioned (PC) and postoptic commissure-sectioned (POC) fish.

RESULTS AND DISCUSSION

Control Fish

The control animals all learned the discrimination within the 68 trials given, and all exhibited interocular transfer. The $^+\text{CD}^{\text{train}}$ and $^+\text{CD}^{\text{test}}$ scores are seen to be very similar, as are the $^\circ\text{CD}^{\text{train}}$ and $^\circ\text{CD}^{\text{test}}$ scores, indicating high levels of interocular transfer. This is confirmed by the TQ scores shown at the bottom of the figure. The somewhat poorer TQ score of fish No. 1 reflects the very good discrimination performance by the trained side.

Tectal commissure-sectioned fish

The tectal commissure-sectioned animals were trained to a criterion of approximately 75% bradycardia (CD = 0.75) to the reinforced stimulus and, by comparing $^+\text{CD}^{\text{train}}$ and $^\circ\text{CD}^{\text{train}}$ scores, a clearly differentiated response is shown at this level. On testing for interocular transfer, good discrimination performance is seen, indicating high levels of interocular transfer. The discrimination performance of the untrained side relative to the trained side of the TC group is not significantly different from that of the controls—a comparison of the TQ scores, using the Mann–Whitney U test (Siegal, 1956) indicates no significant differences ($n_1 = 12, n_2 = 5$, $U = 29, P > 0.1$). Fish No. 7 shows a negative transfer quotient, indicating that the discrimination was performed incorrectly on testing for interocular transfer. It is significant that this animal showed the lowest $^+\text{CD}^{\text{test}}$ score, indicating that a visual deficit on the left side was influencing the absolute, as well as the differential, response levels.

In contrast, therefore, to the instrumental learning studies, the operation of cutting the tectal commissure does not produce significant deficits in the interocular transfer of a classically conditioned discrimination.

Posterior commissure-sectioned fish

Histological examination of the brains of fish Nos. 18–22 revealed that both the dorsal and ventral filaments of the posterior commissure, and the habenular commissure, had been sectioned. All fish are seen to have acquired the discrimination, and interocular transfer is seen to have occurred. Comparing cardiac decelerations of control and PC groups reveals no differences in acquisition or interocular transfer of the discrimination. $^+$CD^{train} and $^{\circ}$CD^{train} values are similar for control and PC groups, ($n_1 = 5, n_2 = 5, U = 9, P \geqslant 0.1; n_1 = 5, n_2 = 5, U = 7, P \geqslant 0.1$ respectively). Levels of the test response to both positive and neutral stimuli—$^+$CD^{test} and $^{\circ}$CD^{test} values—are similar in control and operate groups ($n_1 = 5, n_2 = 5, U = 11, P > 0.1; n_1 = 5, n_2 = 5, U = 12, P > 0.1$, respectively).

However, on comparing TQ values, where differences in responses to both neutral and reinforced stimuli, on training and testing, are combined in a single measure, there is evidence of a small difference between control and operate groups, ($n_1 = 5, n_2 = 5, U = 3, P = 0.028$). This difference is considered to be just significant, and it must be concluded that there is a very slight element of interference with the interocular transfer of the discrimination caused by combined section of the posterior and habenular commissures. The deficit appears to relate to a lack of suppression of the bradycardiac response to the neutral stimulus on testing for interocular transfer, resulting in the slightly poorer discrimination performance. This effect is most noticeable in fish Nos. 21 and 22.

Postoptic commissure-sectioned fish

Fish Nos. 23–27 were found to have complete transection of the horizontal and minor commissures, the two more caudal members of the postoptic commissure group. The third postoptic commissure, the transverse commissure, which lies immediately behind the optic chiasm, was not sectioned in these fish. It can be seen that commissurotomy did not affect acquisition of the discrimination. A comparison of $^+$CD^{train} and $^{\circ}$CD^{train} values for control, and postoptic commissure-sectioned (POC) fish, reveals no significant differences ($n_1 = 5, n_2 = 5, U = 7, P > 0.1; n_1 = 5, n_2 = 5, U = 11, P > 0.1$ respectively).

Testing for interocular transfer, however, revealed that this process had been severely disturbed in the postoptic commissure-sectioned animals. Significant deficits are seen in the magnitude of the bradycardiac responses of the untrained side to the positive test stimulus by comparing $^+$CD^{test} values of control and operate fish ($n_1 = 5, n_2 = 5, U = 0, P = 0.004$). Responses by the untrained side to the neutral test stimulus remained similar to those of control animals ($n_1 = 5, n_2 = 5, U = 11, P > 0.1$). The very low response levels by the untrained side to the positive stimulus are reflected in the significantly poorer TQ scores of the POC group ($n_1 = 5, n_2 = 5, U = 1, P = 0.008$).

It is concluded that interocular transfer of a classically conditioned visual discrimination in the fish is mediated by elements of the postoptic commissure.

Transection of the minor commissure alone does not produce deficits in such interocular transfer (Yeo and Savage, 1976) and it is concluded that the commissure crucial for interocular transfer in the goldfish is the horizontal commissure.

The ability to produce a 'split brain' for classical conditioning allows investigation of the distribution through the brain of the engram of such learning. If a postoptic commissure lesion placed after monocular conditioning is found to have no effect upon lateralisation, then it is reasonable to suppose that, even given unilateral CS input, the engram of monocular conditioning is distributed through both sides of the brain. This finding would suggest that interocular transfer is a process ongoing with acquisition. Alternatively, a postoptic commissure lesion placed after conditioning may have the reverse effect—it may successfully lateralise monocular learning. This finding would suggest that the engram of monocular conditioning is located in the trained side only, and upon testing for interocular transfer, the information passes to, or is accessed by, the untrained side.

In order to establish which of these alternatives may be correct, a group of fish was subjected to postoptic commissure transection after monocular conditioning. On day 0 the fish were implanted with cardiac electrodes. On the following day (day 1) the fish were monocularly conditioned using a block of 68 training trials to the right eye. All apparatus and procedures were as described in the previous experiment. The CD scores of these animals are shown in figure 4.2. To indicate that they are scores on day 1 the suffix '1' has been added—hence, $^{+}CD_1^{\text{train}}$ and $^{\circ}CD_1^{\text{train}}$. Immediately afterwards the fish were anaesthetised and a brain operation was performed. Fish Nos. 28–34 were given a 'sham operation' and fish Nos. 35–40 underwent transection of the postoptic commissure. They were then given a 24-hour postoperative recovery period and, on day 2, they were tested for retention and for interocular transfer. A block of eight unreinforced retention trials was given to the trained side, in the sequence, 0++0+00+. The cardiac decelerations elicited are shown as $^{+}CD_2^{\text{train}}$ and $^{\circ}CD_2^{\text{train}}$. Finally, a block of eight unreinforced interocular transfer test trials was given to the untrained side, again using the 0++0+00+ sequence. The brains were removed, and the commissure lesions were verified histologically.

Control (C) and postoptic commissure-sectioned (POC) groups show no differences in the acquisition of the discrimination on day 1 of the training. This is to be expected, since, at this stage, both groups were in the same, unoperated condition. The retention by the trained sides of C and POC groups on day 2 is seen to be similar—a comparison of $^{+}CD_2^{\text{train}}$ and $^{\circ}CD_2^{\text{train}}$ values for control and operate fish reveals no significant differences ($n_1 = 6, n_2 = 7, U = 14, P > 0.1; n_1 = 6, n_2 = 7, U = 19, P > 0.1$, respectively).

On testing for interocular transfer, the level of responses of the untrained side of the POC group is seen to be significantly lower than that of control fish ($n_1 = 6, n_2 = 7, U = 2, P = 0.002$). In this group, the response of the untrained side to the neutral stimulus was also significantly reduced ($n_1 = 6, n_2 = 7, U = 7, P = 0.026$). This is in contrast to the results of the first experiment, where the deficits in interocular transfer relate specifically to a suppression of responding to the positive test

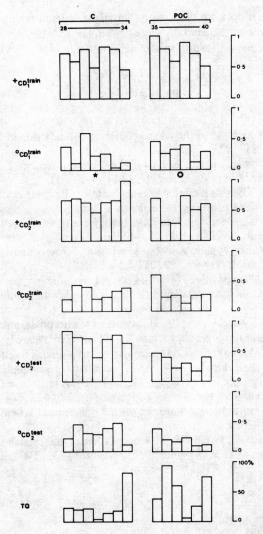

Figure 4.2. Cardiac decelerations (CD) and transfer quotients (TQ) of control (C) and postoptic commissure-sectioned (POC) goldfish. The 'sham operation' was performed at the point marked by the dark asterisk, the commissure transection is denoted by the open asterisk

stimulus. Consequently, the discrimination performance of the untrained side of the POC group remained good, although superimposed upon an overall lower level of responding, and this is reflected in a lack of significant difference between the TQ scores of control and operate groups ($n_1 = 6, n_2 = 7, U = 10, P = 0.069$).

In summary, there is evidence that postoptic commissurotomy, which is sufficient to lateralise monocular conditioning when performed prior to training, does not cause complete lateralisation of learning when performed after monocular conditioning. The inferences must be that substantial elements of the monocular experience are represented bilaterally within the brain, and that the postoptic commisure complex mediates the ipsilateral representation.

REFERENCES

Bernstein, J. J. (1962). Role of the telencephalon in colour vision in fish. *Expl Neurol.*, **6**, 173–85

Bykov, K. M. and Speransky, A. D. (1924). The dog with transected corpus callosum (in Russian). *Proc. Pavlov Physiol. Lab.*, **1**, 44

Mark, R. F. (1966). The tectal commissure and interocular transfer of pattern discrimination in cichlid fish. *Expl Neurol.*, **16**, 215–25

Mark, R. F., Peer, O. and Steiner, J. (1973). Integrative functions in the midbrain commissures in fish. *Expl Neurol.*, **39**, 140–56

McCleary, R. A. (1960). Type of response as a factor in interocular transfer in the fish. *J. comp. physiol. Psychol.*, **53**, 311–21

Overmier, J. B. and Curnow, P. F. (1969). Classical conditioning, pseudoconditioning, and sensitization in 'normal' and forebrainless goldfish. *J. comp. physiol. Psychol.*, **68**, 193–98

Overmier, J. B. and Savage, G. E. (1974). Effects of telencephalic ablation on trace classical conditioning of heart rate in goldfish. *Expl Neurol.*, **42**, 339–46

Roberts, M. G. (1973). Experimental studies on the hypothalamus and related brain regions of the goldfish. *Ph. D. thesis*, University of London

Roberts, M. G., Wright, D. E. and Savage, G. E. (1973). A technique for obtaining the electrocardiogram of fish. *Comp. Biochem. Physiol.*, **44A**, 665–68

Siegal, S. (1956). *Nonparametric Statistics for the Behavioural Sciences*, McGraw-Hill, New York

Yeo, C. H. and Savage, G. E. (1976). Mesencephalic and diencephalic commissures and interocular transfer in the goldfish. *Expl Neurol.*, **53**, 51–63

5

BEHAVIOURAL AND ANATOMICAL ASPECTS OF MONOCULAR VISION IN BIRDS

V. MAIER

VISUAL STRUCTURES AND CONNECTIONS IN BIRDS

In recent years, anatomical and physiological studies have changed our view of the avian visual system. They have revealed a number of similarities in the visual pathways between mammals and birds. At least seven areas receive primary projections from the retina (Cowan *et al.*, 1961; Hirschberger, 1967, 1971). In five of them, efferent connections are still unknown or ill-defined. Hence, attention will be restricted to the two main afferent pathways whose target is the telencephalon.

Most authors agree that the optic chiasm contains only crossed nerve fibres. However, Polyak (1957), Rougeul (1957) and Bons (1969) found some evidence for a small number of uncrossed fibres. The more prominent tectofugal pathway (figure 5.1) passes from retina to optic tectum to nucleus rotundus thalami (Rt) to ecto-striatum telencephali (Karten, 1965; Karten and Hodos, 1970; Karten and Revzin, 1966; Revzin, 1970; Revzin and Karten, 1966; Voneida and Mello, 1975). Hart (1969) and Hunt (1973) claimed an additional connection from optic tectum to the contralateral Rt via the supra-optic decussation (DSO). Thus, interactions between the two tecta may take place via tectal and posterior commissures. For the tectal commissure there is electrophysiological evidence for an intertectal inhibitory influence (Robert and Cuénod, 1968, 1969).

In the thalamofugal pathway (figure 5.1) retinal fibres project directly to the contralateral nucleus opticus principalis of the dorsal thalamus (OPT), which in turn is connected to ipsi- and (via DSO) contralateral nucleus intercalatus hyperstriati accessorii (IHA) of the telencephalic hyperstriatum (Galifret, 1966; Hunt and Webster, 1972; Karten and Nauta, 1968; Karten *et al.*, 1973; Meier, 1973; Meier *et al.*, 1974 Miceli *et al.*, 1975; Parker and Delius, 1972; Repérant, 1973; Repérant and Raffin, 1974; Repérant *et al.*, 1974). Thus, binocular interaction can take place in this area. This view is supported by electrophysiological studies with the pigeon (Perisič *et al.*, 1971) and the owl (Pettigrew and Konishi, 1976a, 1976b). They described cells in the hyperstriatum which could be activated by stimulation from either eye. Mihailovič *et al.* (1974) have shown that the DSO plays a crucial role: in their study, stimulation of the OPT of the pigeon resulted in evoked poten-

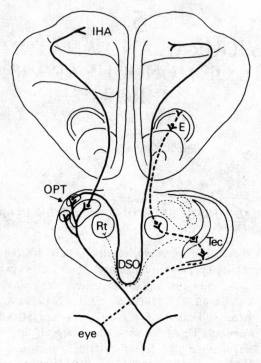

Figure 5.1. Schema of the two main visual pathways in the pigeon (after Hodos and Karten).
————— Thalamofugal pathway; – – – – – – tectofugal pathway. OPT, Rt, DSO see text; Tec =
tectum, E = ectostriatum

tials in both the ipsi- and the contralateral hyperstriatum. If the DSO was cooled or
transected, the contralateral response vanished. These interhemispheric connections
are of special interest because there is no corpus callosum in birds.

The possible homologies of structures in mammals and birds were discussed by
Karten (1969), Campbell and Hodos (1970) and Nauta and Karten (1970). Karten
compared the retino-tecto-rotundo-ectostriate (tectofugal) pathway in birds to the
pathway in mammals passing from retina to superior colliculus to nucleus lateralis
posterior thalami (or pulvinar in higher mammals) to extrastriate cortex. The
retino-thalamo-hyperstriate (thalamofugal) pathway shows many similarities to the
main mammalian visual pathway that passes from the retina to the nucleus geniculatus lateralis dorsalis and into the visual cortex (primary sensory area). Thus, for
example, cells of IHA show some properties that are similar to those of the mammalian visual cortex: small receptive fields, columnal organisation (Revzin, 1969a,
1969b), loss of binocularity after monocular deprivation, selectivity for orientation
and direction of movement, and binocular disparity for straight lines (Pettigrew
and Konishi, 1976a, 1976b). But there is at least a quantitative dissimilarity because
in mammals most retinal fibres project directly to the diencephalon, while in birds
most project to the optic tectum.

VISUAL BEHAVIOUR

There is general agreement that lesions in structures of the tectofugal pathway produces severe visual performance deficits. This was shown for brightness, colour, pattern and localisation problems (Cohen, 1967; Hodos, 1969; Hodos and Fletcher,
1974; Hodos and Karten, 1966, 1970, 1974; Jarvis, 1974; Maier and Tanaka, 1973).
But in most instances the animals can master the problems after prolonged training.

Results after lesions in structures of the thalamofugal pathway show discrepancies: Stettner and Schultz (1967) in the bobwhite quail and Hodos *et al.* (1973) in
the pigeon did not find any deficit in pattern discrimination acquisition or relearning
after they had destroyed the OPT or IHA. However, Zeigler (1963), Pritz *et al.*
(1970) and Maier (1976) described a prolonged training period for similar discrimination tasks. Hodos and Bonbright (1974) found a sustaining elevation of the
brightness difference threshold after OPT lesions. The discrepancies between these
data may well be the result of some visual discrimination not being detailed enough
to reveal a small deficit.

Despite the absence of a corpus callosum and the total crossing of the optic
nerves, interocular transfer of visual information can take place. Positive data are
given for brightness, colour, pattern and movement discriminations (Catania, 1963;
1965; Cherkin, 1970; Diebschlag, 1940; Konermann, 1966; Levine, 1945, 1952;
Mello, 1968; Mello *et al.,* 1963; Menkhaus, 1957; Moltz and Stettner, 1962; Ogawa
and Ohinata, 1966; Schabtach, 1966; Siegel, 1953; St. Claire-Smith, 1966). For
patterned stimuli, a paradoxical transfer of left–right or up–down mirror images was
found. This specific problem will not be discussed here. As possible mediating connections, the tectal and posterior commissures and the DSO were proposed. To
reveal the relevant structure, my colleague, R. E. Meier, transected either the tectal
and posterior commissures or the DSO in pigeons. After operation, the birds were
conditioned in an operant situation where they had to discriminate monocularly
between two simultaneously presented colours or patterns. After they reached the
learning criterion, the untrained eye was exposed and the performance of the bird
tested. In animals with transection of tectal and posterior commissures, interocular
transfer was as good as in normal controls. But in animals with transection of the
DSO, transfer was severely impaired or abolished. This result shows clearly the important role of the DSO for transfer of colour and pattern discriminations (Meier,
1970).

UNILATERAL LESIONS OF VISUAL STRUCTURES AND MONOCULAR VISUAL BEHAVIOUR

Experimental design

To test functional interactions between the tectofugal and thalamofugal pathways,
as well as bilateral interactions, the following experiments were performed (Maier,
1976).

Monocularly pretrained (horizontal versus vertical stripes) pigeons were submitted to unilateral dorsothalamic operations. Stereotactic lesions were placed either in Rt (the thalamic station of the tectofugal pathway), in OPT (the first station of the thalamofugal pathway) or in both structures. In one-half of the birds, an additional transection of the DSO was performed.

After recovery, pattern discrimination abilities were tested, again monocularly, in an operant situation. Each bird learned a second two-choice simultaneous discrimination problem (x versus +) which each eye individually on alternate sessions. Plastic rings into which a small cover could be fitted were attached to the rim of each eye. This restricted vision to one eye during the monocular training sessions.

Anatomical results

After histological verification the birds were divided into eight groups according to their lesions. In figures 5.2 and 5.3, schema of serial reconstructions of the lesions

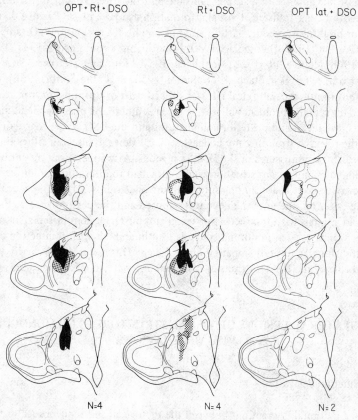

Figure 5.2. Schema of reconstructed thalamic lesions with the DSO transected. Dark area = destroyed tissue, stippled area = retrograde degeneration. Because of the similarity of lesions in a given group, the schema shows a combined picture. For key see p. 66

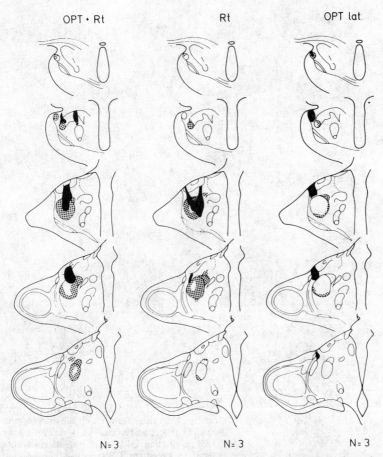

Figure 5.3. Schema of reconstructed thalamic lesions with the DSO intact. Dark area = destroyed tissue, stippled area = retrograde degeneration. For key see p. 66

are presented. In group OPT + Rt, most of Rt as well as parts of OPT are destroyed. For group Rt, the lesions are restricted mainly to Rt, and in group OPT lat destruction involves only most lateral regions of OPT. These lesions are very small (1 mm^3).

Lesions in the corresponding groups with additional transection of the DSO are comparatble (OPT + Rt + DSO, Rt + DSO, OPT lat + DSO) except for group OPT + Rt + DSO, where destruction of OPT is somewhat more prominent. Sham-operated animals (Sh) or, correspondingly, animals with only a transection of the DSO (DSO) served as control groups.

Behavioural results

When testing monocular visual discrimination abilities the following results were

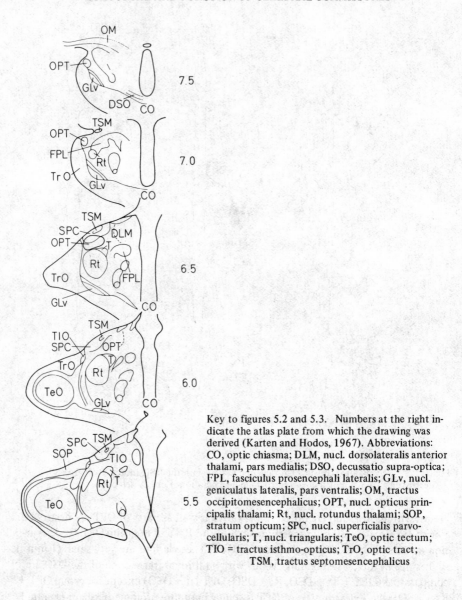

Key to figures 5.2 and 5.3. Numbers at the right indicate the atlas plate from which the drawing was derived (Karten and Hodos, 1967). Abbreviations: CO, optic chiasma; DLM, nucl. dorsolateralis anterior thalami, pars medialis; DSO, decussatio supra-optica; FPL, fasciculus prosencephali lateralis; GLv, nucl. geniculatus lateralis, pars ventralis; OM, tractus occipitomesencephalicus; OPT, nucl. opticus principalis thalami; Rt, nucl. rotundus thalami; SOP, stratum opticum; SPC, nucl. superficialis parvocellularis; T, nucl. triangularis; TeO, optic tectum; TIO = tractus isthmo-opticus; TrO, optic tract; TSM, tractus septomesencephalicus

found. In pre-operative discrimination learning, no performance differences between animals for the different groups were seen. Postoperative retention of this same problem (i.e. vertical versus horizontal stripes) was perfect except for animals of group OPT + Rt + DSO, which failed to perform better than at chance level while using the experimental eye (i.e. the eye in connection with the thalamic lesion). Figures 5.4 and 5.5 summarise results of postoperative discrimination learning.

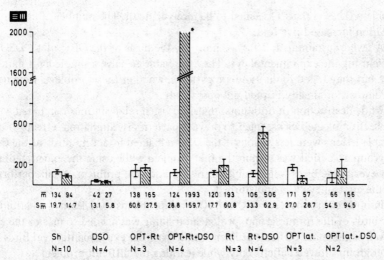

Figure 5.4. Diagram of pattern discrimination abilities after dorsothalamic lesions. Numbers indicate errors to criterion. Open area = control eye, shaded area = experimental eye

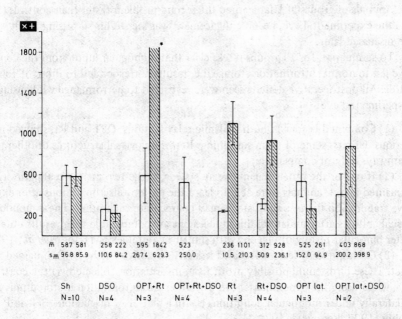

Figure 5.5. Diagram of pattern discrimination abilities after dorsothalamic lesions. Numbers indicate errors to criterion. Open area = control eye, shaded area = experimental eye

For the two control groups, Sh and DSO, the performance did not differ, irrespective of which eye was used. For both groups the second pattern discrimination problem (i.e. x versus +) seemed to be more difficult. The number of errors to criterion increased five-fold.

A severe sustaining deficit was shown by the birds of the OPT + Rt + DSO group while using the experimental eye. They were able to solve a simple light/dark problem, but they failed to discriminate patterns, whether these problems were new to the animals or already learned pre-operatively.

While destruction of both dorsothalamic visual relay stations combined with transection of the DSO seemed to prevent pattern discrimination, effects of comparable lesions were less serious if the DSO remained intact. In birds of the OPT + Rt group no deficit was seen in the first problem while using the experimental eye. However, these birds were unable to solve the second problem. Again, performance via the control eye was undisturbed.

In birds of groups Rt + DSO and Rt, both problems were learned to criterion. For birds of the former group, prolonged training was needed to master the easier as well as the more difficult problem while using the experimental eye. Birds of the latter group showed deficits only while learning the difficult problem.

Data from birds of group OPT lat + DSO were comparable with those of the Rt + DSO animals; also, the first problem was performed somewhat better.

Animals of group OPT lat learned the second problem faster than controls (Sh) via the experimental eye, i.e. an enhancement was seen. This surprising result will be discussed later.

To summarise, for all groups it was clear that monocular input from the control eye led to normal information storage, i.e. results corresponded to those of control birds. All postoperative deficits seen were restricted to performance while using the experimental eye:

(1) Combined lesions in both thalamic relay stations, OPT and Rt, showed most serious deficits, some of them sustaining. Remaining visual structures of other possible pathways did not compensate.

(2) If one or the other thalamic relay station of the two main visual pathways remained intact, animals were able to learn the pattern discriminations after extensive training. So the two subsystems may compensate each other. These monocular visual abilities after unilateral thalamic lesions are comparable with results obtained after binocular testing of pigeons with similar bilateral lesions (Hodos *et al.,* 1973).

(3) Corresponding lesions revealed less serious deficits if the DSO remained intact. These birds could possibly profit from information collected via the control eye while using the experimental eye. (Whether this information is stored uni- or bilaterally under monocular conditions is still a matter of discussion—Bell and Gibbs, 1977; Benowitz, 1974; Greif, 1976).

The result from the animals with OPT lat lesions was quite unexpected. There is confirmation that the enhanced performance after this lesion was a genuine effect rather than an artefact—anatomical studies by Repérant (1973) in the chick and by Streit *et al.* (1974) in the pigeon showed lateral OPT cells (i.e. cells destroyed in our experiment) to project mainly via the DSO to the contralateral telencephalic IHA.

If interruption of the crossed visual input to the IHA enhances monocular performance, DSO controls should be better than Sh controls. In fact, comparison of the results of birds from the two groups revealed a superior performance of the DSO controls (figures 5.4 and 5.5). After lesions of the DSO, monocular input was restricted to one brain hemisphere and information from each eye was handled independently. So, either unilateral (OPT lat) or bilateral (DSO) suppression of binocular interaction (i.e. comparison of probably slightly different information) allows a more effective processing, at least in a monocular situation where binocularity is not needed.

The above results demonstrate again the central role of the DSO for interocular information transfer and interaction. They have to be seen in the general light of performance differences after lesions which result from the combined effects of deficits and excluded inhibitory interactions.

ACKNOWLEDGEMENT

I thank Dr R. D. Oades for reading the English manuscript.

REFERENCES

Bell, G. A. and Gibbs, M. E. (1977). Unilateral storage of monocular engram in day-old chick. *Brain Res.*, **124**, 263–70

Benowitz, L. (1974). Conditions for bilateral transfer of monocular learning in chicks. *Brain Res.*, **65**, 203–13

Bons, N. (1969). Mise en évidence du croisement incomplet des nerfs optiques au niveau du chiasma chez le canard. *C. r. hebd. Séanc. Acad. Sci. Paris*, **268**, 2186–88

Campbell, C. B. G. and Hodos, W. (1970). The concept of homology and the evolution of the nervous system. *Brain, Behav. Evol.*, **3**, 353–67

Catania, A. C. (1963). Techniques for control of monocular and binocular viewing in the pigeon. *J. exp. Anal. Behav.*, **6**, 627–29

Catania, A. C. (1965). Interocular transfer of discriminations in the pigeon. *J. exp. Anal. Behav.*, **8**, 147–55

Cherkin, A. (1970). Eye to eye transfer of an early response modification in chicks. *Nature (Lond.)*, **227**, 1153

Cohen, D. H. (1967). Visual intensity discrimination in pigeons following unilateral and bilateral tectal lesions. *J. comp. physiol. Psychol.*, **63**, 172–74

Cowan, W. M., Adamson, L. and Powell, T. P. S. (1961). An experimental study of the avian visual system. *J. Anat. (Lond.)*, **95**, 545–63

Cuénod, M. (1972). Split-brain studies. Functional interaction between bilateral central nervous structures. In *The Structure and Function of Nervous Tissue*, (G. H. Bourne, ed.), vol. 5, Academic Press, New York, pp. 455–506

Cuénod, M. and Zeier, H. (1967). Transfert interhemisphérique et commissurotomie chez le pigeon. *Schweiz. Arch. Neurol. Neurochir. Psychiatr.*, **100**, 365–80

Diebschlag, E. (1940). Ueber den Lernovorgang bei der Haustaube. *Z. Vergl. Physiol.*, **28**, 67–104

Galifret, Y. (1966). Le système visuel du pigeon: anatomie et physiologie. Correlations psychophysiologiques. *Thèse*, Fac. Sci., Paris

Greif, K. F. (1976). Bilateral memory for monocular one-trial passive avoidance in chicks. *Behav. Biol.*, **16**, 453–63

Hart, J. R. (1969). Some observations on the development of the avian optic tectum. Unpublished thesis, University of Wisconsin

Hirschberger, W. (1967). Histologische Untersuchungen an den primären visuellen Zentren des Eulengehirnes und der retinalen Repräsentation in ihnen. *J. Ornithol.*, **108**, 187–202

Hirschberger, W. (1971). Vergleichend experimentell-histologische Untersuchung zur retinalen Repräsentation in den primären visuellen Zentren einiger Vogelarten. *Thesis*, J. W. Goethe-Univ., Frankfurt

Hodos, W. (1969). Color discrimination deficits after lesions of nucleus rotundus in pigeons. *Brain, Behav. Evol.*, **2**, 185–200

Hodos, W. and Bonbright, J. C. (1974). Intensity difference thresholds in pigeons after lesions of the tectofugal and thalamofugal visual pathways. *J. comp. physiol. Psychol.*, **87**, 1013–31

Hodos, W. and Fletcher, G. V. (1974). Acquisition of visual discrimination after nucleus rotundus lesions in pigeons. *Physiol. Behav.*, **13**, 501–506

Hodos, W. and Karten, H. J. (1966). Brightness and pattern discrimination deficits in the pigeon after lesions of nucleus rotundus. *Expl Brain Res.*, **2**, 151–67

Hodos, W. and Karten, H. J. (1970). Visual intensity and pattern discrimination deficits after lesions of ectostriatum in pigeons. *J. comp. Neurol.*, **140**, 53–68

Hodos, W. and Karten, H. J. (1974). Visual intensity and pattern discrimination deficits after lesion of the optic lobe in pigeons. *Brain, Behav. Evol.*, **9**, 165–94

Hodos, W. Karten, H. J. and Bonbright, J. C. (1973). Visual intensity and pattern discrimination after lesions of the thalamofugal visual pathway in pigeons. *J. comp. Neurol.*, **148**, 447–67

Hunt, S. P. (1973). A study of forebrain visual areas in the pigeon. *Ph.D. thesis*, University College, London

Hunt, S. P. and Webster, K. E. (1972). Thalamo-hyperstriate interrelations in the pigeon. *Brain Res.*, **44**, 647–51

Jarvis, C. D. (1974). Visual discrimination and spatial localisation deficits after lesions of the tectofugal pathway in the pigeon. *Brain, Behav. Evol.*, **9**, 195–228

Karten, H. J. (1965). Projections of the optic tectum of the pigeon (*C. livia*). *Anat. Rec.*, **151**, 369

Karten, H. J. (1969). The organizaiton of the avian telencephalon and some speculations on the phylogeny of the amniote telencephalon. *Ann. N. Y. Acad. Sci.*, **167**, 164–79

Karten, H. J. and Hodos, W. (1967). *A Stereotaxic Atlas of the Brain of the Pigeon (Columba livia)*, The Johns Hopkins Press, Baltimore

Karten, H. J. and Hodos, W. (1970). Telencephalic projections of the nucleus rotundus in the pigeon *(C. livia)*. *J. comp. Neurol.*, **140**, 35–52

Karten, H. J. and Nauta, W. J. H. (1968). Organization of retinothalamic projections in the pigeon and owl. *Anat. Rec.*, **160**, 373

Karten, H. J. and Revzin, A. M. (1966). The afferent connections of the nucleus rotundus in the pigeon. *Brain Res.*, **2**, 368–77

Karten, H. J., Hodos, W., Nauta, W. J. H. and Revzin, A. M. (1973). Neural connections of the visual wulst of the avian telencephalon. Experimental studies in the pigeon *(C. livia)* and owl *(Speotyto cunicularia). J. comp. Neurol.*, **150**, 253–78

Konermann, G. (1966). Monokulare Dressur von Hausgänsen zum Teil mit entgegengesetzter Merkmalsbedeutung für beide Augen. *Z. Tierpsychol.*, **23**, 555–80

Levine, J. (1945). Studies in the interrelations of central nervous structures in binocular vision. I. The lack of bilateral transfer of visual discriminative habits acquired monocularly by the pigeon. *J. genet. Psychol.*, **67**, 105–29

Levine, J. (1952). Studies on the interrelations of central nervous structures in binocular vision. II. The conditions under which interocular transfer of discriminative habits take place in the pigeon. *J. genet. Psychol.*, **67**, 131–42

Maier, V. (1976). Effekte unilateraler telencephaler und thalamischer Läsionen auf die monokulare Musterdiskriminationsfähigkeit kommissurotomierter Tauben. *Rev. Suisse Zool.*, **83**, 59–82

Maier, V. and Tanaka, M. (1973). Monocular pattern discrimination deficits in pigeons after unilateral lesions of the dorsolateral region of the thalamus. *Brain Res.*, **49**, 497

Meier, R. E. (1970). Interhemisphärischer Transfer visueller Zweifachwahlen bei kommissurotomierten Tauben. *Psychol. Forsch.*, **34**, 220–45

Meier, R. E. (1973). Autoradiographic evidence for a direct retinohypothalamic projection in the avian brain. *Brain Res.*, **53**, 417–21

Meier, R. E., Mihailović, J. and Cuénod, M. (1974). Thalamic organisation of the retino-thalamo-hyperstriatal pathway in the pigeon *(C. livia). Expl Brain Res.*, **19**, 351–64

Mello, N. K. (1968). Interhemispheric transfer of a discrimination of moving patterns in pigeon. *Brain Res.*, **7**, 390–98

Mello, N. K., Erwin, F. R. and Cobb, S. (1963). *Bol. Inst. Estud. Med. Biol. (Méx.)*, **21**, 519–33

Menkhaus, J. (1957). Versuche über einäugiges Lernen und Transponieren beim Haushuhn. *Z. Tierpsychol.*, **14**, 210–30

Miceli, D., Peyrichoux, J. and Repérant, J. (1975). The retino-thalamo-hyperstriatal pathway in the pigeon *(C. livia). Brain Res.*, **100**, 121–25

Mihailović, J., Perisić, M., Bergonzi, R. and Meier, R. E. (1974). The dorsolateral thalamus as a relay in the retino-wulst pathway in pigeon *(C. livia). Expl Brain Res.*, **21**, 229–40

Moltz, H. and Stettner, L. (1962). Interocular mediation of the following response after patterned light deprivation. *J. comp. physiol. Psychol.*, **55**, 626–32

Nauta, W. J. H. and Karten, H. J. (1970). A general profile of the vertebrate brain, with sidelights on ancestry of cerebral cortex. In *The Neurosciences* (F. O. Schmidt, ed.), Second Study Program, The Rockefeller University Press, New York

Ogawa, T. and Ohinata, S. (1966). Interocular transfer of color discrimination in a pigeon. *Ann. Anim. Psychol.*, **16**, 1–9

Parker, D. M. and Delius, J. D. (1972). Visual evoked potentials in the forebrain of the pigeon. *Expl Brain Res.*, **14**, 198–209

Perisić, M., Mihailović, J. and Cuénod, M. (1971). Electrophysiology of contralateral and ipsilateral visual projections to the wulst in the pigeon *(C. livia). Int. J. Neurosci.,* **2**, 7-14

Pettigrew, J. D. and Konishi, M. (1976a). Neurons selective for orientation and binocular disparity in the visual wulst of the barn owl *(Tyto alba). Science*, **193**, 675-77

Pettigrew, J. D. and Konishi, M. (1976b). Effect of monocular deprivation on binocular neurons in the owl's visual wulst. *Nature (Lond.),* **264**, 753

Polyak, S. (1957). *The Vertebrate Visual System,* University of Chicago Press

Pritz, M. B., Mead, W. R. and Northcutt, R. G. (1970). The effects of wulst ablations on color, brightness and pattern discrimination in pigeons *(C. livia). J. comp. Neurol.,* **140**, 81-100

Repérant, J. (1973). Nouvelles données sur les projections visuelles chez le pigeon *(C. livia). J. Hirnforschung,* **14**, 151-87

Repérant, J. and Raffin, J.-P. (1974). Les projections visuelles chez le goéland argenté*(Larus argentatus argentatus)*et le goéland brun *(L. fucus graellsii). C. r. hebd. Seanc. Acad. Sci. Paris,* ser D. **278**, 2335-38

Repérant, J. Raffin, J.-P. and Miceli, D. (1974). La voie rétino-thalamo-hyperstriatale chez le poussin *(Gallus domesticus L.). C. r. hebd. Séanc. Acad. Sci. Paris,* ser. D, **279**, 279-82

Revzin, A. M. (1969a). A specific visual projection area in the hyperstriatum of the pigeon *(C. livia). Brain Res.,* **15**, 246-49

Revzin, A. M. (1969b). Some characteristics of a visual projection area in the owl *(Speotyto conicula). Fedn. Proc.,* **28**, 395

Revzin, A. M. (1970). Some characteristics of wide-field units in the brain of the pigeon. *Brain, Behav. Evol.,* **3**, 195-204

Revzin, A. M. and Karten, H. J. (1966). Rostral projections of the optic tectum and the nucleus rotundus in the pigeon. *Brain Res.,* **3**, 264-76

Robert, F. and Cuénod, M. (1969). Electrophysiology of the intertectal commissures in the pigeon. I. Analysis of the pathway. II. Inhibitory interaction. *Expl Brain Res.,* **9**, 116-36

Rougeul, A. (1957). Exploration oscillographique de la voie visuelle du pigeon. *Thèse,* Fac. Med., Paris

Schabtach, G. (1966). Interocular and interhemispheric transfer in the domestic chick. Unpubl. Ph. D. thesis, Johns Hopkins University, Baltimore

Siegel, A. L. (1953). Deprivation of visual form definition in the ring dove. 1. Discrimination learning. *J. comp. physiol. Psychol.,* **46**, 249-52

St. Claire-Smith, R. (1966). Interocular transfer in the pigeon. The effect of monocular training on a behavior established monocularly with the opposite eye. Paper read at Eastern Psychol. Ass. Meetings, New York

Stettner, L. J. and Schultz, W. J. (1967). Brain lesions in birds: effects on discrimination, acquisition and reversal. *Science,* **155**, 1689-92

Streit, P., Knecht, E., Burkhalter, A. and Cuéned, M. (1974). Retrograde axonal tracing of thalamo-telencephalic connections. *Experientia,* **30**, 684

Voneida, T. J. and Mello, N. K. (1975). Interhemispheric projections of the optic tectum in pigeon. *Brain, Behav. Evol.,* **11**, 91-108

Zeigler, H. P. (1963). Effects on endbrain lesions upon visual discrimination learning in pigeons. *J. comp. Neurol.,* **120**, 161-82

6

DO TRAINING CONDITIONS AFFECT INTEROCULAR TRANSFER IN THE PIGEON?

J. A. GRAVES and M. A. GOODALE

INTRODUCTION

Despite the fact that pigeons in many situations show excellent interocular transfer of visual discrimination habits, there have been a number of reports of failure of transfer under certain training conditions. One of the most striking examples of failure of interocular transfer was reported by Levine (1945a, 1945b, 1952) using a modified Lashley jumping-stand. When the discriminanda were presented vertically in front of the pigeon, he found that birds trained monocularly on a brightness, colour or pattern discrimination showed no evidence of learning when tested with the 'naive' eye.

However, Catania (1965) found that with the stimuli located in the same position relative to the bird, there was complete interocular transfer of brightness, colour and pattern discriminations. But instead of using a jumping-stand, Catania trained the birds using an operant conditioning method employing transilluminated keys and a pecking response. His findings have been replicated by a large number of investigators (Cuénod and Zeier, 1967; Maier, 1976; Meier, 1971; Ogawa and Ohinata, 1966).

Catania (1964) suggested that one possible explanation for the discrepancy in these two sets of findings could be derived from the characteristics of the pigeon's visual system. He argued that the pigeon is laterally far-sighted and anteriorly near-sighted. Thus, in order to view the stimuli at the distance required in the jumping-stand, the pigeons had to cock their heads to one side and so bring the stimuli into the lateral visual field. Since the direction in which the head would be cocked would depend on which eye was covered, the jumping response in each case could also have been affected. Thus, switching the eye cover would involve a change in posture which could have interfered with any interocular transfer that was present.

Nevertheless, it is still possible that Levine's results do represent a genuine failure of interocular transfer. Almost without exception, subsequent investigations of interocular transfer in the pigeon have used transilluminated keys and the pecking response. For this reason, we felt it important to re-examine Levine's findings using the same jumping-stand situation but employing a more sensitive reversal training procedure.

MONOCULAR TRAINING

Jumping-stand experiments

The training situation we used is fully described in Graves and Goodale (1977). Briefly, we attempted to reproduce a jumping-stand (figure 6.1) of the same dimen-

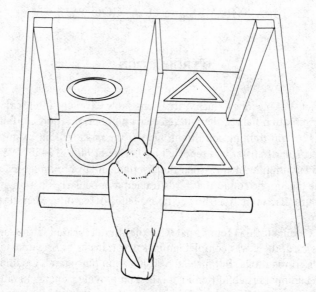

Figure 6.1. Schematic of jumping-stand showing position of platforms, perch and stimuli

sions as that used by Levine (1945a) and Halstead and Yacorzynski (1938). A rotating perch 45 cm in length was constructed from a 2.5 cm diameter rod and was covered with rough cloth. Two collapsible platforms measuring 19 x 14 cm were located 7 cm in front of and 5 cm below the perch. Each platform could be made secure or allowed to collapse when a bird landed on it. A 10 cm partition separated the two platforms allowing a pigeon to jump to one or the other but not to both platforms at once. In the first experiment, stimulus cards measuring 19 x 14 cm were positioned on the surface of the platforms themselves as well as vertically on the wall of the apparatus directly behind the platforms. In all other jumping-stand experiments the stimulus cards were located in only the vertical position.

In the experiments described below, each pigeon was given 20 trials a day on the jumping-stand, with one eye covered with a cloth blindfold. On each trial, the pigeon was placed on the perch which was then rotated forcing it to jump to one of the two platforms. If the pigeon jumped on to the correct platform, it was allowed to stay there for 15 s. If it jumped on to the incorrect one, the platform would collapse and the pigeon would fall 20 cm into a pile of hay placed in the bottom of the apparatus. The pigeon was then picked up immediately. A non-correction procedure was employed with an intertrial interval of approximately 30 s in which the bird was held in the experimenter's hand outside the apparatus. The stimulus cards were switched from right to left in accordance with a pseudo-random sequence. Training was continued on each discrimination task until the criterion of 18 trials correct in one day was reached.

Experiment 1

We first trained and tested 6 pigeons monocularly on a triangle–circle discrimination. The training of each bird took place in four stages. Both eyes were trained successively to criterion on the triangle versus circle discrimination, and then both eyes were trained successively to criterion on the reversal of that discrimination. This procedure is summarised for one of the pigeons in figure 6.2. As this figure shows,

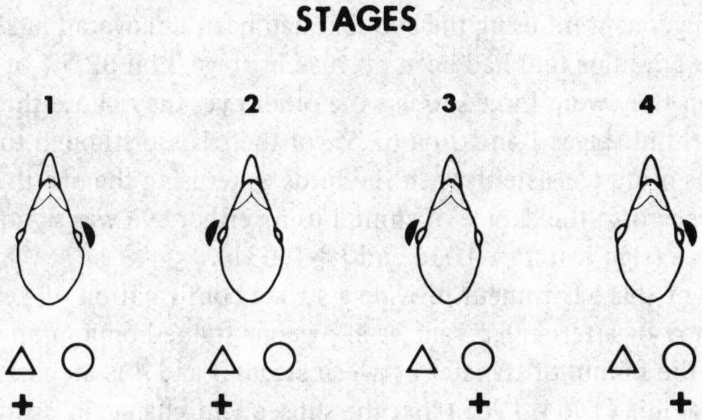

STAGES

Figure 6.2. The training procedure

during stage 1 this bird was trained with the right eye covered and triangle positive until it reached criterion. During stage 2, the left eye was covered and the bird was trained with triangle positive again. After reaching criterion, the bird was shifted to stage 3, in which the left eye was still occluded, but now the circle was the positive stimulus. In stage 4, the blindfold was switched back to the right eye, and the bird was trained with the circle positive once more.

   The results of experiment 1 are summarised in table 6.1. In agreement with Levine, we found no significant difference between the number of errors or days required to reach criterion in stages 1 and 2. The pigeons took as long to learn the task with the second eye as they did with the first. A similar relationship exists between stages 3 and 4. However, the birds made significantly more errors ($q = 3.70$, $P < 0.05$) and took significantly longer ($P < 0.05$) to learn the reversal task in stage 4, than they did to learn the original discrimination in stage 1.

Table 6.1

Pigeon	Stage 1		Stage 2		Stage 3		Stage 4	
	errors	days	errors	days	errors	days	errors	days
7	292	36	194	24	295	33	283	37
8	197	25	196	22	257	32	187	25
9	259	33	256	33	380	43	368	39
10	190	22	196	24	223	25	286	32
11	173	21	87	15	310	33	341	38
12	189	22	202	24	230	29	267	28
$\overline{X}$	216.7	26.5	188.5	23.7	282.5	32.5	288.7	33.2

We also interpolated a retention test between stages 3 and 4 to discover whether the pigeons had, at that point, formed conflicting discrimination habits dependent on which eye was covered. During this test, both platforms were secured and the blindfold was switched from side to side in blocks of five trials.

When the pigeons were using the eye that had been uncovered in stages 2 and 3, they chose the stimulus that had been positive in stage 3 on 82.5% of the jumps. However, when they were forced to use the other eye, they chose the stimulus that had been correct in stages 1 and 2 on 62.5% of the trials. Although the pattern of responding was more consistent when the birds were using the eye that had been trained most recently, the choice of stimuli using either eye was significantly different from chance (sign test; $P = 0.016$ and $P = 0.031$).

The results of this experiment provide a strong confirmation of Levine's earlier reports of failure of interocular transfer in pigeons trained on a jumping-stand. Furthermore, the failure of transfer between stages 3 and 4 is inconsistent with the proposal by Catania (1964, 1965) that the subsequent change in posture following switching of eye covers is responsible for the poor performance of the discrimination habit. During stage 4, the pigeons were using the eye that they had already used on a large number of trials during stage 1 and were well accustomed to the apparatus. Nevertheless, contrary to what Catania might have predicted, these birds failed to learn the discrimination reversal in stage 4 any faster than they had in stage 3 using the other eye. Indeed, the performances in both these stages were highly similar and during the early portion of both stages, the pigeons jumped towards the previously positive stimulus a considerable number of times before they began to jump to the correct platform.

The results of the retention test administered between stages 3 and 4 also indicate that in the jumping-stand situation there is no evidence for interocular transfer in the pigeon. When tested with the eye that had been uncovered during stage 1, the pigeons jumped towards the stimulus that had been negative during stage 3, even though they had not been trained with that eye for an average of 1120 trials. In fact, in the last 660 of those trials, they had been trained with the other eye not to jump towards that stimulus, but towards the other one.

Experiment 2

The question arises whether other visual discrimination tasks will show failure of transfer in the jumping-stand situation.

The triangle–circle discrimination is much more difficult for pigeons to learn than brightness or colour discriminations. A number of investigators (Ingle, 1968; Zeier, 1976) have suggested that difficult discriminations transfer far less readily than easy ones. Therefore, we decided to test pigeons on a simple red–green discrimination using the same four-stage design (figure 6.2) that we used in experiment 1.

Table 6.2

Pigeon	Stage 1		Stage 2		Stage 3		Stage 4	
	errors	days	errors	days	errors	days	errors	days
71	85	10	26	5	111	11	75	9
81	33	4	37	6	71	11	71	10
121	21	4	71	10	150	17	91	11
22	21	4	15	3	129	15	67	8
$\overline{X}$	40	5.5	37.25	6	115.25	13.5	76	9:5

The results of this experiment, which are summarised in table 6.2, were very similar to those obtained with the triangle–circle discrimination. Even though the red–green discrimination was learned much more quickly, there was still no evidence of transfer between stages 1 and 2 or stages 3 and 4. Although the stage 4 scores were lower than those of stage 3, this difference was not significant. Moreover, during the first 40 trials of stage 4, all the pigeons persisted in jumping towards the stimulus that had been positive in stage 1, even though it was no longer rewarded.

The retention test results were also similar to those of the triangle–circle experiment. Using the eye that was uncovered in stage 3 the pigeons chose the stimulus that had been correct during that stage on 80% of the retention-test trials. With the other eye, they chose the stimulus that had been positive in stage 1 on 68.7% of the trials.

Thus it would appear that even simple visual discrimination habits do not show interocular transfer on the jumping-stand.

Experiment 3

During the retention tests administered in experiments 1 and 2, the pigeons' performances using the eye that had last been trained in stage 1 fell to 62.5% and 68.7%, respectively, significantly lower than their performances with the other eye. It could be argued that this decrease in performance was due to interhemispheric transfer of conflicting information from the other eye-hemisphere system, rather than a function of the amount of time elapsed between the first stage of training and testing. We tested this possibility by training eight pigeons on a new yellow–blue discrimination. One group of four birds was trained through stages 1, 2 and 3 as usual, but the remaining four birds were trained with one eye on stage 1 and were then given irrelevant training on a horizontal–vertical discrimination with the second eye for the same number of days as stages 2 and 3 took for the first group. Both groups were then given the retention test on the yellow–blue discrimination. There was no significant difference between the performance of the two groups using the eye trained during stage 1 ($U = 4.5$). Furthermore, there was no evidence of interocular transfer of the yellow–blue discrimination in the four birds given irrelevant training, i.e. they performed at chance level on the retention test using the eye that had learned the horizontal–vertical discrimination.

These results suggest that the poor retention-test performance of the pigeons using the eye trained during stage 1 in experiments 1 and 2 cannot be interpreted in terms of interhemispheric transfer of a conflicting habit. Instead, the scores probably reflect a simple deterioration of habit retention over time.

Key-pecking experiments

The preceding three experiments provide strong support for Levine's original conclusion that interocular transfer does not occur in pigeons trained monocularly on a jumping-stand. But Catania has also suggested that one reason why he found transfer when the stimuli were positioned vertically in front of the birds, whereas Levine did not, could have been due to a difference in the number of responses demanded in the two situations. Levine's jumping-stand experiments (and our own) required only a few hundred responses from the birds, whereas Catania's operant task required several thousand. The resultant overtraining might have facilitated transfer.

Experiment 4

In order to test Catania's overtraining hypothesis, we carried out an experiment in which the number of responses required to reach criterion on a key-pecking task was made comparable to the number of responses demanded in the jumping-stand situation. This was accomplished by requiring only a single peck for reinforcement and a correction procedure, rather than the 3-min VI schedule used by Catania. The situation was made even more comparable with the jumping-stand by using a two-choice simultaneous discrimination instead of the successive discrimination procedure used by Catania.

Using this procedure, five birds were trained monocularly on a red–green discrimination following the same four-stage design illustrated in Figure 6.2. Each bird was given 100 trials a day until it reached a criterion performance of 90% correct trials in one day. Both initial and perseverative errors were separately recorded.

As table 6.3 clearly shows, the number of responses required to reach criterion on stages 1 and 3 of this experiment were comparable to or less than those obtained

Table 6.3

Pigeon	Stage 1		Stage 2		Stage 3		Stage 4	
	perseverative errors	days	perseverative errors	days	perseverative errors	days	perseverative errors	days
1	21	1	6	1	67	2	22	2
2	49	2	3	1	197	4	42	3
3	84	2	5	1	91	2	9	1
6	37	2	12	1	171	2	8	1
21	62	2	25	2	217	4	5	1
$\overline{X}$	50.6	1.8	10.2	1.2	148.6	2.8	17.2	1.6

on the jumping-stand. Yet the pigeons showed good interocular transfer between stages 1 and 2 and stages 3 and 4. This high level of transfer from the trained eye to the naive eye is consistent with other studies using key-pecking and simultaneous discrimination training (Maier, 1976; Meier, 1971).

The results of this experiment indicate that Catania's overtraining suggestion does not adequately explain the discrepancy between the jumping-stand data and those obtained from key-pecking experiments. Even when the number of responses in the two situations were made comparable, there was still transfer in one situation but not in the other.

Experiment 5

There are a number of factors that could possibly account for this difference in interocular transfer. All the jumping-stand experiments involved the use of a non-correction training procedure, whereas in the preceding experiment we allowed the birds to correct following an error. The possibility exists that what 'transferred' in this experiment was not the visual discrimination habit *per se* but rather the correction strategy. Perhaps more important, the discriminanda on the jumping-stand were separated from one another by a 10 cm deep partition, whereas there was no partition between the keys in experiment 4. The presence of the partition may have affected the scanning strategy and viewing distance used by the bird and thus influenced the amount of interocular transfer in the situation. We designed a key-pecking experiment to investigate the possible effect of these two factors on interocular transfer in the Skinner box. Five birds were trained monocularly on a triangle-circle discrimination using a non-correction training procedure. The keys themselves were separated from one another by a 10 cm deep partition running from the ceiling of the training chamber down to the central feeding aperture.

As table 6.4 shows, despite the use of non-correction training and the presence of

Table 6.4

Pigeon	Stage 1		Stage 2		Stage 3		Stage 4	
	errors	days	errors	days	errors	days	errors	days
2	285	7	10	1	354	11	133*	5*
17	623	15	60	3	389	10	38	3
23	211	8	106	3	238	8	132	4
24	134	4	30	2	229	5	20	2
$\bar{X}$	313.25	8.5	51.5	2.25	302.5	8.5	80.75	3.5

*There was an unavoidable 10-day hiatus during the training of stage 4.

the partition, all birds showed good interocular transfer between stages 1 and 2 and stages 3 and 4.

It seems then that neither of Catania's suggested explanations (postural habits or difference in the number of responses) can account for the failure of transfer in the jumping-stand or its success in the operant conditioning apparatus. The results indicate that monocularly learned visual discriminations do not transfer to the other eye on the jumping-stand, whereas they do in the Skinner box.

BINOCULAR TRAINING

In addition to his observation of failure of interocular transfer following monocular training, Levine (1945a) reported an even more startling finding. He found that pigeons trained on the jumping-stand with both eyes uncovered apparently learned the discrimination with only one eye. That is, when tested monocularly after reaching criterion, they performed at the criterion level with one eye uncovered, but at chance with the other eye. Levine was able to demonstrate that this effect was not due to the continuous dominance of one eye. Also binocular discrimination training and its reversal failed to disrupt the discrimination habits previously acquired by each eye separately.

Experiment 6

On the basis of these results we decided to see if pigeons would alternate the use of their two eyes to learn successive reversals in binocular training. Therefore, we trained six pigeons binocularly on a red–green discrimination on the jumping-stand. Following this training, each bird was given four days of monocular testing, two days with double reward, followed by two days of testing in which the positive stimulus was the reverse of the one used in the preceding training. Eye covers were switched in blocks of five trials for 20 trials a day. After the four-day test period, all the birds were trained with both eyes uncovered on the reversal of the original discrimination and a further four days of testing followed this reversal training. Throughout training and testing, cine film records were made of the scanning behaviour (head movements and postural changes) of the birds immediately before they jumped towards one of the platforms.

The performance of the birds in the two test periods is summarised in table 6.5. As Levine might have predicted, on the two days of testing following the original training, five of the six birds showed markedly better performance with one eye than the other. However, there was considerable variation from bird to bird on the amount of difference between the performance of the two eyes. No. 17, for example, performed at near criterion levels with either eye, whereas No. 13 performed at criterion using its right eye but at chance using its left eye. By using the film records it was possible to compare the amount of time the stimulus cards were within the

Table 6.5

Percentage of jumps to the positive stimulus

| | Post-discrimination retention tests | | | | Post-reversal retention tests | | | |
| | Double reward | | Single reward | | Double reward | | Single reward | |
Pigeon	left eye	right eye	left eye	right eye	left eye	right eye	left eye	right eye
11	95	65	80	50	50	65	55	70
13	45	90	60	70	70	50	75	50
14	80	55	65	60	100	60	65	70
17	90	80	60	50	85	75	70	60
18	70	40	55	55	95	45	85	55
19	70	50	50	50	70	60	60	50

visual field of each eye. A ratio of the amount of time the positive stimulus was within the visual field of the left eye or the right eye could then be correlated with a ratio of the performance using each eye. This correlation was +0.84, indicating that during binocular training the more a bird used a particular eye to view the stimulus cards the more likely it was to have learned with that eye. Since it has already been shown that there is no interocular transfer of visual discrimination habits learned monocularly, it is not surprising that having learned with one eye the bird cannot use the other eye to perform the task.

Although most of the birds in our experiment learned the original discrimination with only one eye, they did not always learn the reversal of the discrimination with the other eye. Instead, as table 6.5 shows, four of the six birds learned the reversal in much the same way as they had learned the original discrimination. In these birds the high score on the second retention test was obtained with the same eye that produced the high score on the original retention test. On the other hand, the scores of the other two birds suggest that they had switched eyes to learn the reversal. Interestingly, the birds which did seem to use an eye-switching strategy did not learn the reversal more quickly than those that learned the reversal with the same eye as the original discrimination.

The finding that pigeons learn a discrimination with only one eye even though they are trained binocularly is not unique. In a closely related species, the Barbary dove, Friedman (1976) has reported a similar finding. When the doves were trained binocularly to select one type of seed out of the two types available on the floor of a cage, he found that there were short-term preferences in the use of the left and right visual fields for selecting the next seed. Although trained binocularly, the birds showed a clear difference between the performance of each eye when tested monocularly. When the eye tested was the one used preferentially during the preceding binocular training, the birds pecked significantly more often at the type of seed they had been trained to select. When the other eye was tested the discrimination broke down.

CONCLUSION

The present series of experiments has demonstrated a clear and striking difference between the interocular transfer observed in pigeons trained on a jumping-stand and in a Skinner box. Moreover, the experiments have shown that this difference is not due to the amount of training nor is it a function of task difficulty. The results of the present jumping-stand experiments also eliminate Catania's earlier suggestion that the learning of new postural habits interferes with normal interocular transfer.

Catania's argument about posture on the jumping-stand was dependent on the assumption that pigeons use their lateral fields to view distant stimuli and their frontal binocular field to view stimuli nearby. There is some support for this assumption in the physiological observations, by Nye (1973), of the optics of the pigeon's eye. He found that pigeons are indeed laterally hypermetropic and frontally myopic.

However, it should be emphasised that he also found that the pigeon's eye is capable of accommodating very near objects in the lateral field.

Despite these observations, the pigeons in our own experiments do not appear to have been consistently using their lateral visual fields to view the stimuli on the jumping-stand. On many of the trials, in both monocular and binocular training conditions, the birds jumped correctly even though the stimuli did not fall laterally beyond 40° from the beak of the animal.

However, this does not mean that the birds are not using their eyes differently in the two training situations. One of the several differences between the Skinner box and the jumping-stand experiments is that the pigeons are using a different part of the retina to view the stimuli in the two situations. This does not seem to be a difference between anterior and lateral visual fields, but between the superior and inferior quadrants of the posterior half of the retina. In the Skinner box, when the pigeon is pecking directly at the stimulus key, the stimuli are viewed with the superior temporal quadrant of the retina (Delius *et al.,* 1974; Romeiskie and Yager, 1976). But when the pigeons are on the jumping-stand with the stimuli vertically in front of them, they do not view the stimuli with this quadrant. Our observations show that when they are standing on the perch preparing to jump they hold their heads in their usual positions, with an angle between beak and horizon of about 25° down (Duijm, 1951). In this position the stimuli fall on the lower posterior quadrant of the retina.

Interestingly, the superior temporal quadrant of the pigeon's eye contains the 'red area', an additional area of specialisation in the retina. It is known to be morphologically and functionally differentiated from the rest of the retina (Galifret, 1968; Nye, 1973; Yazulla, 1974). It also has a high tectal magnification factor and a higher retinal ganglion cell density, suggesting an area of acute vision (Binggeli and Paule, 1969; Clarke and Whitteridge, 1976; Whitteridge, 1965) comparable with the fovea itself.

It may well be that discriminative stimuli must fall on the red area in order for interocular transfer to take place—a hypothesis which accords well with Levine's original conclusions. He found, in two experimental situations, that when the stimuli were placed vertically in front of the pigeons there was no interocular transfer, but when the same stimuli were located horizontally under the beak, then there was interocular transfer. In the latter position the stimuli would be falling on the red area.

Thus the discrepancy in the findings of Levine and Catania may be due to the difference in the way the pigeons use their eyes in the two situations. Although Catania placed the discriminative stimulus in the same position as Levine did relative to the bird, the stimulus nevertheless fell on a different part of the retina.

Other obvious differences between the two sets of experiments include the type of response required, the type of reinforcement and whether the pigeons are responding freely or in discrete trials. (Beritov and Chichinadze (1936) did report a failure of transfer in a go/no-go task using a food reward.) However, speculation that these factors or the red area are necessarily involved in interocular transfer must await further behavioural and physiological investigations.

REFERENCES

Beritov, U. S. and Chichinadze, N. (1936). Localization of visual perception in the pigeon. *Bull. Biol. Med. Exp. URSS,* **20**, 105–107

Binggeli, R. L. and Paule, W. J. (1969). Pigeon retina: quantitative aspects of the optic nerve and ganglion cell layer. *J. comp Neurol.,* **137**, 1–18

Catania, A. C. (1964). On the visual acuity of the pigeon. *J. exp. Anal. Behav.,* **7**, 361–66

Catania, A. C. (1965). Interocular transfer of discriminations in the pigeon. *J. exp. Anal. Behav.,* **8**, 147–55

Clarke, P. G. H. and Whitteridge, D. (1976). The projection of the retina, including the 'red area' on to the optic tectum of the pigeon. *Q. J. exp. Physiol.,* **61**, 351–58

Cuénod, M. and Zeier, M. (1967). Transfer interhemisphérique et commissurotomie chez le pigeon. *Schweiz. Arch. Neurol. Psychiat.,* **100**, 365–80

Delius, J. D., Perchard, R. V. and Emmerton, J. (1976). Polarized light discrimination by pigeons and an electroretinographic correlate. *J. comp. physiol. Psychol.,* **90**, 560–71

Duijm, M. (1951). On the head positions in birds and its relation to some anatomical features. *Proc. koninklijke Nederlandse akad. van wetensch.,* **54C**, 202–11

Friedman, M. B. (1975). How birds use their eyes. In *Neural and Endocrine Aspects of Behaviour in Birds* (P. Wright, P. G. Caryl and D. M. Vowles, eds), Elsevier, Amsterdam

Galifret, Y. (1968). Les diverses aires fonctionelles de la rétine du pigeon. *Z. Zellforsch.,* **86**, 535–45

Graves, J. A. and Goodale, M. A. (1977). A failure of interocular transfer in the pigeon (*Columba livia*). *Physiol. Behav.* **19**(3), 425–28

Halstead, W. and Yacorzynski, G. (1938). A jumping method for establishing differential responses in pigeons. *J. genet. Psychol.,* **52**, 227–31

Ingle, D. (1968). Interocular integration of visual learning by goldfish. *Brain, Behav. Evol.,* **1**, 58–85

Levine, J. (1945a). Studies in interrelations of central nervous structures in binocular vision. Lack of bilateral transfer of visual discrimination habits acquired monocularly by the pigeon. *J. genet. Psychol.,* **67**, 105–29

Levine, J. (1945b). Studies in interrelations of central nervous structures in binocular vision. II. Conditions under which interocular transfer of discrimination habits takes place in the pigeon. *J. genet. Psychol.,* **67**, 131–42

Levine, J. (1952). Studies in interrelations of central nervous structures in binocular vision. III. Localization of memory trace as evidenced by lack of inter and intraocular habit transfer in the pigeon. *J. genet. Psychol.,* **81**, 19–27

Maier, V. (1976). Effekte unilateraler telencephaler und thalamisher Läsionen auf die monokulere Masterdiskriminations fähigkeit kommissurotomierter Tauben. *Rev. Suisse Zool.,* **83**, 59–82

Meier, R. E. (1971). Interhemisphärischer Transfer visueller Zweifachwahlen bei kommissurotomierten Tauben. *Psychol. Forsch.,* **34**, 220–45

Nye, P. W. (1973). On the functional differences between frontal and lateral visual fields of the pigeon. *Vision Res.,* **13**, 559–74

Ogawa, T. and Ohinata, S. (1966). Interocular transfer of colour discrimination in the pigeon. *A. Anim. Psychol. Tokyo,* **16**, 1-9

Romeiskie, M. and Yager, D. (1976). Psychophysical studies of pigeon color vision. I. Photopic spectral sensitivity. *Vision Res.,* **16**, 501-505

Whitteridge, D. (1965). Geometrical relations between the retina and the visual cortex. In *Mathematics and Computer Science in Biology and Medicine,* Medical Research Council, London

Yazulla, S. (1974). Intraretinal differentiation in the synaptic organization of the inner plexiform layer of the pigeon retina. *J. comp. Neurol.,* **153**, 309-24

Zeier, H. (1975). Interhemispheric interactions. In *Neural and Endocrine Aspects of Behaviour in Birds* (P. Wright, P. G. Caryl and D. M. Vowles, eds.). Elsevier, Amsterdam

7

INTERHEMISPHERIC INTEGRATION OF VISUAL INFORMATION IN THE PIGEON — A BEHAVIOURAL STUDY

M. GRAF and H. ZEIER

INTRODUCTION

The optic nerves of birds cross completely at the optic chiasm and the eye movements are independent of each other (Cowan *et al.*, 1962). Nevertheless, there is complete interocular transfer of intensity, colour and form discriminations (Catania, 1965). Lesion studies have revealed the central position of the supra-optic decussation (DS) as a commissural pathway for interhemispheric transfer (Meier, 1971; Cuénod, 1974). The DS is part of the retinothalamohyperstriatal system (Nauta and Karten, 1970; Miceli *et al.*, 1975).

The first findings of interocular reversal (paradoxical transfer) of left–right mirror images in the pigeon (Mello, 1965), in the goldfish (Ingle, 1967) and in the monkey (Noble, 1968), were questioned by further studies (Mello, 1966, 1967b; Hamilton *et al.*, 1973). Hamilton *et al.* proposed the 'masking hypothesis' as a possible explanation of the previous findings. Corballis and Beale (1970) and Palmers (1972) also criticised the paradoxical transfer studies and recent investigations argue against an anatomical basis for paradoxical transfer (Tieman *et al.*, 1974; Voneida and Mello, 1975).

Mello (1967b) investigated paradoxical transfer in the binocular situation. But she did not concern herself with the question how pigeons respond to the simultaneous presentation of different information to each eye separately. Palmers (1972) was the first to investigate this question thoroughly. Out of the two principal possibilities, (a) to analyse the input to both eyes simultaneously (simultaneous binocular integration) or (b) to suppress the input to one eye (interhemispheric suppression), he found interhemispheric suppression in a simultaneous discrimination of colour, and this finding was supported by further experiments (Palmers and Zeier, 1974).

However, there was still no evidence of a capacity for simultaneous binocular vision or, as it is called, interhemispheric integration of visual information in pigeons. This had been questioned for non-mammals by Walls (1963), by Walk (1965) and by Mello (1967). To answer this question we chose visual patterns, restriction of visual input and reinforcement contingencies in a way that enabled pigeons to learn the presented discrimination exclusively in the case of simultaneous analysis of the visual input to both hemispheres. In other words, subjects had to learn a discrimination for which no successful monocular strategy exists. Under these circumstances, the hypothesis that 'pigeons are able to learn such a discrimination' becomes identical to the hypothesis that 'pigeons are capable of simultaneous binocular or interhemispheric integration'.

The patterns presented consisted of either parallel bars or non-parallel ones (see top row in figure 7.2). The presentation of parallel bars indicated 'no reward' (no-go), whereas presentation of non-parallel bars meant 'reward' (go). The left half of the pattern was red and the right half green. As the animals were trained on a successive go/no-go discrimination, this meant that they were exposed to only one pattern display on any occasion. The pigeon wore goggles (figure 7.1) with a red filter over the left eye and a green filter over the right eye. Therefore, each eye saw only the left or right half of the display. Thus the animal could only decide whether the pattern had parallel or non-parallel lines by integrating the information from both retinal images in the central nervous system.

METHODS

Subjects

Twelve pigeons (*Columba livia*) were used as subjects. Eight were trained under interhemispheric conditions. The final data are presented in detail on two animals.

Apparatus

To restrict the input to the visual system, goggles were attached by collodium and anchored by acrylic cement (figure 7.1). Such goggles had already been used earlier (Catania, 1963; Mello, 1967a; Palmers, 1972). They allowed fixation of red and green filters (Kodak Wratten No. 92, red; No. 65, green) in front of the eyes. The filters were fixed during the sessions in the operant conditioning chamber. Glass covers protected the gelatine filters against the influence of humidity on the side of the eyes.

The same filters were used for the construction of the slides, which were projected by a Kodak Carousel S-RA (150 W lamp in a distance of 40 cm) on to the pecking key (ϕ, 30 mm). Additionally a 0.6 neutral density filter (Kodak Wratten No. 96) assimilated the intensity of the red part of the slides to the intensity of the green parts (Hodos, 1969). Figure 7.2 shows the stimuli as they were visible on the pecking key. To increase the probability that the stimuli would be appropriate for the analysis, two pattern sets were used (figure 7.2), but we never changed between the fine and the heavier stripes within one bird.

A stimulus was set by a control apparatus connected to a PDP-8/e laboratory

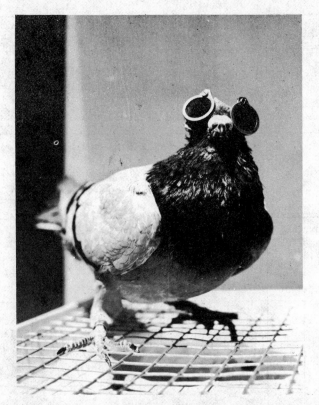

Figure 7.1. A pigeon with the filters fixed on to the goggles, ready for the session in the operant conditioning chamber

computer, which also controlled food reinforcement, the projector lamp and the recording of time and pecking responses. The methods including the SKED software used for the programs are explained elsewhere (Zeier, 1973).

Procedure

Pigeon AM1

The pigeon was shaped in the experimental chamber situation by an autoshaping program. Consecutively, the programs were adjusted to a variable interval schedule of 20 s (VI 20 s) and finally to a VI 1 (Ferster and Skinner, 1957), first without goggles, then with goggles.

During the main training *correct stimuli* (S^+) were reinforced by a 6 s access to grains for responses according to a 1 min variable interval schedule. An S^+ was always presented for 5 min. Incorrect stimuli (S^-) were never reinforced, and were

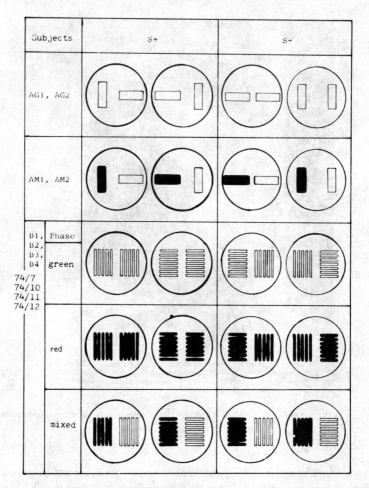

Figure 7.2. The stimuli as they were visible on the pecking key; black means red and framed white means green

removed *only* after a 1 min period without pecking. The presentation of a new stimulus according to a pseudo-random sequence was accompanied by a 10 s blackout. Such a reinforcement schedule was also used by Mello (1967b), and is a chained schedule (chain DRO VI 1). The discrimination was a successive go/no-go discrimination. During the main training and during all tests we used no additional light in the experimental chamber. After 60 rewards the program stopped and the session ended. Pigeon AM1 was trained during 45 sessions on the discrimination of the bar displays, partly red and partly green (mixed), wearing a red filter in front of the left eye and a green filter in front of the right—aligning the colour of the mixed patterns.

The main training was followed by an extinction test. Each of the four stimuli were three times presented for 2 min. The responses were recorded for each stimulus and for each presentation separately. No food rewards were available. The extinction test should show how far the subject is under stimulus control. During a second extinction session the filters were crossed compared with the training situation.

After a short retraining, a 'blank' test, run under the training program but without any patterns projected on to the pecking key, was administered to reveal possible sequential control.

Pigeon 74/12

Pretraining was the same as described for pigeon AM1, but without goggles. Pigeon 74/12 was then first trained—still without any goggles— during 15 sessions on the patterns with the fine stripes partly red and partly green and given two resistance-to-extinction tests followed by a 'blank' test. This gives a within-subjects control in the situation where the information was available for both eyes at the same time. Four other sessions, performed *with goggles* without filters, enabled the pigeon to get accustomed to the goggles.

Then, green stimuli were presented and green filters covered both eyes during 23 sessions. Again, two extinction tests and the blank test followed. This phase should reveal any impairment possibly caused by the restriction of the lateral visual fields and by the filters.

After retraining (under the double green conditions), red and green stimuli were presented and, correspondingly, the left eye was covered by a red filter and the right eye by a green filter. In this phase, pigeon 74/12 was trained for 20 sessions before testing.

RESULTS

Considerable individual differences were found between subjects. Therefore, averaging of learning curves and of test results or statistical analysis did not seem adequate. Instead, the final data of two subjects, AM1 and 74/12, are presented in detail.

Pigeon AM1

Figure 7.3 shows the learning curve of pigeon AM1. The solid line represents the percentage of responses to S^+; the broken line indicates the percentage of presence of S^+. This variable is, on the one hand, also dependent on the behaviour but, on the other, may be seen as a kind of chance level. The dotted line shows the time needed for 60 rewards. The *star* shows the percentage of responses to S^+ during the extinction test and the *asterisk* during the extinction test with the filters reversed.

Figure 7.4 represents the distribution of the responses of pigeon AM1 to the two

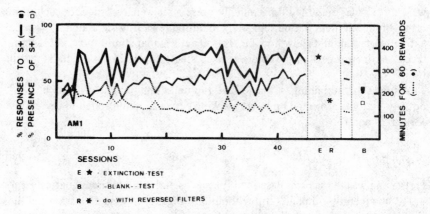

Figure 7.3. Learning curve of pigeon M1 (for explanations see text)

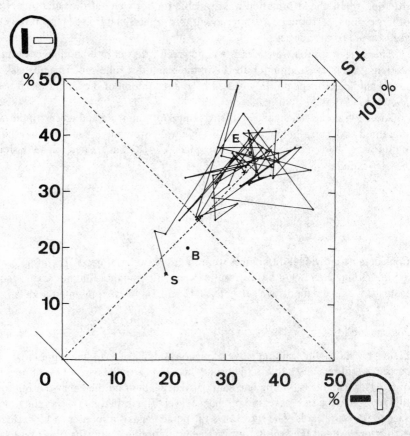

Figure 7.4. Distribution of the responses of pigeon AM1 to the two different patterns used as S[+]. Percentage of total responses to all patterns. (For further explanations see text)

different patterns used as S⁺. S indicates the start of training, E the result of the extinction test and B the result of the blank test.

Pigeon 74/12

In the same manner as described for AM1, figures 7.5 (a) and 7.5 (b) show the success of 74/12 during the different phases of the training procedure described above.

The results of the two resistance-to-extinction tests of 74/12 are reported in detail in table 7.1 and in figure 7.6. The difference between the responses to S⁺ and

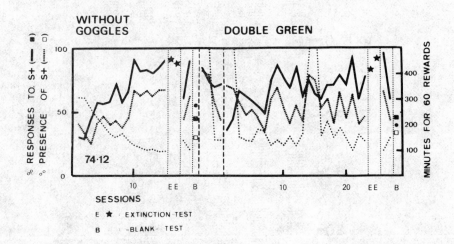

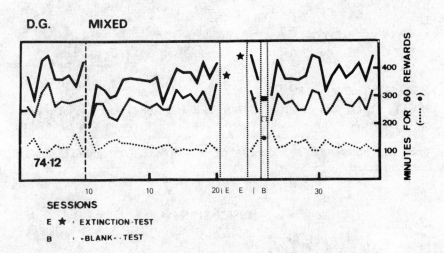

Figure 7.5 (a)   Learning curve of pigeon 74/12 part I (for explanations see text); (b) learning curve of pigeon 74/12 part II (for explanations see text)

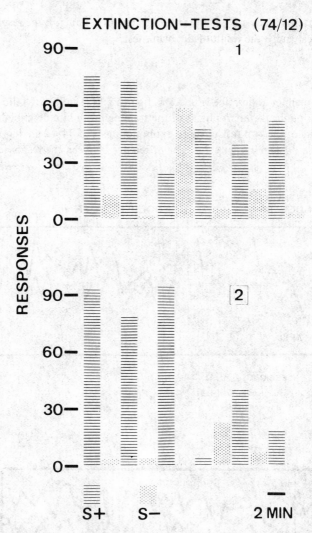

Figure 7.6. Extinction tests of pigeon 74/12, mixed phase. Striped blocks mean responses to an S$^+$ pattern, dotted blocks mean responses to an S$^-$ pattern. (See also table 7.1 and text)

to S$^-$ are significant ($P < 0.05$) according to the Wilcoxon test and to the binomial distribution test.

DISCUSSION

Five out of eight pigeons, trained under interhemispheric conditions, learned the discrimination reasonably well. The results in the extinction tests (E) of AM1 and

Table 7.1

Distribution of the responses of pigeon 74/12 during the two resistance-to-extinction tests in the mixed phase (see also figure 7.6 and text). The differences between the responses to S^+ and to S^- are significant ($P < 0.05$) according to the Wilcoxon test and to the binomial distribution test

Extinction test	Presentation	S_1^+	S_1^-	S_2^+	S_2^-
I	1	75	13	73	2
	2	14	59	47	6
	3	39	16	52	3
	1 + 2 + 3	128	88	172	11
II	1	92	4	78	4
	2	94	1	4	23
	3	40	7	18	1
	1 + 2 + 3	226	12	100	28
I + II		354	100	272	39

of 74/12 are significant ($P < 0.05$, Wilcoxon test). The failure of the three unsuccessful subjects and the long-lasting acquisition (see figure 7.3) show the difficulty of the discrimination task. The distribution of the responses of pigeon AM1 to the two different patterns used as S^+ (see figure 7.4) shows the development of the stimulus control and of binocular vision. In the case of a monocular strategy, such an analysis would lead to a distribution along the other diagonal.

The learning curve of AM1 (presented in figure 7.3) shows the direct acquisition of the discrimination under binocular conditions without any previous experience on discrimination tasks with this type of pattern. On the contrary, pigeon 74/12 first had additional training. Without any goggles, the discrimination on the red and green patterns is learned well and rapidly (see figure 7.5a). Colour is an irrelevant aspect of the discrimination. The relevant aspect is whether or not the orientation of the lines on one half of the stimulus matches the orientation of the lines on the other half. Attaching goggles with green filters in front of each eye and presenting completely green stimuli had already led to some impairment of performance, but finally the pigeon performed well, as results of the extinction tests show. The initial impairment may be due to the new colour of the right part of the stimulus and/or to the restriction of the lateral visual fields. Proceeding to the binocular conditions reveals (see figure 7.5b) that, to some extent, transfer from the binocular double-green situation to the performance under red–green conditions takes place.

A good performance is finally reached, which is underlined by the results of the two resistance-to-extinction tests (figure 7.6 and table 7.1). Significantly successful discrimination proves—according to our hypothesis—that pigeons are capable of interhemispheric integration. Our experiment does not show the way nor the manner in which this integration occurs, but probably the supra-optic decussation, through which fibres cross from the thalamic relay nucleus to the contralateral hyperstriatum, might be involved. This could be investigated by lesion studies.

Our behavioural study gives support to the view that the avian brain is organised at a higher level than supposed earlier, supporting investigations about the visual cortex in the owl (*Tyto alba*) by Pettigrew and Konishi (1976) and the electron microscope study in the pigeon's optic tectum by Angaut and Repérant (1976).

REFERENCES

Angaut, P. and Repérant, J. (1976). Fine structure of the optic fibre termination layers in the pigeon optic tectum: a Golgi and electron microscope study. *Neuroscience*, **1**, 93–105

Catania, A. C. (1963). Techniques for the control of monocular and binocular viewing in the pigeon. *J. exp. Anal. Behav.*, **6**, 627–29

Catania, A. C. (1965). Interocular transfer of discriminations in the pigeon. *J. exp. Anal. Behav.*, **8**, 147–155

Corballis, M. C. and Beale, I. L. (1970). Monocular discrimination of mirror-image obliques by pigeons: evidence for lateralized stimulus control. *Anim. Behav.*, **18**, 563–66

Cowan, W. M., Adamson, L. and Powell, T. S. P. (1962). An experimental study of the avian visual system. *J. Anat.*, **95**, 545–63

Cuénod, M. (1974). Commissural pathways in interhemispheric transfer of visual information in the pigeon. In *The Neurosciences*, 3rd Study Program, MIT Press, Cambridge, Massachusetts

Ferster, C. B. and Skinner, B. F. (1957). *Schedules of Reinforcement*, Appleton, New York

Hamilton, C. R., Tieman, S. B. and Brody, B. A. (1973). Interhemispheric comparison of mirror-image stimuli in chiasm sectioned monkeys. *Brain Res.*, **58**, 415–25

Hodos, W. (1969). Colour discrimination deficits after lesions of the nucleus rotundus in pigeons. *Brain, Behav. Evol.*, **2**, 185–200

Ingle, D. (1967). Two visual mechanisms underlying the behavior of fish. *Psychol. Forsch.*, **31**, 44–51

Meier, R. E. (1971). Interhemisphärischer Transfer visueller Zweifachwahlen bei kommissurotomierten Tauben. *Psychol. Forsch.*, **34**, 220–45

Mello, N. K. (1965). Interhemispheric reversal of mirror-image oblique lines following monocular training in pigeons. *Science*, **148**, 252–54

Mello, N. K. (1966). Concerning the interhemispheric transfer of mirror-image patterns in pigeon. *Physiol. Behav.*, **1**, 293–300

Mello, N. K. (1967a). A method for restricting stimuli to the frontal or lateral visual field of each eye separately in pigeon. *Psychonom. Sci.*, **8**, 15–16

Mello, N. K. (1967b). Interhemispheric comparison of visual stimuli in the pigeon. *Nature (Lond.)*, **214**, 144–45

Miceli, D., Peyrichoux, J. and Repérant, J. (1975). The retino-thalamo-hyperstriatal pathway in the pigeon *(Columba livia)*. *Brain Res.*, **100**, 125–31

Nauta, W. J. H. and Karten, H. J. (1970). A general profile of the vertebrate brain, with sidelights on the ancestry of cerebral cortex. In *The Neurosciences* (F. O. Schmitt, ed.), 2nd Study Program, New York, The Rockefeller University Press, pp. 7-26

Noble, J. (1968). Paradoxical interocular transfer of mirror-image discriminations in the optic chiasm sectioned monkey. *Brain Res.*, **10**, 127-51

Palmers, C. (1972). Interhemisphärische Suppression bei der Taube. *Unveröffentlichte Doktorarbeit,* Universität Wien

Palmers, C. and Zeier, H. (1974). Hemispheric dominance and transfer in the pigeon. *Brain Res.*, **76**, 537-41

Pettigrew, J. D. and Konishi, M. (1976). Neurons selective for orientation and binocular disparity in the visual wulst of the barn owl *(Tyto alba). Science,* **193**, 675-78

Tieman, S. B., Tieman, D. G., Brody, B. A. and Hamilton, C. R. (1974). Interocular reversal of up-down mirror-images in pigeons. *Physiol. Behav.,* **12**, 615-20

Voneida, T. J. and Mello, N. K. (1975). Interhemispheric projections in the optic tectum in pigeon. *Brain, Behav. Evol.,* **11**, 91-108

Walk, R. D. (1965). *The Study of Visual Depth and Distance Perception in Animals,* Academic Press, New York

Walls, G. L. (1963). *The Vertebrate Eye and its Adaptive Radiation,* Hafner, New York

Zeier, H. (1973). Programmierung und Auswertung von Lernexperimenten mit einem Prozessrechner. *Neue Technik,* **4**, 3-7

8
EFFECTS OF EARLY VISUAL DEPRIVATION ON PATTERN DISCRIMINATION LEARNING AND INTEROCULAR TRANSFER IN THE PIGEON *(COLUMBA LIVIA)*

A. BURKHALTER and M. CUÉNOD

INTRODUCTION

The organisation of the visual pathways in the pigeon provides an opportunity to study the effects of sensory deprivation upon the higher visual centres. The pigeon, as an experimental animal, has the advantage over mammals that the fibre tracts leading from either eye to the visual areas of binocular convergence are segregated and thus easily accessible to surgery. At the chiasma the optic nerve fibres are almost completely distributed to the contralateral side of the brain (Cowan *et al.,* 1961; Repérant *et al.,* 1973; Streit, private communication). The retinotectal pathway sends its fibres to the optic tectum (Hunt and Webster, 1975; Karten, 1965; Karten and Revzin, 1966) from where it ascends via the nucleus rotundus of the thalamus to the ectostriatum in the telencephalon (Benowitz and Karten, 1976; Karten and Hodos, 1970; Karten and Revzin, 1966). Although quantitatively less powerful, the retinothalamohyperstriatal pathway plays a role in pattern discrimination. It relays in the dorsolateral thalamus (DLLd, DLLv) from where fibres project to the contralateral nucleus intercalatus hyperstriatum accessorium (IHA), and by means of recrossing fibres via the dorsal aspect of the supra-optic decussation (DSO) to the ipsilateral IHA of the visual Wulst (Hunt and Webster, 1972; Karten *et al.,* 1973; Meier *et al.,* 1974). Units recorded in the visual Wulst were activated by photic stimulation of either eye (Perišić *et al.,* 1971). Thus, this gives evidence that despite the almost complete crossing of the optic nerve fibres at the chiasma, binocular convergence of visual input takes place in the visual wulst.

As established in a number of vertebrate species (Cuénod, 1972) the ability to perform with the untrained eye a visual discrimination learned through the other eye, has also been observed in the pigeon. Transection of the DSO was shown to confine monocularly learned differential behaviour to one side (Meier, 1971).

The purpose of the present study was to investigate the effects of different kinds of visual deprivation on pattern discrimination learning and interocular transfer. Monocular deprivation in pigeons, after DSO section, allows a comparison of (1) the visual behaviour while using a visually completely naive eye with the behaviour while using a visually experienced eye within the same animal, and (2) the effects of monocular deprivation in animals with and without the possibility of DSO-mediated binocular interaction.

METHODS

Forty-nine pigeons (*Columba livia*) were divided into three deprivation groups: (1) binocular deprivation (BD, $n = 11$), (2) monocular deprivation (MD, $n = 26$), and (3) monocular deprivation with additional section of the DSO (MD + DSO, $n = 12$). According to the order of monocular discrimination training, both monocular deprivation groups MD and MD + DSO were divided each into two subgroups: MED (experienced eye trained first), MDE (deprived eye trained first), MED + DSO and MDE + DSO. Three groups served as control groups: (1) unoperated control (CO, $n = 10$), (2) section of the DSO in the adult animal (DSOad, $n = 12$), and (3) section of the DSO in the newly hatched pigeon (DSOjuv, $n = 9$).

Rearing

Immediately after hatching, but before natural eye opening, the eyelids were painted with a black plastic colour (Shiny Eye-liner[R], Max Factor) and additionally covered by a sprayed film of Nobecutan[R] (Bofors, Nobel-Pharma, Sweden). The birds grew up in the nest under the care of their parents. When the squabs were two weeks old the plastic patches were replaced by opaque PVC caps, which were glued on the sprouting feathers. The deprivation lasted for 87–185 days. During that time BD animals were force fed through a special pigeon-feeding syringe.

  Ophthalmological examinations at the end of the deprivation revealed clear optic media, a well preserved corneal surface and no lens aberrations. The pupillary response was normal.

Surgery

In the young animals surgical intervention was performed at the third or fourth day of life. The adult animals underwent surgery at the age of at least three months.

  To transect the DSO two versions of the same instrument were used. For the young animals it was a miniaturised type of that described earlier (Cuénod and Zeier, 1967). Under anaesthesia (young animals: 0.02 ml/10 g bodyweight, Equithesin[R]; adult animals: 0.25 ml/100 g bodyweight) the head of the animals was fixed in a head holder, allowing stereotaxically lowering of the instrument through a little hole in the skull (for details see Burkhalter and Cuénod, 1978).

Training

Pigeons were trained in a standard operant conditioning apparatus placed in a soundproof chamber. The stimuli were projected from behind directly on to two pecking keys, mounted at the front panel. Misplaced pecks were registered by a special device. Through an aperture 16 cm below the keys, animals had access to hemp seed which was delivered through an automatic dispenser. The training apparatus was controlled and data collected by a PDP-8 computer.

Pretraining on a light–dark discrimination began after termination of the deprivation, following one week of normal visual experience. Food deprived animals (75–85% free-feeding weight) had to learn to peck the illuminated key monocularly. Every correct response was rewarded by 3.5 s access to food. The position of the positive stimulus was changed according to a Gellermann sequence (Gellermann,

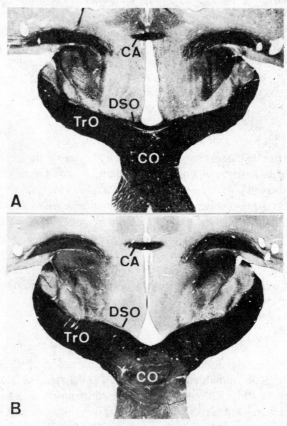

Figure 8.1. Frontal section through the mesodiencephalic region: (A) unoperated control, (B) section of the DSO in the newly hatched pigeon (DSOjuv). The decussating fibres are completely degenerated. CA, commissura anterior; CO, chiasma opticum; DSO, decussatio supra-optica; TrO, tractus opticus

1933). Pretraining of the left and right eye was alternated and continued until the animals reached criterion (50 correct responses on 3 successive sessions) with each eye separately.

Each animal had to learn with one eye (first eye) two pattern discriminations. The discriminanda were presented simultaneously and the animals learned to discriminate successively between ||| and ≡, then between + and ×. To counteract position preferences a correction procedure was programmed. Daily sessions of 60 rewarded trials proceeded to three different criteria: $C_1 \geqslant 90\%$ correct responses on 3 successive sessions, $C_2 \geqslant 90\%$ correct on 3 sessions, $C_3 \geqslant 90\%$ correct for the first time. Interocular transfer was tested in a 40-trial session under extinction conditions (retention test).

The interocular transfer was estimated in four different ways: (1) number of correct choices with the transfer eye in the retention test, (2) percent correct trials with the transfer eye in the first training session, (3) number of trials to criterion with the transfer eye in percent of the number of trials to criterion with the eye trained first (intra-individual comparison), and (4) trials to criterion with the transfer eye in percent of the trials to criterion with the eye trained first of the control (CO) (inter-individual comparison).

Histology

At the end of the experiment the brains of commissurotomised animals (DSOad, DSOjuv) were histologically controlled. The extent of the DSO lesion was measured out on Weil pictures. Only animals with at least 80% of the DSO fibres cut were retained in the groups.

The pictures obtained from the DSOjuv animals differed from those of the DSOad animals. Where the sectioned myelinated fibres were still visible in the adult cases (DSOad), they completely disappeared in the juvenile animals (DSOjuv) (figure 8.1).

RESULTS

Pecking accuracy

It is known that visual deprivation disintegrates the well-coordinated visuomotor action of pecking behaviour in the chicken (Kovach, 1969). To estimate pecking accuracy in the visually deprived pigeon the ratio R_a was calculated (R_a is the number of pecks beside the key versus number of pecks on the key).

Comparison of the R_a values of the first with the second eye in any group revealed no statistically significant difference, except in the MDE group (Mann-Whitney U test; $|||/\equiv$ $U = 37, P < 0.05$; $+/\times$ $U = 37, P < 0.05$). However, compared with the monocular pecking accuracy of the control animals (CO), pecking with the deprived eye (MDE) was not significantly less accurate.

To know whether high pecking accuracy correlates with good discrimination performance, the R_a values obtained at the beginning of the acquisition (first training session) were compared with those at the end of the acquisition (last training session). The result did not confirm the assumption of a training-dependent amelioration of pecking accuracy. Therefore, we conclude that the precision of the key peck did not reduce the discrimination performance, at least in the testing situation used in the present study.

Acquisition and interocular transfer of pattern discriminations

Control group (CO)

Pigeons required more trials to learn the $+/\times$ discrimination than the $|||/\equiv$ discrimination (figure 8.2). The initial interocular transfer of the $+/\times$ task was present, although it was poorer than for the $|||/\equiv$ problem. With the eye trained in the second position, the animals learned the $|||/\equiv$ discrimination significantly faster

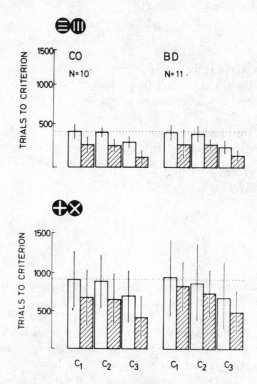

Figure 8.2. Mean number of trials to criterion (C_1, C_2, C_3) with the first (open columns) and the second (hatched columns) trained eye of the $|||/\equiv$ and the $+/\times$ discrimination. CO, control group; BD, binocular deprivation group

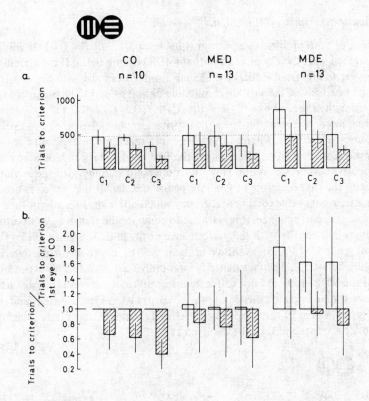

Figure 8.3. (a) Mean number of trials to criterion (C_1, C_2, C_3) on the |||/≡ discrimination. First trained eye, open columns; second trained eye, hatched columns. CO, control group; MED, monocular deprivation group (experienced eye trained first); MDE, monocular deprivation group (deprived eye trained first). (b) Inter-individual comparison of the trials to criterion required with the eye in first (open columns) and in second (hatched columns) position with the first eye of the control group (CO). Values below 1.0 indicate interocular transfer

($P < 0.01$) according to each of the three criteria. For the +/× problem significant savings ($P < 0.05$) were obtained in C_3 only. In the present chapter we concentrate on the results of the |||/≡ discrimination.

Binocular deprivation (BD)

On the |||/≡ discrimination, binocularly deprived pigeons (BD) performed as well as control animals (CO) with normal visual experience (figure 8.2). With the exception of interocular transfer this statement holds for the +/× discrimination, too. It should be pointed out that learning curves, as judged by the three criteria in both the CO and BD groups, showed an identical time course. The interocular transfer of the +/× discrimination, already poor in the CO group, is completely absent in the BD group.

Monocular deprivation (MED, MDE)

Learning of both problems was slower ($|||/\equiv P < 0.01$, $+/\times P < 0.01$) if animals were trained with their deprived eye first (MDE) (figure 8.3a). If the training succession was reversed (MED) the animals learned normally with the deprived eye: they performed the $|||/\equiv$ discrimination almost as perfectly as control animals (CO) using their second eye ($C_1 P < 0.1$, $C_2 P < 0.2$, $C_3 P < 0.1$).

Initial interocular transfer from the deprived to the experienced eye (MDE) was completely absent, whereas from the experienced to the deprived eye (MED) the mean score of 71% correct trials in the first training session indicated substantial interocular transfer. Conventionally, the more rapid learning with the second eye than with the first is assigned to an interocular transfer. If this notion is used to differentiate between experimental groups which differ significantly in their monocular learning performance, it is essential to compare the transfer eye's performance inter-individually with the performance of the initially trained eye of the control group (CO). Thus, as shown in figure 8.3 (b), interocular transfer is indicated by values below 1.0. The fact that this inter-individual ratio for the experienced eye of the MDE group did not differ significantly from 1.0 was taken as further evidence for a complete absence of interocular transfer. On the other hand, in the MED group, values of the deprived eye below 1.0 demonstrate interocular transfer from the experienced to the deprived eye.

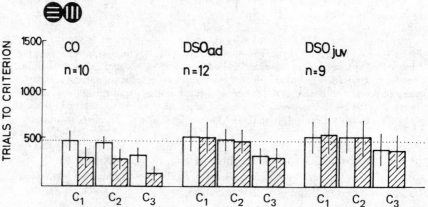

Figure 8.4. Mean number of trials to criterion (C_1, C_2, C_3) required by the first (open columns) and the second (hatched columns) eye in the adult (DSOad) and the young (DSOjuv) DSO-sectioned animals

Section of the DSO in newly hatched pigeons

Interocular transfer of pattern discriminations can be prevented by section of the supra-optic decussation in the adult pigeon (Meier, 1971). This observation was confirmed in the present study (DSOad) and extended to animals where the DSO was sectioned early in life (3rd-4th day) (figure 8.4). This showed that in the developing animal no alternative pathway took over interocular transfer.

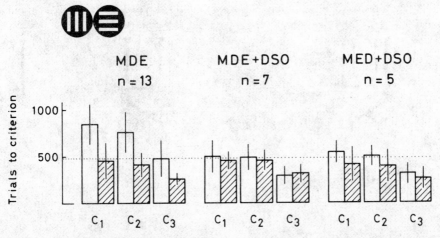

Figure 8.5. Mean number of trials to criterion (C_1, C_2, C_3) with the first (open columns) and the second (hatched columns) trained eye of monocularly deprived animals with additional section of the DSO just after hatching (MDE + DSO, MED + DSO)

Monocular deprivation with additional section of the DSO

The impairment in pattern discrimination learning already described for monocularly deprived animals using the deprived eye first (MDE) did not occur in monocularly deprived animals which had their DSO cut just after hatching (MDE + DSO, MED + DSO) (figure 8.5). With respect to learning velocity there was complete compatibility with the CO, DSOad and DSOjuv animals. As can be expected from the results of the DSOad and DSOjuv animals, no sign of interocular transfer was observed.

DISCUSSION

The experiments reported here present evidence for a behavioural change in the pigeon, following early monocular deprivation. Combining this with the observation that simultaneous deprivation of both eyes did not affect the pigeons' discrimination supports the hypothesis of a competition between left and right eye afferents for terminal space in the central regions of binocular convergence (Guillery, 1970; Wiesel and Hubel, 1963, 1965a). In an attempt to eliminate competition in the monocularly deprived animals from the beginning of the post-natal period, the supra-optic decussation (DSO) was surgically cut just after hatching (group MED + DSO and MDE + DSO). This was shown to result in a normalisation of pattern discrimination learning with the deprived eye as well as in a complete blockage of interocular transfer. Therefore, the fact that the deprivation-dependent impairment failed to appear in the MED + DSO and MDE + DSO group supports

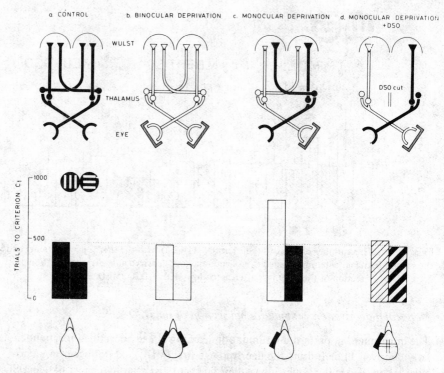

Figure 8.6. Schematic representation of the hypothetical deprivation induced modification in the retinothalamohyperstriatal system. (a) Unoperated control (CO). (b) No measurable behavioural changes after simultaneous deprivation in both eyes (BD). (c) Impaired learning with the deprived eye, possibly corresponding to an asymmetrical development of the afferents from each eye after monocular deprivation (MD). Interocular transfer from the deprived to the experienced eye is deficient. (d) Early DSO section prevents the learning deficit induced by monocular deprivation: this could be related to the elimination of the binocular interaction in the wulst (MED + DSO, MDE + DSO)

the hypothesis that this impairment was related in some way to the asymmetry of the binocular input. Cutting the DSO prevents the asymmetry (figure 8.6).

Because of important methodological differences between the present and previous studies about the effects of visual deprivation on the behaviour in birds, a comparison of the results is difficult. Binocular deprivation of comparable duration in ring doves (Siegel, 1953) and the chicken (Tucker, 1957) was found to impair visual acquisition performance and interocular transfer. On the other hand, monocular deprivation failed to create behavioural deficits in the chicken (Tucker, 1957). Since it was shown that ring doves trained in a jumping-stand failed to transfer pattern discriminations (Graves and Goodale, 1977), the conflicting results of the ring dove study, obtained in a similar apparatus, are probably due to methodological differences. The results of the chicken study suggest that in addition to methodological discrepancies (successive presentation of triangles and circles in a horizontal position) one has to think of ontogenetic differences between the precocial chicken and the altricial pigeon, which may account for the heterogeneity of observations.

The investigations about changes in the visual system due to environmental influences have indicated a certain parallelism between behavioural and physiological modifications (Dews and Wiesel, 1970; Ganz and Fitch, 1968; Ganz et al., 1968; Ganz et al., 1972; Ganz and Haffner, 1974; Hirsch, 1972; Movshon, 1976a, 1976b; Muir and Mitchell, 1975; Wiesel and Hubel, 1965b). From these results in the cat it was inferred that highly selective cells are important for normal pattern vision. A recent study reported the loss of the deprived eye's ability to activate neurons with small receptive fields and a high degree of orientation specificity, whereas cells with large receptive fields and little orientation preference preserve their binocularity (Leventhal and Hirsch, 1977). The generalisation of this finding for the interpretation of the low perceptual capacity of monocularly deprived pigeons is a matter of speculation. Although binocularly activated cells have not yet been observed in any other visual structure of the pigeon than in the IHA of the visual Wulst (Perišić et al., 1971), nothing is known about their receptive fields and their response properties after monocular deprivation.

However, recordings from neurons with small receptive fields (2-10°) and some degree of orientation selectivity (Revzin, 1969) in the same area of pigeon's visual wulst, revealed some similarity to neuronal properties known of the visual cortex of the cat. More direct evidence for a functional similarity of avian and mammalian visual centres derives from the owl, where recordings in the IHA characterised binocular, disparity and orientation sensitive cells with small receptive fields (Pettigrew, 1976). Furthermore, the analysis of the effect of monocular deprivation on binocular neurons in the owl's visual Wulst (Pettigrew and Konishi, 1976) gave results similar to those obtained in the cat: binocularly activated cells were lost, neurons driven by the experienced eye had orientation-selective properties and there were cells with the receptive field in the deprived eye with poor orientation preferences. It seems that at least highly binocular animals share the susceptibility of binocular neurons to environmental modifications. The results of the present study suggest that similar processes take place in the pigeon, where the binocular visual field is comparatively narrow (24°) (Catania, 1964).

The convergence between the afferences of the two eyes in the visual wulst is likely to involve units whose receptive fields are located in the binocular segment of the visual field, similar to what has been shown for the owl (Pettigrew, 1976). Thus, the deficit induced by monocular deprivation according to the competition hypothesis would be restricted to the binocular visual field. This implies that the pigeon normally relies mainly on the binocular field for pattern discrimination (Nye, 1973), and that the deficit is an expression of its need to adjust to, or to use, the lateral monocular visual field.

The supra-optic decussation (DSO) is an important pathway for the interocular exchange of visual shape and colour information not only in the pigeon but also in the goldfish (Ingle and Campbell, 1977; Yeo and Savage, 1976). The finding that DSO-sectioned, monocular-deprived pigeons (MED + DSO, MDE + DSO) learned pattern discriminations with equal ease as undeprived animals favours structures which receive binocular input via the DSO as locus for neuronal change. At present two likely candidates are the nucleus rotundus which receives inputs from both ipsilateral and contralateral tectum (through the ventral aspect of the DSO (Benowitz and Karten, 1976; Hunt and Künzle, 1976)) and the visual Wulst. Compared with the nucleus rotundus with its large receptive fields (90–120°) (Giorgetti de Britto, 1975), the visual Wulst is more likely to play a role in binocular vision in the pigeon. Thus, applying the concept of binocular competition between the endings of the crossed and uncrossed afferents in the visual Wulst (figure 8.6), the result of the MED + DSO and MDE + DSO animals can be explained by an elimination of binocular competitive interaction via the DSO. Thus a central lesion such as the transection of the DSO in the pigeon prevents damage caused by visual deprivation in the centres of binocular convergence. A similar finding was shown earlier by placing retinal lesions in the normal eye of a monocularly deprived cat (Sherman et al., 1974).

ACKNOWLEDGEMENTS

The authors are grateful to Professor K. Akert for his generous support, to Dr P. Streit for valuable advice, to Dr U. Wyss and F. Terrenghi for computer programming and maintenance, to Miss E. Knecht, A. Fäh, A. Fidéler, J. B. Frei and R. Kägi for excellent technical assistance, and to Dr J. H. J. Allum for helping to improve the English.

This work was supported by Grants 3.636.75 and 3.744.76 from the Swiss National Science Foundation and the Dr Eric Slack-Gyr-Foundation.

REFERENCES

Benowitz, L. I. and Karten, H. J. (1976). The organization of the tectofugal pathway in the pigeon: a retrograde transport study. J. comp. Neurol., 167, 503–20

Burkhalter, A. and Cuénod, M. (1978). Changes in pattern discrimination learning induced by visual deprivation in normal and commissurotomized pigeons. Expl Brain Res., 31, 369–85

Catania, A. C. (1964). On the visual acuity of the pigeon. J. exp. Anal. Behav., 7, 361–6

Cowan, W. M., Adamson, L. and Powell, T. P. S. (1961). An experimental study of the avian visual system. J. Anat., 95, 545–63

Cuénod, M. (1972). Split-brain studies. Functional interaction between bilateral central nervous structures. In The Structure and Foundation of Nervous Tissue, vol. 5, (G. H. Bourne, ed.), Academic Press, New York pp. 455-506

Cuénod, M. and Zeier H. (1967). Transfer interhémisphérique et commissurotomie chez le pigeon. *Schweizer. Arch. Neurol. Psychiat.*, **100**, 365-380

Dews, P. B. and Wiesel, T. N. (1970). Consequences of monocular deprivation on visual behaviour in kittens. *J. Physiol., Lond.*, **206**, 437-55

Ganz, L. and Fitch, M. (1968). The effect of visual deprivation on perceptual behaviour. *Expl Neurol.*, **22**, 638-60

Ganz, L., Fitch, M. and Satterberg, J. A. (1968). The selective effect of visual deprivation on receptive field shape determined neurophysiologically. *Expl Neurol.*, **22**, 614-37

Ganz, L. and Haffner, M. E. (1974). Permanent perceptual and neurophysiological effects of visual deprivation in the cat. *Expl Brain Res.*, **20**, 67-87

Ganz, L., Hirsch, H. V. B. and Tieman, S. (1972). The nature of perceptual deficits in visually deprived cats. *Brain Res.*, **44**, 547-68

Giorgetti de Britto, L. R., Brunelli, M., Francesconi, W. and Magni, F. (1975). Visual response pattern of thalamic neurons in the pigeon. *Brain Res.*, **97**, 337-43

Graves, J. F. and Goodale, M. A. (1977). Failure of interocular transfer in the pigeon (*Columba linia*). *Physiol. Behav.*, **19**, 425

Gellermann, L. W. (1933). Change orders of alternating stimuli in visual discrimination experiments. *J. genet. Psychol.*, **42**, 206-8

Guillery, R. W. (1970). Binocular competition in the control of geniculate cell growth. *J. comp. Neurol.*, **144**, 117-30

Hirsch, H. V. B. (1972). Visual perception in cats after environmental surgery. *Expl Brain Res.*, **15**, 405-23

Hunt, S. P. and Künzle, H. (1976). Observations on the projections and intrinsic organization of the pigeon optic tectum; An autoradiographic study based on anterograde and retrograde, axonal and dendritic flow. *J. comp. Neurol.*, **170**, 153-72

Hunt, S. P. and Webster, K. E. (1972). Thalamo-hyperstriate interrelations in the pigeon. *Brain Res.*, **44**, 647-51

Hunt, S. P. and Webster, K. E. (1975). The projections of the retina upon the optic tectum of the pigeon. *J. comp. Neurol.*, **162**, 433-46

Ingle, D. and Campbell, A. (1977). Interocular transfer of visual discriminations in goldfish after selective commissure lesions. *J. comp. physiol. Psychol.*, **53**, 311-21

Karten, H. J. (1965). Projections of the optic tectum of the pigeon (Columba livia). *Anat. Rec.*, **151**, 369

Karten, H. J. and Hodos, W. (1970). Telencephalic projections of the nucleus rotundus in the pigeon (*Columba livia*). *J. comp. Neurol.*, **140**, 35-52

Karten, H. J., Hodos, W., Nauta, W. J. H. and Revzin, A. M. (1973). Neural connections of the 'visual Wulst' of the avian telencephalon. Experimental studies in the pigeon (*Columba livia*) and the owl (*Speotyto cunicularia*). *J. comp. Neurol.*, **150**, 253-78

Karten, H. J. and Revzin, A. M. (1966). The afferent connections of the nucleus rotundus in the pigeon. *Brain Res.*, **2**, 368-77

Kovach, J. K. (1969). Development of pecking behaviour in chicks: Recovery after deprivation. *J. comp. physiol. Psychol.*, **68**, 516-23

Leventhal, A. G. and Hirsch, H. V. B. (1977). Effects of early experience upon orientation sensitivity and binocularity of neurons in visual cortex of cats. *Proc. natn Acad. Sci. U.S.A.*, **74**, 1272-6

Meier, R. E. (1971). Interhemisphärischer Transfer visueller Zweifachwahlen bei kommissurotomierten Tauben. *Psychol. Forsch.*, **34**, 220-45

Meier, R. E., Mihailovic, J. and Cuénod, M. (1974). Thalamic organization of the retino-thalamo-hyperstriatal pathway in the pigeon (*Columba livia*). *Expl Brain Res.*, **19**, 351-64

Movshon, J. A. (1976a). Reversal of the physiological effects of monocular deprivation in the kitten's visual cortex. *J. Physiol., Lond.*, **261**, 125-74

Movshon, J. A. (1976b). Reversal of behavioural effects of monocular deprivation in the kitten. *J. Physiol., Lond.*, **261**, 175-87

Muir, D. W. and Mitchell, D. E. (1975). Behavioral deficits in cats following early selected visual exposure to contours of a single orientation. *Brain Res.*, **85**, 459-77

Nye, P. W. (1973). On the functional differences between frontal and lateral visual fields of the pigeon. *Vision Res.*, **13**, 559-74

Perišić, M., Mihailovic, J. and Cuénod, M. (1971). Electrophysiology of contralateral and ipsilateral visual projections to the Wulst in the pigeon (*Columba livia*). *Int. J. Neurosci.*, **2**, 7-14

Pettigrew, J. D. (1976). Neurons selective for orientation and binocular disparity in the visual Wulst of the barn owl (*Tyto alba*). *Science*, **193**, 675-8

Pettigrew, J. D. and Konishi, M. (1976). Effect of monocular deprivation on binocular neurones in the owl's visual Wulst. *Nature*, **264**, 753-4

Repérant, J. (1973). Nouvelles données sur les projections visuelles chez le pigeon (*Columba livia*). *J. Hirnforsch.*, **14**, 151-88

Revzin, A. M. (1969). A specific projection area in the hyperstriatum of the pigeon (*Columba livia*). *Brain Res.*, **15**, 246-249

Revzin, A. M. (1970). Some characteristics of wide-field units in the brain of the pigeon. *Brain, Behav. Evol.*, **3**, 195-204

Siegel, A. I. (1953). Deprivation of visual form definition in the ring dove. II. Perceptual-motor transfer. *J. comp. physiol. Psychol.*, **46**, 249-252

Sherman, M. S., Guillery, R. W., Kaas, J. H. and Sanderson, K. J. (1974). Behavioral, electrophysiological and morphological studies of binocular competition in the development of the geniculo-cortical pathways of cats. *J. comp. Neurol.*, **158**, 1-18

Tucker, A. (1957). The effect of early light and form deprivation on the visual behaviors of the chicken. Unpublished doctoral dissertation, University of Chicago

Wiesel, T. N. and Hubel, D. H. (1963). Single responses in striate cortex of kittens deprived of vision in one eye. *J. Neurophysiol.*, **26**, 1003-17

Wiesel, T. N. and Hubel, D. H. (1965a). Comparison of the effects of unilateral and bilateral eye closure on cortical unit responses in kittens. *J. Neurophysiol.*, **28**, 1029-40

Wiesel, T. N. and Hubel, D. H. (1965b). Extent of recovery from the effects of visual deprivation in kittens. *J. Neurophysiol.*, **28**, 1060-72

Yeo, Ch. H. and Savage, G. E. (1976). Mesencephalic and diencephalic commissures and interocular transfer in the goldfish. *Expl. Neurol.*, **53**, 51-63

9
EXPERIENCE AND PLASTICITY IN THE CENTRAL NERVOUS SYSTEM*

G. HORN, S. P. R. ROSE and P. P. G. BATESON

INTRODUCTION

The neural mechanisms involved in learning have always excited great interest, but such are the complexities which surround their study that their analysis seemed virtually impossible. In recent years, however, there has been a great increase in knowledge of the central nervous system (CNS), and many new techniques have become available for its study. These advances have generated an upsurge of research activity into the neural bases of learning, and the field has become one of the most exciting in biology.

In this chapter we inquire whether the morphological, physiological and biochemical properties of the CNS are modified by experience. (The terms 'experience' and 'plasticity' will not be defined rigorously. We use 'experience' in the general sense used by Schneirla (1956): the effects of extrinsic stimulation on development and behaviour. The term 'plasticity' is used to refer to relatively long-lasting changes in the organisation of the nervous system associated with experience or physiological stimulation.) Since learning is a special result of experience, we go on to consider whether any neural changes have been observed which may be related exclusively to the acquisition and storage of information.

When we consider learning we restrict ourselves to the biochemical correlates, not only because our own efforts have been in this area, but also because the difficulties of interpretation are particularly well defined. We do not discuss other biochemical approaches to the study of learning, such as the use of inhibitors of protein synthesis, or attempts to transfer learning biochemically, or electrophysiological correlates of learning, since all these areas have been reviewed (Adám, 1971; Ansell and Bradley, 1973; Gaito and Bonnet, 1971; Glassman, 1969; Greenough and Maier, 1972; Horn, 1971a; John, 1972; Lajtha, 1971; Rose, 1970; Ungar, 1970).

We discuss experiments that illustrate some of the problems that arise in attempt-

*This chapter was first published in *Science,* **181**, 506–14; Copyright 1973 by the American Association for the Advancement of Science.

111

ing to relate a neural change to the processes responsible for particular and lasting changes in behaviour and go on to consider our own work on imprinting in the light of these problems. In conclusion we discuss whether the evidence for plasticity in the CNS can provide guidelines for further analysis of learning and memory.

GENERAL EFFECTS OF EXPERIENCE ON THE CNS

Fibres in the optic nerve of vertebrates make highly specific connections with neurons in the optic tectum. The formation of these linkages does not appear to depend on visual function, and the connections, once established, do not appear to exhibit any capacity for functional adaptation (Sperry, 1943, 1944). Are all neurons and their connections of this kind, or are some capable of being modified by experience? Attempts to answer these questions have largely been made by studying the effects on the CNS of varying the visual experience of young animals.

EFFECTS OF VARYING VISUAL EXPERIENCE

One method of modifying the visual experience of animals is to rear them in darkness. Such treatment affects the morphology of neurons in the visual pathways (Chow et al., 1957; Globus and Scheibel, 1967; Guillery, 1972; Gyllensten, 1959; Ruiz-Marcus and Valverde, 1969; Valverde, 1967, 1971; Weiskrantz, 1958; Wiesel and Hubel, 1963a). For example, neurons in the outer layers of the visual cortex of dark-reared mice are smaller and more densely packed than those in light-reared controls (Gyllensten, 1959). In this cortical area, there is also a reduction in the number of spines (regions of synaptic contact—Gray, 1959; Gray and Guillery, 1963) per unit length of the apical dendrites of large pyramidal cells (Ruiz-Marcus and Valverde, 1969; Valverde, 1967, 1971) and, in cats, a reduction in the density of the neuropil (Coleman and Riesen, 1968). Light deprivation may not, however, be the only difference between light- and dark-reared animals; there may also be differences in the pattern and amount of locomotor activity and in general metabolism. These factors, rather than light deprivation as such, might be responsible for the histological changes in the cerebral cortex. Indeed, similar histological changes have been described in the cerebral cortex of rats thyroidectomised shortly after birth or reared on a restricted diet (Cragg, 1970, 1972; Eayrs, 1955; Eayrs and Horn, 1955; Eayrs and Taylor, 1951; Horn, 1955; Sugita, 1978). These general factors cannot, however, be solely responsible for the changes described in the cortex of the dark-reared animals. This is because rearing in the dark, unlike thyroid deficiency or inanition, appears differentially to affect the visual cortex (Gyllensten et al., 1966; Valverde, 1967, 1971).

Morphological changes can also be demonstrated in dark-reared animals that have been exposed to light. The changes affect both presynaptic and postsynaptic structures. When dark-reared rats are exposed to light for as little as 3 h at the age of 3 weeks, changes occur in the diameter of synaptic terminals in the visual cortex (Cragg, 1967). Alterations in the morphology of synaptic knobs also occur in the lateral geniculate nucleus and retina of dark-reared rats exposed to light (Cragg,

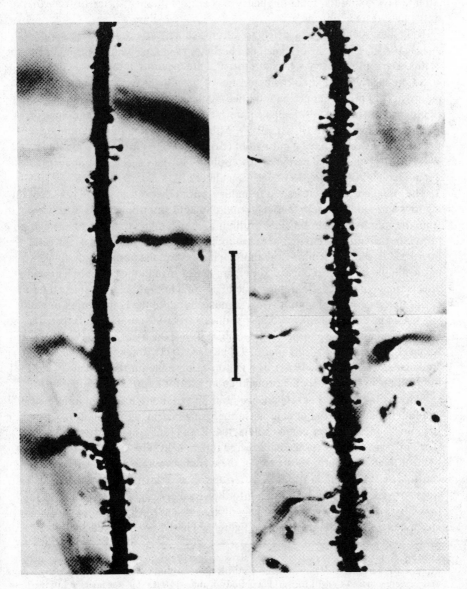

Figure 9.1. Segments of apical dendrites in the visual cortex of mice raised in darkness for 20 days and then allowed to live under normal conditions for 4 days (left) and 10 days (right). Scale, 20 μm. (From Valverde, 1971)

1968, 1969). When mice reared in darkness are exposed to light 20 days after birth, there is an increase in the number of dendritic spines per unit length of the apical dendrites of pyramidal cells in layer 5 of the cortex. Valverde (1971) found that the frequency of spines varied with the duration of light exposure (figure 9.1). After 4 days' exposure, spine frequency was not significantly different from that of the light-reared controls.

If the lids of one eye of a kitten are sutured shortly after birth (Wiesel and Hubel, 1963b, 1965), the occluded eye becomes functionally disconnected from the cortex. During these early weeks of postnatal life, neurons in the visual cortex of the kitten are highly sensitive to characteristics of the visual environment, and their receptive field properties can be modified by the changes in this environment (Barlow and Pettigrew, 1971; Blakemore and Cooper, 1970; Hirsch and Spinelli, 1970, 1971; Spinelli and Hirsch, 1971). Although the period of maximum susceptibility of many cells may be quite brief (Blakemore and Mitchell, 1973; Hubel and Wiesel, 1970), the actual period of susceptibility of the visual cortex appears to extend beyond three months of age (Spinelli et al., 1972).

The visual cortex of rats raised from birth with other rats in a large cage containing toys and running tracks (enriched environment) differs in a number of ways from that of rats brought up alone without such playthings (impoverished environment). In the enriched environment group, the visual cortex is thicker, the cell bodies are larger, the dendrites are more branched and the postsynaptic thickenings in the middle layers of the visual cortex are longer than in the controls. These effects, some of which also occur in the brains of adult rats, are not solely a result of differences in the amount of visual stimulation, since the visual cortex of blind rats reared in the enriched environments differs from the cortex of rats reared in the impoverished environment (Bennett et al. 1964; Diamond et al., 1964, 1972; Krech et al., 1963; Møllgaard et al., 1971; Riege, 1971: Rosenzweig et al., 1969; Volkmar and Greenough, 1972). The factors responsible for these changes and the mechanisms by which they are brought about are not known.

Since variations in visual experience result in variations in some morphological and functional properties of neurons in the visual system, we might also expect that biochemical changes could be detected. Rose (1967), in a study parallel to that of Cragg (1967), exposed dark-reared rats to light. The incorporation of [³H] lysine into acid-insoluble substances in these animals was compared with that in controls that remained in the dark. After up to 3 h of light exposure there was a transient elevation of incorporation into the visual cortex. This elevation was followed by a depression, which gradually disappeared as the length of exposure was increased to 4 days. Similar changes (figure 9.2) have been observed at the retina

Figure 9.2. Incorporation of [³H]lysine following first exposure to light. Specific activities are expressed as percentage of those of dark controls. Littermate rats, reared in the dark to 50 days of age, were exposed to light for varying periods of time. [³H]Lysine was injected intraperitoneally 60 min before killing of animals and separation of the various brain regions. Values are mean ± standard error from between 5 and 14 pairs at each time point. Significant differences compared with dark controls: *, $P < 0.01$; **, $P < 0.001$

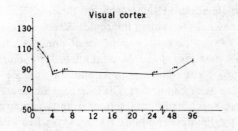

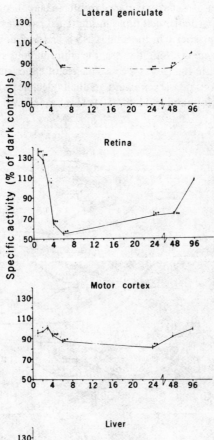

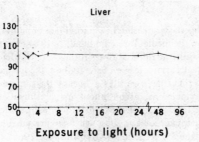

Exposure to light (hours)

and lateral geniculate nucleus (Richardson and Rose, 1972; Rose, 1967). This biphasic response may help to explain the contradictory reports on the biochemical consequences of varying the visual experience of animals (Altman *et al.,* 1966; Appel *et al.,* 1967; Brattgård, 1952; Metzger *et al.,* 1967; Singh and Talwar, 1969; Talwar *et al.,* 1966). Elevated incorporation in the first phase is confined to a cell fraction enriched in nerve cell bodies. The increased incorporation into protein is not general. Certain specific protein fractions from the retina and visual cortex are affected differently. Incorporation into fractions enriched with glial cells is not elevated (Richardson and Rose, 1973a, b; Sinha and Rose, 1972). These experiments suggest that the onset of visual experience results in an enhanced synthesis of specific proteins, in particular cell types in the visual pathways.

The evidence for plasticity in the adult CNS is less well documented than for the developing nervous system. None the less, the adult nervous system is capable of long-lasting and specific changes as a consequence of experience, inasmuch as transmission through various neural pathways gradually declines when the stimulus is repeatedly applied (Horn and Hinde, 1970). This change, which has many features

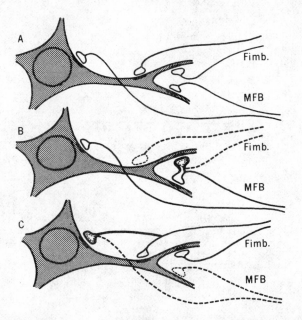

Figure 9.3. Plastic changes after a lesion in the forebrain of adult rats. (A) In the normal situation, afferent fibres from the medial forebrain bundle (MFB) terminate in boutons on the cell soma and on dendrites while the fimbrial fibres (Fimb.) are restricted in termination to the dendrites. (B) Several weeks after a lesion of the fimbria, the medial forebrain bundle fibre terminals extend across from their own sites to occupy the vacated sites, thus forming double synapses; degenerated connections, discontinuous line; presumed plastic changes, heavy black line. (C) Several weeks after a lesion of the medial forebrain bundle, the fimbrial fibres now give rise to terminals occupying somatic sites, which are presumably those vacated as a result of the former lesion. (After Raisman, 1969)

in common with behavioural habituation (Horn, 1965, 1967; Thompson and Spencer, 1966) is found in vertebrates and invertebrates; in the latter, the change in transmission may last for many hours or days and possibly longer (Bruner and Tauc, 1966; Carew *et al.,* 1972; Castelluci *et al.,* 1970; Horn and Rowell, 1968a, 1968b). The adult CNS also retains a capacity for morphological adaptation that, although only demonstrated in pathological conditions, is potentially of great interest for studies of the effects of the environment on the brain. Raisman (1969) has shown that neurons in the septal nuclear complex in the forebrain of adult rats receive afferent synaptic terminals from two sources, each of which can selectively be destroyed (figure 9.3). The distribution of the terminals from the two sources is different. When one source of afferents is damaged, it appears that afferents from the other source sprout (Liu and Chambers, 1958; McCouch *et al.,* 1958; Moore *et al.,* 1971; Williams and Palay, 1967) and form synaptic terminals in the spaces previously occupied by the other afferent fibres.

BIOCHEMICAL CHANGES ASSOCIATED WITH LEARNING

There is strong evidence, then, that the CNS is modified by experience. But is there evidence that these or similar modifications underlie learning? After all, experience frequently has general or short-lived behavioural effects that would not ordinarily be attributed to learning. Broadly speaking, learning refers to the processes involved in acquisition and storage when a particular experience exerts a specific and relatively lasting effect on behaviour. Admittedly, a diverse collection of phenomena— ranging from habituation to the most complex types of problem-solving—are lumped under the general category of learning (Hinde, 1970; Razran, 1971; Thorpe, 1963). Nevertheless, without prejudging whether unity exists in mechanisms underlying learning, we can ask if any one of these phenomena is implicated when experience gives rise to changes in the CNS. In this section we discuss the problems of interpreting experiments relating biochemical changes in the nervous system to learning procedures and changes in behaviour. Learning is commonly identified in terms of a *change* in behaviour. Frequently what is measured, however, is not a change of a subject's behaviour, but a *difference* between groups of subjects that have been treated differently. For example, the responsiveness of a group that has previously been exposed to the stimulus may be compared with that of another group which has not been exposed in this way before the experiment. For brevity we have referred throughout the chapter to learning producing a change in behaviour, even though a difference between groups may have been measured. We do so because it has often been assumed without adequate evidence that such biochemical changes are an exclusive part of the acquisition or storage mechanisms. We then describe our own work and indicate how we have attempted to deal with some of these problems.

The difficulties of finding a direct and exclusive link between a neural change and a learning process are formidable. Procedures used to train animals may have a variety of side effects that are themselves responsible for measurable changes (Bateson, 1970a; Glassman, 1969). For example, a shock avoidance technique is likely to lead to massive changes in concentrations of hormones associated with stress. Furthermore, a problem arises because learning processes are not directly observed; they are inferred from the behavioural changes associated with a training procedure. While it is first necessary to establish that a neural change is part of the nexus of events directly linking training conditions with a lasting and specific change of behaviour, the relations between the neural change and learning may not be exclusive. The change may also be involved in many other processes. For example, even though the acquisition of a visual discrimination is dependent on changes in state of photoreceptors, it would be absurd to argue that such changes are involved only in learning. Problems of this kind are raised in more subtle and varied forms by all reductionist studies of learning.

While the goals of analysis are clear, they are extraordinarily difficult to attain. For example, Kerkut and his collaborators (Kerkut *et al.,* 1970a, 1970b, 1971, 1972; Oliver *et al.,* 1971) have been conducting extensive biochemical studies on a cockroach preparation first devised by Horridge (1962). The cockroach is decapitated and arranged so that when one of the metathoracic legs hangs down it dips into saline, completes an electrical circuit and the preparation receives a shock. The preparations are highly variable, but in many the leg is eventually retracted for a sustained period so that it no longer dips into the saline and therefore avoids further shocks. Descriptively, the adaptive behaviour of the leg is very similar to avoidance conditioning in intact animals, since yoked controls, which receive shock at the same time as the experimentals regardless of leg position, do not retract their legs for sustained periods. Kerkut and his colleagues have found numerous biochemical differences between the ganglia of experimentals, yoked controls and undisturbed preparations, and suggest that some of these differences might be the basis of memory. However, the differences between experimental and yoked control preparations may lie in the extent to which the metathoracic leg was retracted. Hoyle (1965) found that after the preparation was trained, the coxal adductor muscles, which keep the leg in a retracted position, showed a continuous discharge at a high frequency. The possibility that the biochemical measures are related to the maintained discharge in the coxal adductors is strengthened by the observation that acetylcholinesterase activity, which fell as the leg received fewer shocks, began to rise as the effects of training wore off and the muscles relaxed. At present it would be unwise to assume that the biochemical differences between experimentals and yoked cockroach preparations are specifically related to the acquisition process.

Variants of the yoked control procedure have been widely used and are superficially elegant. The results are, however, not so unambiguous as might at first appear. An animal that can actively control its environment is likely to be in a different state than one that cannot. The experimental animal might, for example, be more alert, and this might be responsible for any biochemical or physiological differences between it and its control. Furthermore, subtle forms of data selection may arise from the yoked control procedure. If an experimental animal does not learn, it might be tempting to exclude it from the analysis. However, non-specific factors making learning possible might also influence directly the biochemical or physiological measures. Since the capacity of the yoked controls to learn is not measured, it is not possible to exclude those in which the relevant factors are absent. Consequently, a spurious difference between experimentals and yoked controls could arise from the selection of experimental animals.

Comparable problems are raised by the well-known work of Hydén and Lange and their co-workers (Haljamäe and Lange, 1972; Hydén and Lange, 1968, 1970a, 1970b, 1970c; Yanagihara and Hydén, 1971). In recent years they have used rats that prefer to use one forepaw rather than the other when reaching for food pellets in a tube. In the training situation, the tube containing the food was placed against the wall so that each rat was forced to use its non-preferred forepaw if it was to reach the food. Hydén and his collaborators concluded that in one region of the hippocampus, synthesis of S 100 protein (an acidic, brain-specific protein of molecular weight 21 000) increased during initial training. Synthesis remained high when training was resumed 2 weeks afterwards, but returned to the level of the control group at subsequent training after 4 weeks. Such experiments suggest that enhanced protein synthesis is correlated with acquisition rather than with maintained performance of the activity. Furthermore, injection of an antiserum specific to S 100 protein 4 days after the beginning of training blocks further acquisition. The number of reaches that rats made with the non-preferred paw levelled off, whereas a control group continued to improve their performance. While these results strongly implicate the hippocampus and S 100 protein in the processes involved in acquiring a new skill with the forepaw, the question remains: are these processes exclusively involved in learning a new skill? May they not also be involved in many other situations that require, say, the animal's focused attention, but do not involve learning? For example, would a rat that is forced by suitable penalties or rewards to wait for a particular signal before responding—and, hence, forced to maintain a high level of vigilance—show high rates of synthesis during performance as well as during acquisition? Nothing that has been done so far provides a clear answer on this point.

BIOCHEMICAL CHANGES DURING IMPRINTING

In our work in this area (Bateson, 1972; Bateson et al., 1969, 1973; Horn et al., 1971, 1973; Rose et al., 1970), we have examined the sequence of biochemical changes that occur during imprinting of young chicks. The recently hatched chick will quickly form a social attachment to a conspicuous object as a result of being exposed to it (Bateson, 1966; Sluckin, 1972). The original conception of 'imprinting' was as a process responsible for restricting both the young bird's preference for social companions early in life and its adult sexual preference. Recent evidence suggests, however, that in many species early experience determining initial social attachments is not sufficient to determine subsequent sexual preferences. Furthermore, while the term has been applied to the acquisition of a wide variety of preferences and habits by all kinds of animals, many of the original defining characteristics of imprinting have been questioned. Consequently, the term is no longer used with much precision. In this article we use it for the learning process that restricts the filial behaviour of young birds to a familiar object. This learning process is called imprinting and involves the first significant visual experience for the birds. We argued that the resulting cellular changes were likely to be greater than those produced by comparable visual experience later in life.

At the stage of development when learning occurs most readily, the birds show an astonishing responsiveness to conspicuous objects. They will attempt to approach for hours on end, even though they receive no additional reward for doing so. For example, in one experiment, day-old chicks were placed in running wheels from which they could see a rotating, flashing light. The chicks were positioned in this way for 12 sessions for 20 min interspersed with 20-min rest periods in the dark. Even after 4 h of training, their readiness to approach showed no signs of diminishing (figure 9.4). The birds' continued responsiveness is useful, because it is maintained long after they have learned the characteristics of the stimulus to which they are exposed. Some of the general behavioural changes, such as increased attentiveness and motor activity, that are frequently confounded with learning can thus be dissociated from the processes involved in acquisition. The recently hatched chick has an additional advantage for *in vivo* work in that the blood-brain barrier has not yet fully developed (Key and Marley, 1962).

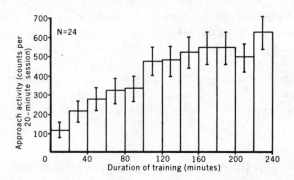

Figure 9.4.   Chick approach activity (mean ± S.E.) in successive 20-min training procedures. Each day-old chick was placed for 20-min periods in an activity wheel 50 cm from a flashing rotating light. Successive training sessions were separated by 20 min in the dark. Four counts were obtained for each complete revolution of the wheel, and 400 counts is equivalent in distance to movement of approximately 100 m, N, number of animals

In the first series of experiments, the incorporation of [^{3}H] lysine into acid-insoluble substances was studied. Eggs were incubated and hatched in the dark. Chicks from the early part of the hatch were maintained in the dark until the start of behavioural procedures, 14–19 h later. Chicks from each batch were divided into

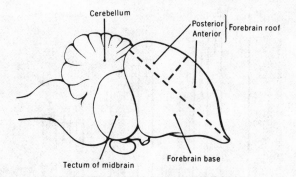

Figure 9.5.   Lateral view of chick brain. The forebrain was divided as shown into two parts, the plane indicated by the longer broken line. In some experiments the roof was divided, as shown, into two parts. The midbrain was separated from the forebrain and from the hindbrain by vertical incisions immediately anterior and posterior to the tectum. The cerebellum and hindbrain were discarded

three groups. One group of chicks was maintained in the dark (dark controls), another group was exposed to overhead illumination (light controls) and another group (experimentals) was also exposed to a flashing orange light known (Bateson and Reese, 1969) to be highly effective as an imprinting stimulus. The period of exposure was 105 min. Each chick received an injection in the heart region of $20\,\mu c$ of $[^3H]$lysine 90 min before death.

At the end of the experiment, each chick was killed, and the brain was divided into three regions—the forebrain roof, the forebrain base and the midbrain, which includes the optic tectum (figure 9.5). The brain regions were frozen on dry ice until they were assayed for acid-insoluble radioactivity. The specific activity measure (disintegrations per minute of acid-insoluble radioactivity per mg of protein) was standardised for bodyweight and normalised between experiments. This measure is referred to as the standardised specific activity (SSA). The acid-insoluble together with the acid-soluble fractions are referred to as the 'pool'. All assays were done without knowledge of the behavioural treatment the chick had received.

A significant elevation of incorporation in the experimentals compared with the dark control birds occurred in the forebrain roof region; incorporation in this region for the light control group was intermediate between values for the other two groups (figure 9.6). No significant differences in incorporation were found in the other brain regions, and there were no significant differences in pool values for any region among the three groups of chicks.

If these results reflect changes of incorporation into protein, we might reasonably expect a change in the incorporation of a labelled base into RNA. If this occurred, it would not only enhance the confidence with which we might regard the results with lysine, but it might also prove a more sensitive measure of change of biochemical activity, because the rate of incorporation of RNA precursor into acid-insoluble material was much lower. After 90 min, 60–70% of the $[^3H]$lysine

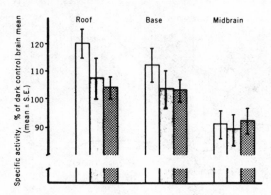

Figure 9.6. Standardised specific activities for radioactive lysine incorporated into acid-insoluble substances in the forebrain roof, forebrain base and midbrain. Open bars refer to experimental chicks (N = 17); light stippled bars, to light controls (N = 18); and heavy stippled bars, to dark controls (N = 17). Incorporation into the forebrain roof was significantly higher ($P <$ 0.05) in the experimentals than in the dark controls. (From Bateson *et al.*, 1969)

was in the acid-insoluble fraction and hence, presumably, bound to macromolecules, whereas only 4-6% of the [^{3}H] uracil was bound in this way.

In another series of experiements, chicks were again divided into dark control, light control and experimental groups; each chick received an injection of 20 μCi of [^{3}H]uracil 150 min before death. The periods of exposure of the experimental and light controls were 38 min, 76 min and, in a separate experiment, 160 min. The SSAs were expressed as a percentage of the mean for the dark controls. The earliest significant change (figure 9.7) was an elevated incorporation into the forebrain roof of the experimental chicks after 76 min of exposure to the flashing light. After 160 min of exposure, incorporation was elevated in all brain regions of both experimental and light controls. The largest change, occurring in the experimentals, was in the midbrain. This region contains the optic tectum, in which prolonged activation by photic stimulation may, for example, create a greater demand for transmitter substances than in other regions of the brain.

Two effects can therefore be distinguished. One of these occurred in all brain regions after prolonged exposure to light and may be a non-specific consequence of stimulation; the other appeared in the forebrain roof after 76 min of exposure to the imprinting stimulus.

The enzyme RNA polymerase is necessary for the synthesis of RNA, so an enhanced level of activity of this enzyme might be expected before the enhancement of incorporation into RNA. The RNA polymerase activity in the forebrain roof of chicks exposed to a flashing light for only 30 min was 34% higher than that of the dark controls (Haywood *et al.*, 1970). The differences between groups for the other regions were not significant. No differences were found after 45 min of stimulation. This effect is obtained on an enzyme system that can be assayed *in vitro* and has the advantage of eliminating problems associated with fluctuations of pool size

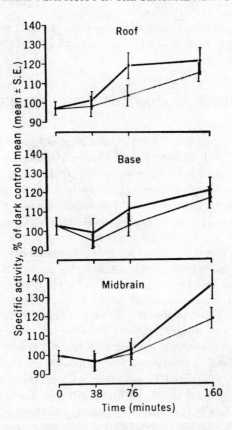

Figure 9.7. Standardised specific activities (mean ± S.E.) of presumed RNA from the forebrain roofs, bases and midbrains of differently treated chicks. The experimental birds (heavy line) were exposed to a flashing light, and the light controls (dotted line) to a continuous light. Twelve experimentals and 12 light controls received 38 min of exposure, 19 experimentals and 19 light controls received 76 min of exposure, and 18 experimental and 18 light controls received 160 min of exposure; 35 chicks were dark controls. (From Rose *et al.*, 1970)

in incorporation studies *in vivo*, as discussed below. The activity of the enzyme adenylate cyclase was also measured *in vitro*. This is a predominantly membrane-bound enzyme necessary for the synthesis of adenosine 3', 5'-monophosphate (cyclic AMP). The activity of adenylate cyclase was increased in the forebrain roof of experimental chicks compared with either light or dark controls after 60 min of exposure to the respective conditions (Hambley and Rose, 1973). The relatively long time course of the change in adenylate cyclase is difficult to relate to the changes in RNA polymerase and enhanced incorporation into presumed RNA and presumed protein. One possible explanation for the late change in adenylate cyclase is that it is occurring at synaptic terminals, known in other species (de Robertis *et al.*, 1967) to be rich in the enzyme. The increased activity of the enzyme might result from conformational changes brough about by earlier events initiated in the nucleus. Such changes might influence synaptic transmission over short periods of time.

SOME BIOCHEMICAL AMBIGUITIES OF INTERPRETATION

Before looking in more detail at the behavioural implications of these data, it is necessary to consider their biochemical significance. Although in the battery of changes that we have observed the change in each variable lends support to the others, there is an ambiguity of interpretation which is central to the incorporation data that we (and others) have presented. This rests in the neat elision by which incorporation of labelled precursor tends to be equated with 'net synthesis'. At best, incorporation of precursor is a measure of turnover and not of net synthesis. Another difficulty is that the actual precursor to the macromolecule is intracellular, whereas the label is injected into the bloodstream, the peritoneal cavity or the cerebrospinal fluid. Variations in regional blood flow (which is affected by sensory stimulation—Bondy and Morelos, 1971), in uptake mechanisms across cell membranes, and in the pool of the unlabelled precursor (Rose, 1972), all complicate interpretation. In an attempt to avoid these difficulties, it has becomes the practice to normalise the results by calculating 'relative activity', i.e. the ratio of bound radioactivity to total radioactivity, bound and unbound, or of bound radioactivity to unbound radioactivity. Indeed, in some cases, such as in the transfer of handedness experiments (Hydér and Lange, 1968), the effect of training is only apparent when this procedure is used (Bowman and Harding, 1969).

Another example of the use of the relative activity measure is provided in the work of Glassman and Wilson and their colleagues (Adair et al., 1968; Coleman et al., 1971; Kahan et al., 1970; Zemp et al., 1966, 1967). In the experimental situation that they have most commonly used, mice were presented with a light and sound for 3 s before an electric shock was delivered through the metal grid floor of their cage. The experimental mice continued to receive shocks until they jumped on to a ledge. Yoked control mice were presented with the same sequence of stimuli as the experimental animals, but were unable to escape from the shock. Among other things, the incorporation of isotopically labelled uridine into nuclear and ribosomal RNA was higher in the brains of experimental animals compared with the yoked controls, especially in the diencephalon and hippocampus. More recent studies (Entingh et al., 1972), under slightly different experimental conditions, including precursor injection by the subcutaneous route rather than the intracranial route, have led to a reassessment of these results. They are now interpreted not in terms of changes in the synthesis of macromolecules, but in terms of a reduction in the labelling of uridine monophosphate, the precursor used as the 'normalising' factor in the earlier work. The results of a further study, in which significantly increased phosphorylation of non-acid extractable nuclear proteins was found in brains of experimentals but not of yoked controls, would not appear to be affected by these complications, although other difficulties of interpretation remain.

Even when the uncertainty over the precursor is resolved, the relative activity measure is still only partially adequate. This is because it is calculated at a single point in time, whereas incorporation studies measure the sum of events occurring over a period during which there may be considerable fluctuation in pool between experimental and control animals. The interpretation of the ratio becomes even more difficult when the relation between bound and unbound radioactivity is complex (Bateson, 1972).

It is not only uptake that may change. There may also be changes in metabolism of the precursor along other pathways. Thus, it has recently become apparent that when tritiated leucine, lysine, uracil or uridine are used as precursors, within 1 h of injection up to 50% of the free radioactivity may be found not in the precursor but in other small molecules or in water (Banker and Cotman, 1971). Provided that the rate of dissociation is not affected by the training procedure, this phenomenon cannot account for quantitative differences in incorporation between experimental and control groups. However, in double labelling experiments in which one group receives $[^{14}C]$-labelled precursors and the other receives $[^{8}H]$-labelled precursors, differences between experimental and control groups could result from differences in rates of dissociation of the isotopes from the precursors (Ramirez et al., 1972). All experiments with $[^{3}H]$-labelled precursors are open to question: if the dissociated tritium exchanges with hydrogen in other precursors, the radioactivity may appear in many acid-insoluble molecules (such as protein, RNA or DNA). As a result, the identity of the macromolecules containing the isotope will be in doubt unless collateral evidence is available.

Yet another complicating factor may be introduced by changes in low-molecular-weight precursors other than the labelled one. Thus, in the dark-reared rat there are changes in the concentrations of a number of amino acids in the free pool which might conceivably affect protein synthesis rates (Rose, 1972). Unequivocal interpretation of incorporation data would require continuous monitoring of intracellular pool sizes and specific activities, a criterion that has not been achieved in any of the experiments reviewed here. Many of these objections disappear, of course, if differential labelling between protein or RNA fractions is observed, for it is difficult to interpret such effects as being caused by changes at the precursor level. The fact that such differential labelling has been found for proteins of the retina and visual cortex in the dark-reared rat (Richardson and Rose, 1973a, b) lends confidence to the other data. Similarly, changes in enzyme activity are not open to this criticism although they are subject to others, such as interpretation in terms of activation or induction. Changed enzyme activities represent a snapshot of the situation at a particular time; incorporation measures the sum of a cumulative sequence.

SOME BEHAVIOURAL AMBIGUITIES OF INTERPRETATION

If, with appropriate caution, the biochemical data are accepted at face value, we still have to consider their relation to processes responsible for a change in behaviour.

The imprinting experiments we have reported so far do not go very far to meet the criticism outlined above concerning the non-specific effects of the training procedure on brain biochemistry. Many factors could account for the biochemical differences between the experimental group exposed for 76 min and the other chicks. The groups may, for example, have differed in the amount of motor activity and in the levels of stress to which they were subjected. Protein and RNA metabolism in the central nervous sytem may be affected by motor activity (Hydén, 1943; Jakoubek *et al.,* 1968; Tiplady, 1972), by stress (Altman and Das, 1966; Semiginovsky *et al.,* 1970), and by exogenous adrenocorticotrophic hormone (Jakoubek *et al.,* 1971, 1972) or corticosterone (Azmitia and McEwen, 1969). The experiments with exogenous hormones suggest that any procedure that modifies the endogenous concentration of these substances may have repercussion on RNA and protein synthesis in the brain. Such general effects can largely be allowed for by effectively restricting input to one side of the brain during the training procedures. If any biochemical differences exist between the 'trained' and 'untrained' sides of the brain, it is reasonable to ascribe them to differences in visual experience. They are unlikely to result from general changes in hormonal levels as a consequence of stress, from differences in non-visual sensory stimulation or from differences in motor activity between the corresponding sides of the body. The supra-optic commissure of 12 chicks was divided shortly after hatching (Horn *et al.,* 1971, 1973). After they had recovered from the operation, each chick had one eye covered with a patch and was exposed to a flashing yellow light for 60 min. The chick was then given two choice tests between the familiar flashing yellow light and an unfamiliar flashing red light, first with its trained eye exposed and then with its untrained eye uncovered. All of the chicks approached the familiar light with the originally trained eye uncovered, but not with the other eye uncovered. The incorporation of [^{3}H]uracil into acid-insoluble substances was higher in the trained side of the forebrain roof than in the untrained side. No other regional differences between trained and untrained sides were observed (figure 9.8). No significant regional differences in pool size were found between the two sides of the brain. This rules out the possibility that incorporation of the labelled base into macromolecules can be ascribed to asymmetric changes in pool size—resulting, for example, from differences in cerebral blood flow, which can be affected by patterned visual stimulation (Bondy and Morelos, 1971). There are good grounds for supposing that both sides of the brain of the intact chick are trained when input is restricted to one side (Bateson, 1970b; Cherkin, 1970; Moltz and Stettner, 1962—an exception has been described by Zeier (1970)). We therefore expected and found no differences in incorporation of [^{3}H]uracil between the two sides of the brain of intact chicks after monocular exposure to a flashing light (Horn *et al.,* 1973).

We concluded from the 'split-brain' studies that the effects of our imprinting procedure on the incorporation of uracil cannot be attributed to some of the general consequences of training. The split-brain preparation does not, however, eliminate all such non-specific effects (Bateson, 1970a), and it remains possible that the biochemical changes are caused by sensory stimulation as such and are not the exclu-

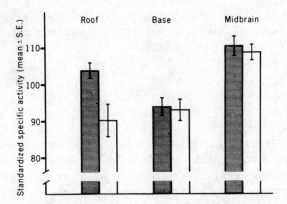

Figure 9.8. Standardised specific activities (mean ± S.E.) of presumed RNA from trained sides (hatched bars) and untrained sides (open bars) of forebrain roofs, forebrain bases and midbrains of split-brain chicks. The trained side was contralateral to the exposed eye. (From Horn *et al.*, 1971)

sive effects of training. In the next series of experiments (Bateson *et al.*, 1973) we attempted to examine this possibility.

Chicks were trained for 60 min on the second day after hatching, after having been trained for 20, 60, 120 or 240 min on the first day. We reasoned that if incorporation in some regions was specifically related to learning, birds that had been exposed for a longer period on the first day and had learned more of the characteristics of the stimulus object would show a lower rate of incorporation in those regions on the second day. In this hypothesis it is assumed that the extent to which further learning takes place diminishes as the length of training increases. We found, in the anterior part of the forebrain roof, that as the length of exposure on the previous day increased, incorporation of [^{3}H]uracil into acid-insoluble substances decreased (figure 2 of Bateson *et al.*, 1973). No such relationship was found in any other region of the brain. As with other studies, it could be argued that the biochemical changes in the forebrain roof are correlated with vigilance on the part of the young birds as they learn. This view would have some plausibility if the chicks trained for longer periods on the first day after hatching were less responsive than other chicks to the familiar stimulus on the second day. However, if anything, they approached more vigorously than the other chicks; therefore, it does not seem likely that the lower rate of incorporation in the anterior roof region of their forebrains can be explained in terms of reduced attentiveness. While these results confirmed our expectations, the data can also be interpreted in terms of a general effect on the rate of neural development (Bateson *et al.*, 1973).

Taken together, the results of all our experiments are consistent with the view that the rapidly occurring biochemical changes in the forebrain roof are specifically related to the training procedure, although the evidence is not yet conclusive. By degrees, we have been able to rule out a number of strong alternatives that might have explained the biochemical results. We are optimistic, therefore, about the possibility of discovering whether the biochemical changes are necessary for the development of a preference and are exclusively related to the training procedure.

CONCLUSIONS

Strong evidence indicates that the morphological and functional organisation of parts of the CNS in many species can be modified by changes in internal and external environments. Many biochemical variables are also affected; in particular, the connectivity of neurons can be altered by experience. The evidence that any of these changes is intimately involved in learning is suggestive but remains inconclusive. Does the analysis of learning pose altogether new and different neurobiological problems, or has the investigation of the general neural effects of experience offered models for the further pursuit of learning? The answer lies, in part, in the relations at the behavioural level between learning and other processes with less specific outcomes.

In defining learning at the behavioural level, various distinctions are drawn to separate the effects of learning from those of other processes. Probably the most important criterion is behavioural specificity. Consider exposure of a mammal to an intense sound that destroyed part of the basilar membrane. If, as a result, no behaviour patterns could subsequently be elicited by sounds of that pitch, these non-specific effects on behaviour would not usually be explained in terms of learning. A more subtle example of an effect of experience on behaviour which would not normally be attributed to learning is that of exposing young kittens with both eyes open to vertical lines. Shortly after exposure, such kittens are said to be unresponsive to lines place at right angles to the familiar orientation (Blakemore and Cooper, 1970). Consequently, all behaviour patterns dependent on the detection of lines with unfamiliar orientation would presumably no longer occur. It is assumed, of course, that the cat does not rotate its head when inspecting the unfamiliar lines. If it did, the image that fell on the retina might come to have the familiar orientation and so be detected. This result differs from the effects of imprinting young birds, even though the procedures are rather similar. Whereas the chicks cease to respond socially to objects that differ in certain characteristics from those to which they were exposed, these chicks have no difficulty in detecting unfamiliar conspicuous objects, which they actively avoid (Bateson, 1966; Sluckin, 1972).

The criterion of specificity of effect on behaviour, used for identifying learning, is easy enough to apply when classifying extreme cases, but intermediates may pose considerable problems; the distinctions may be entirely arbitrary. Consequently, it is by no means obvious that sharp discontinuities exist between behaviour changes supposedly dependent on learning and behaviour changes that are accompanied by lasting changes in other behaviour patterns.

The possibility of continuities at the behavioural level raises the question of whether the neural mechanisms underlying behavioural change at one end of this spectrum can be related to those at the other end. Changes occur in the morphological and functional properties of neurons during ontogeny. The direction of these changes is such that neurons progressively lose their plasticity. The factors responsible for the termination of plasticity may be local (Detwiler, 1936, 1949; Spemann, 1938; Spemann and Mangold, 1924); may be remote but internal, as with changes in hormone levels (Harris and Levine, 1965); or may be external, such as visual experience (Blakemore and Cooper, 1970; Gaze et al., 1970; Hirsch and Spinelli, 1970, 1971; Keating and Gaze, 1970; Wiesel and Hubel, 1965). Spinelli et al. (1972) found that once the receptive field of a neuron in the visual cortex of a kitten had been modified, the receptive field was not subsequently changed by other visual experiences. Despite the diverse ways that changes are brought about, the end result is that the functional and morphological properties of the affected neurons become rigorously defined, with a concomitant loss of plasticity.

Could similar changes underlie learning? A neuron may be functionally connected to many others, but the number of connections may become restricted as a consequence of synaptic activity initiated by the training procedure. The combinations of synaptic inputs necessary to terminate connectional plasticity might be expected to have varying grades of complexity. This view is based on studies in the mammalian visual and auditory systems, in which the features of external stimuli necessary to fire a cell are more complex as recordings are made successively from first-order to fifth-order sensory neurons. Some neurons concerned in storage would have the necessary combinations of synaptic inputs provided by relatively simple external stimuli, so these neurons would cease to be plastic quite early in life. For other modifiable neurons, the necessary combinations of input may have such a low likelihood of occurring that the connections remain plastic for a large part of the animal's life cycle.

At the biochemical level, similarities may be found between the effects of hormones on target organs (Tata, 1967) and the effects of experience on specific changes in behaviour. Impulses generated in the CNS by stimuli falling on receptor surfaces during a training procedure change the membrane potential of many neurons. At modifiable neurons, such electrical changes in the membrane may lead to a changed phosphorylation of nuclear proteins (Glassman, 1969; Glassman and Wilson, 1972), to the methylation of DNA bases (Griffith and Mahler, 1969), or to both. With either change, modification of gene expression would occur and would lead to activation of RNA polymerase. This would be followed by enhanced synthesis of messenger RNA, polysome formation and synthesis of particular proteins. These proteins may be involved in the modification of connectivity either by affecting synapses directly or by affecting them indirectly through enzyme action on other cell constituents, such as lipids or transmitter molecules.

If the training procedures modify the connectivity of neurons in those parts of the CNS which are necessary for the analysis of common features of the environment, such as lines and angles, the sensory capacities of the animal would be restricted. As a result the animal would not be able to discriminate certain stimuli, and all behaviour patterns dependent on the detection of these stimuli would be affected. The results of this experience would be long lasting but non-specific. If the neural changes occur in parts of the CNS which are not used to extract common features of the environment, there might be no change in the sensory capacities of the animal. In this case, the effects of the experience would be much more like the effects of training in a conventional learning situation. In behavioural terms, the consequences of a procedure having a general effect and of one having a specific effect are different. The cellular changes might, however, be identical in the two situations, although the sites of the changes in the CNS would have to differ.

Nevertheless, it is unwise to assume that one cellular mechanism underlies storage in all learning situations; there is no reason to suppose that the constraints on the storage of acquired information are nearly so limited as those on the storage of genetic information. Within one animal, storage could take place by different means. For example, storage may be represented by a growth of synaptic terminals (Cajal, 1911; Hebb, 1949; Young, 1964), a change in the number of receptor sites on the postsynaptic membrane (Horn, 1962), the inactivation of synaptic transmission (Bruner and Tauc, 1966; Cragg, 1971; Dawkins, 1971; Horn, 1970, 1971b; Mark, 1970; Rosenzweig *et al.*, 1972), and so on. If the capacity to learn has evolved independently in a number of taxonomic groups (e.g. cephalopods and vertebrates) and meets a variety of biological needs, it may be that storage takes place in diverse ways throughout the animal kingdom.

ACKNOWLEDGEMENTS

We thank Ann Horn and Arun Sinha for their contributions to the imprinting studies from their inception, and the Medical and Science Research Councils for financial support.

REFERENCES

Adair, L., Wilson, J. E. and Glassman, E. (1968). *Proc. natn Acad. Sci. U.S.A.*, **61**, 917

Adám, G., ed. (1971). *Biology of Memory*, Akademiai Kiado, Budapest

Altman, J. and Das, G. D. (1966). *Phys. Behav.*, **1**, 105

Altman, J., Das, G. D. and Chang, J. (1966). *Physiol. Behav.*, **1**, 111

Ansell, G. B. and Bradley, P. B., eds. (1973). *Macromolecules and Behaviour*, Macmillan, London

Appel, S. H., Davis, W. and Scott, S. (1967). *Science*, **157**, 836

Azmitia, E. C., Jnr. and McEwen, B. S. (1969). *Science*, **116**, 1274

Banker, G. and Cotman, C. W. (1971). *Archs Biochem. Biophys.*, **142**, 565

Barlow, H. B. and Pettigrew, J. D. (1971). *J. Physiol. Lond.*, **218**, 98

Bateson, P. P. G. (1966). *Biol. Rev.*, **41**, 177

Bateson, P. P. G. (1970a). In *Short-Term Changes in Neural Activity and Behaviour* (G. Horn and R. A. Hinde, eds.), Cambridge University Press, pp. 553–64

Bateson, P. P. G. (1970b).Unpublished data

Bateson, P. P. G. (1972). *Brain Res.,* **39**, 449

Bateson, P. P. G. and Reese, E. P. (1969). *Anim Behav.,* **17**, 692

Bateson, P. P. G., Horn, G. and Rose, S. P. R. (1969). *Nature (Lond.),* **223**, 534

Bateson, P. P. G., Rose, S. P. R. and Horn, G. (1973). *Science,* **181**, 576

Bennett, E. L., Krech, D. and Rosenzweig, M. R. (1964). *J. comp. physiol. Psychol.,* **57**, 440

Blakemore, C. and Cooper, G. F. (1970). *Nature (Lond.),* **228**, 447

Blakemore, C. and Mitchell, D. F. (1973). *Nature (Lond.),* **241**, 467

Bondy, S. C. and Morelos, B. S. (1971). *Expl Neurol.,* **31**, 200

Bowman, R. E. and Harding, R. (1969). *Science,* **164**, 199

Brattgård, S. O. (1952). *Acta Radiol.,* suppl. 96, 1

Bruner, J. and Tauc, T. (1966). *Nature,* **210**, 37

Cajal, S. R. (1911). *Histologie du Système Nerveux,* Maloine, Paris

Carew, T. J., Pinsker, H. M. and Kandel, E. R. (1972). *Science,* **175**, 451

Castelluci, V., Kupferman, I., Pinsker, H. M. and Kandel, E. R. (1970). *Science,* **167**, 1445

Cherkin, A. (1970). *Nature (Lond.),* **227**, 1153

Chow, K. L., Riesen, A. H. and Newell, F. W. (1957). *J. comp. Neurol.,* **107**, 27

Coleman, P. D. and Riesen, A. H. (1968). *J. Anat.,* **102**, 363

Coleman, M. S., Pfingst, B., Wilson, J. E. and Glassman, E. (1971). *Brain Res.,* **26**, 349

Cragg, B. G. (1967). *Nature (Lond.),* **215**, 251

Cragg, B. G. (1968). *Proc. R. Soc., Ser. B.,* **171**, 319

Cragg, B. G. (1969). *Brain Res.,* **15**, 79

Cragg, B. G. (1970). *Brain Res.,* **18**, 297

Cragg, B. G. (1971). In *Structure and Function of Nervous Tissue* (G. H. Bourne, ed.), Academic Press, New York, pp. 1–60

Cragg, B. G. (1972). *Brain,* **95**, 143

Dawkins, R. (1971). *Nature (Lond.),* **229**, 118

Detwiler, S. R. (1936). *Neuroembryology: An Experimental Study,* Macmillan, New York

Detwiler, S. R. (1949). *J. exp. Zool.,* **111**, 79

Diamond, M. C., Krech, D. and Rosenzweig, M. R. (1964). *J. comp. Neurol.,* **123**, 111

Diamond, M. C., Rosenzweig, M. R., Bennett, E. L., Lindner, B. and Lyon, L. (1972) *J. Neurobiol.,* **3**, 47

Eayrs, J. T. (1955). *Acta Anat.,* **25**, 160

Eayrs, J. T. and Horn, G. (1955). *Anat. Rec.,* **121**, 53

Eayrs. J. T. and Taylor, S. H. (1951). *J. Anat.,* **85**, 350

Entingh, D., Entingh, T., Glassman, E. and Wilson, J. E. (1972). In *Abstr. 2nd Ann. Mtg, Soc. Neurosci,* Houston, p. 122

Gaito, J. and Bonnet, K. (1971). *Psychol. Bull.,* **75**, 109

Gaze, R. M., Keating, M. J., Székely, G. and Beazley, L. (1970). *Proc. R. Soc. Ser. B.,* **175**, 107

Glassman, E. (1969). *Ann. Rev. Biochem.,* **38**, 605

Glassman, E. and Wilson, J. E. (1972). In *Macromolecules and Behaviour* (G. B. Ansell and P. B. Bradley, eds.), Macmillan, London, pp. 81-92

Globus, A. and Scheibel, A. B. (1967). *Expl Neurol.*, **19** , 331

Gray, E. G. (1959). *J. Anat.*, **93**, 420

Gray, E. G. and Guillery, R. W. (1963). *J. Anat.*, **97**, 389

Greenough, W. T. and Maier, S. F. (1972). *Psychol Bull.*, **78**, 480

Griffith, J. S. and Mahler, H. R. (1969). *Nature (Lond.)*, **233**, 580

Guillery, R. W. (1972). *J. comp. Neurol.*, **144**, 117

Gyllensten, L. (1959). *Acta Morphol. Neer. Scand.*, **2**, 331

Gyllensten, L., Malmfors, T. and Norrlin, M. -L. (1966). *J. comp. Neurol.*, **126**, 463

Haljamäe, H. and Lange, P. W. (1972). *Brain Res.*, **38**, 131

Hambley, J. and Rose, S. P. R. (1973). Paper read at Int. Soc. Neurochemistry, Tokyo

Harris, G. W. and Levine, S. (1965). *J. Physiol., Lond.*, **181**, 379

Haywood, J., Rose, S. P. R. and Bateson, P. P. G. (1970). *Nature (Lond.)*, **228**, 373

Hebb, D. O. (1949). *The Organisation of Behaviour*, Wiley, New York

Hinde, R. A. (1970). *Animal Behaviour*, 2nd ed., McGraw-Hill, New York

Hirsch, H. V. B. and Spinelli, D. N. (1970). *Science*, **168**, 869

Hirsch, H. V. B. and Spinelli, D. B. (1971). *Expl Brain Res.*, **13**, 509

Horn, G. (1955). *Anat. Rec.*, **121**, 63

Horn, G. (1962). In *Viewpoints in Biology*, vol. 1 (J. D. Carthy and C. L. Duddington, eds.), Butterworths, London, pp. 242-85

Horn, G. (1965). *Adv. Stud. Behav.*, **1**, 155

Horn, G. (1967). *Nature*, **215**, 707

Horn, G. (1970). In *Short-Term Changes in Neural Activity and Behaviour* (G. Horn and R. A. Hinde, eds.), Cambridge University Press, pp. 567-606

Horn, G. (1971a). *Activ. Nerv. Super.*, **13**, 119

Horn, G. (1971b). In *Biology of Memory* G. Adám, ed.), Akademiai Kiado, Budapest, pp. 267-86

Horn, G. and Hinde, R. A., eds. (1970). *Short-Term Changes in Neural Activity and Behaviour*, Cambridge University Press

Horn, G. and Powell, C. H. F. (1968a). *J. exp. Biol.*, **49**, 143

Horn, G. and Powell, C. H. F. (1968b). *J. exp. Biol.*, **49**, 171

Horn, G., Horn, A. L. D., Bateson, P. P. G. and Rose, S. P. R. (1971). *Nature (Lond.)*, **229**, 131

Horn, G., Rose, S. P. R. and Bateson, P. P. G. (1973). *Brain Res.*, **56**, 227

Horridge, G. A. (1962). *Prog. R. Soc. Ser. B.*, **157**, 33

Hoyle, G. (1965). In *The Physiology of the Insect Nervous System* (J. E. Treherne and J. W. L. Beament, eds.), Academic Press, London, pp. 203-32

Hubel, D. H. and Wiesel, T. N. (1970). *J. Physiol. Lond.*, **206**, 419

Hydén, H. (1943). *Acta physiol. scand.*, **6**, suppl. 17

Hydén, H. and Lange, P. W. (1968). *Science*, **159**, 1370

Hydén, H. and Lange, P. W. (1970a). *Proc. natn Acad. Sci. U.S.A.*, **65**, 898

Hydén, H. and Lange P. W. (1970b). *Proc. natn Acad. Sci. U.S.A.*, **67**, 1959

Hydén, H. and Lange, P. W. (1970c). *Brain Res.*, **22**, 423

Jakoubek, B., Horăckova, M. and Gutman, E. (1968). *Proc. Int. Un. Physiol. Sci.*, **7**, 215

Jakoubek, B., Semiginovsky, B. and Dědičová, A. (1971). *Brain Res.*, **25**, 133

Jakoubek, B., Burešová, M., Hajek, I. Etrychová, J., Pavlik, A. and Dědičová, A. (1972). *Brain Res.*, **43**, 417

John, E. R. (1972). *Science*, **177**, 850

Kahan, B. E., Krigman, M. R., Wilson, J. E. and Glassman, E. (1970). *Proc. natn Acad. Sci. U.S.A.*, **65**, 300

Keating, M. J. and Gaze, R. M. (1970). *Brain, Behav. Evol.*, **3**, 102

Kerkut, G. A., Oliver, G., Rick, J. T. and Walker, R. J. (1970a). *Nature (Lond.)*, **227**, 722

Kerkut, G. A., Oliver, G., Rick, J. T. and Walker, R. J. (1970b). *Comp. gen. Pharmac*, **1**, 437

Kerkut, G. A., Beesley, P., Emson, P., Oliver, G. and Walker, R. J. (1971). *Comp. Biochem. Physiol.*, **39B**, 423

Kerkut, G. A., Emson, P. C. and Beesley, P. W. (1972). *Comp. Biochem. Physiol.*, **41B**, 635

Key, B. J. and Manley, B. (1962). *Electroenceph. clin Neurophysiol.*, **14**, 90

Krech, D., Rosenzweig, M. R. and Bennett, E. L. (1963). *Arch Neurol.*, **8**, 403

Lajtha, A., ed. (1971). *Handbook of Neurochemistry*, vol. 6, Plenum, New York

Liu, C. N. and Chambers, W. W. (1958). *Archs Neurol.*, **79**, 46

Mark, R. F. (1970). *Nature (Lond.)*, **225**, 178

McCouch, G. P., Austin, G. M. and Liu, C. N. (1958). *J. Neurophysiol.*, **21**, 205

Metzger, H. P., Cuénod, M., Grybaum, A. and Waelsch, H. (1967). *J. Neurochem.*, **14**, 183

Møllgaard, K., Diamond, M. C., Bennett, E. L., Rosenzweig, M. R. and Lindner, B. (1971). *Int. J. Neurosci.*, **2**, 113

Moltz, H. and Stettner, L. J. (1962). *J. comp. physiol Psych.*, **55**, 626

Moore, R. Y., Björklund, A. and Stevens, V. (1971). *Brain Res.*, **33**, 13

Oliver, G. W., Taberner, P. V., Rick, J. T. and Kerkut, G. A. (1971). *Comp. Biochem. Physiol.*, **38B**, 529

Raisman, G. (1969). *Brain Res.*, **14**, 25

Ramirez, G., Levitan, I. B. and Mushnyski, W. E. (1972). *Brain Res.*, **43**, 309

Razran, G. (1971). *Mind in Evolution*, Houghton Mifflin, Boston

Richardson, K. and Rose, S. P. R. (1972). *Brain Res.*, **44**, 299

Richardson, K. and Rose, S. P. R. (1973a). *J. Neurochem.*, **21**, 521

Richardson, K. and Rose, S. P. R. (1973b). *J. Neurochem.*, **21**, 531

Riege, W. H. (1971). *Devl. Pyschobiol.*, **4**, 157

Robertis, E. de, Amaiz, G. R., Alberice, M., Butcher, K. W. and Sutherland, E. W. (1967). *J. biol. Chem.*, **242**, 3487

Rose, S. P. R. (1967). *Nature*, **215**, 253

Rose, S. P. R. (1970). In *Short-Term Changes in Neural Activity and Behaviour* (G. Horn and R. A. Hinde, eds.), Cambridge University Press, pp. 517-55

Rose, S. P. R. (1972). *Brain Res.*, **38**, 171

Rose, S. P. R., Bateson, P. P. G., Horn, G. and Horn, A. L. D. (1970). *Nature (Lond.)*, **225**, 650

Rosenzweig, M. R., Bennett, E. L., Diamond, M. C., Wu, S. -Y., Slagle, R. W. and Saffran, E. (1969). *Brain Res.*, **14**, 427

Rosenzweig, M. R., Møllgaard, K., Diamond, M. C. and Bennett, E. L. (1972). *Pyschol. Rev.*, **79**, 93

Ruiz-Marcus, A. and Valverde, F. (1969). *Exp. Brain Res.,* **8**, 284

Schnierla, T. C. (1956). *L'Indistinct dans le Compartment des Animaux et de l'Homme,* Fondation Singer-Polignac, Masson et Cie, Paris

Semiginovsky, B., Jakoubek, B., Krauss, M. and Erdössová, R. (1970). *Brain Res.,* **23**, 298

Singh, U. B. and Talwar, G. P. (1969). *J. Neurochem.,* **16**, 951

Sinha, A. K. and Rose, S. P. R. (1972). *Life Sci.,* **11**(2), 665

Sluckin, W. (1972). *Imprinting and Early Learning,* 2nd ed., Methuen, London

Spemann, H. (1938). *Embryonic Development and Induction,* Yale University Press, New Haven

Spemann, H. and Mangold, H. (1924). *Arch. Mikr. Anat. Entwicks, Mech.,* **100**, 599

Sperry, R. W. (1943). *J. comp. Neurol.,* **79**, 33

Sperry, R. W. (1944). *J. Neurophys.,* **7**, 57

Spinelli, D. N. and Hirsch, H. V. B. (1971). *Fedn Proc.,* **30**, 615

Spinelli, D. N., Hirsch, H. V. B., Phelps, R. W. and Metzler, J. (1972). *Expl Brain Res.,* **15**, 289

Sugita, N. (1918). *J. comp. Neurol.,* **29**, 177

Talwar, G. P., Chopra, S. P., Goel, B. K. and D'Monte, B. (1966). *J. Neurochem.,* **13**, 109

Tata, J. R. (1967). *Biochem. J.,* **104**, 1

Thompson, R. F. and Spencer, W. A. (1966). *Psychol. Rev.,* **173**, 16

Thorpe, W. H. (1963). *Learning and Instinct in Animals,* 2nd ed., Methuen, London

Tiplady, B. (1972). *Brain Res.,* **43**, 215

Ungar, G., ed. (1970). *Molecular Mechanisms in Memory and Learning,* Plenum, New York

Valverde, F. (1967). *Expl Brain Res.,* **3**, 337

Valverde, F. (1971). *Brain Res.,* **33**, 1

Volkmar, F. R. and Greenough, W. T. (1972). *Science,* **176**, 1445

Weiskrantz, L. (1958). *Nature (Lond.),* **181**, 1047

Wiesel, T. N. and Hubel, D. H. (1963a). *J. Neurophys.,* **26**, 978

Wiesel, T. N. and Hubel, D. H. (1963b). *J. Neurophys.,* **26**, 1003

Wiesel, T. N. and Hubel, D. H. (1965). *J. Neurophys.,* **28**, 1029

Williams, T. H. and Palay, S. L. (1967). *J. Anat.,* **101**, 603

Yanagihara, T. and Hydén, H. (1971). *Expl Neurol.,* **31**, 151

Young, J. Z. (1964). *A Model of the Brain,* Oxford University Press

Zeier, H. (1970). *Nature (Lond.),* **225**, 708

Zemp, J. W., Wilson, J. E., Schlesinger, K., Boggan, W. O. and Glassman, E. (1966). *Proc. natn Acad. Sci. U.S.A.,* **55**, 1423

Zemp, J. W., Wilson, J. E. and Glassman, E. (1967). *Proc. natn Acad. Sci. U.S.A.,* **58**, 1120

10
MAMMALIAN NEOCORTICAL COMMISSURES

L. J. GAREY

The object of this chapter is to serve as an introduction to the part of the text devoted to structure and function of cerebral commissures in the mammal. It will attempt to give a brief review of some of the work to date and to outline some of the problem areas which face workers in this field today. For fuller treatment of some aspects of the subject the papers of Berlucchi (1972) and Doty and Negrão (1973) are recommended.

The organisation of the afferent and efferent connections of the neocortex has been studied with many techniques, both anatomical and physiological, but in recent years it is probably true to say that the introduction of new anatomical methods has been particularly rapid. In addition to methods based on degeneration, both anterograde and retrograde, we now have at our disposal new techniques for pathway tracing based on axonal transport. The two techniques most frequently used at the moment are the autoradiographic demonstration of anterograde transport of radioactive precursors (Cowan *et al.*, 1972) and the histochemical demonstration of retrograde transport of enzymes, especially horseradish peroxidase (Kristensson and Olsson, 1971; LaVail and LaVail, 1972). These techniques have been much used recently in the study of the connections of the neocortex, and in the chapters which follow many examples will be given of their use to study mammalian commissural systems.

The corpus callosum is the main pathway connecting the cortices of the two cerebral hemispheres. It reaches its highest development in man, where it is said to contain 200 million fibres (Tomasch, 1954). The diameter of the axons is small, mostly between 0.5 and 1 μm, and about 40% are unmyelinated (Fleischhauer and Wartenberg, 1967). The relative importance of the callosum to man is indicated by noting that the mouse has only 300 000 callosal axons and that the ratio of its callosal fibres to those in its pyramidal tract is 5 to 1, while in man this ratio is 100 to 1 (Tomasch and MacMillan, 1957).

Yet, in human cases of agenesis of the corpus callosum or callosal section for intractable epilepsy, clinical deficits are, on superficial examination, few or none (Bridgman and Smith, 1945). This rather remarkable negative finding was bound to provoke an experimental attack on callosal function. In pioneering work, Myers and Sperry (1953) and Myers (1956) transected the optic chiasma, effectively disconnecting the input of each eye to the contralateral visual cortex, and then trained cats to perform visual discrimination through one eye, the other being covered. When tested with the trained eye covered, the cat could still discriminate: there had been interhemispheric transfer. Transfer was abolished by section of the corpus callosum and the anterior commissure, the second interhemispheric commissure of the mammalian brain. Similar results were obtained by Downer (1959) in the monkey. Myers and Henson (1960) later extended these observations to the somatosensory system, showing that, in the chimpanzee, unilaterally acquired tactile discrimination could not be transferred in the absence of the corpus callosum and anterior commissure. Myers (1959) also showed that visual transfer was in the posterior part of the callosum, the splenium, and tactile transfer in anterior parts.

It is in its relationship to the visual system that we have the most information about the corpus callosum. Its importance in depth discrimination and stereoscopic vision has been stressed (Mitchell and Blakemore, 1970). It is known that some visual cortical receptive fields cross the vertical meridian of the visual field, and it has been suggested that the callosum helps to synthesise such receptive fields (Berlucchi, 1972; Choudhury et al., 1965; Hubel and Wiesel, 1967). However, Leicester (1968) found intact fields across the vertical meridian even after callosal section and Stone (1965) showed that ganglion cells in a central strip of retina project bilaterally. Thus, one aspect of suggested callosal function is open to further investigation.

Sperry and his colleagues succeeded in demonstrating the subtle deficits in humans with callosal sections (see Gazzaniga and Sperry, 1967; Sperry, 1966). For example, when a discrimination was learned with the dominant hemisphere, usually the left one, the subject could talk and write about his task, whereas a right-sided learning situation was not transferred to the other side and could not be expressed in verbal form.

There could be endless speculation about the human implications of the 'split brain' and, indeed, about the *two* brains which a man possesses, but it is on the anatomical implications of the early experimental work that I shall concentrate. For further discussion of the problem of the split brain, the work of Gazzaniga (1970) is recommended.

Many studies have used the anterograde degeneration technique with staining of degenerated axons by various modifications of the Nauta method to determine the distribution of axons crossing in the corpus callosum. From these results it was soon clear that not all parts of the neocortex received commissural connections. For example, most of area 17, the primary visual cortex, together with the hand and foot areas of the somatosensory cortex and parts of the auditory cortex were free of degeneration after large contralateral cortical lesions or callosal sections (Diamond et al., 1968; Ebner and Myers, 1965; Garey et al., 1968; Jones and Powell, 1968, 1969; Myers, 1962; Pandya et al., 1971; Wilson, 1967)—see figure 10.1. Otherwise, a small lesion in a cortical area gives a region of degeneration in the opposite cortex in an approximately homotopic site. The situation is not quite as simple as this, however, for Jones and Powell (1969) showed that primary somatosensory cortex (SI) projected to SI and the secondary area (SII) contralaterally,

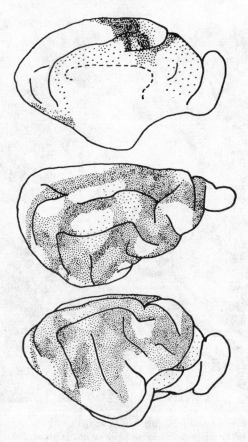

Figure 10.1. Medial, dorsal and lateral surface reconstructions of a cerebral hemisphere of the cat to show the site of degenerating axons after section of the corpus callosum and anterior commissure. Note the absence of commissural connections in the primary visual cortex and the hand and foot areas of the somatosensory cortex. (From Ebner and Myers (1965), by courtesy of the authors and the *Journal of Comparative Neurology*)

whereas SII projected to SII but only a restricted part of SI. A somewhat similar situation exists in auditory cortical commissural connections (Diamond *et al.,*1968).

However, different authors have arrived at different conclusions about the real extent of the callosal projection into primary sensory areas away from the 'midline', represented for example by the border of areas 17 and 18 in visual cortex and the face area of somatosensory cortex. Shoumura (1974) described a quite wide extension of callosal terminals into area 17, and Hubel and Wiesel (1967) found 'simple' units in the callosum of the cat, also presumably axons from area 17. There is also physiological evidence that the cat callosum carries information from the forepaws (Innocenti *et al.,* 1974). One specialised part of the rodent SI, the 'barrel' field containing the representation of the mystacial vibrissae (Woolsey and Van der Loos,

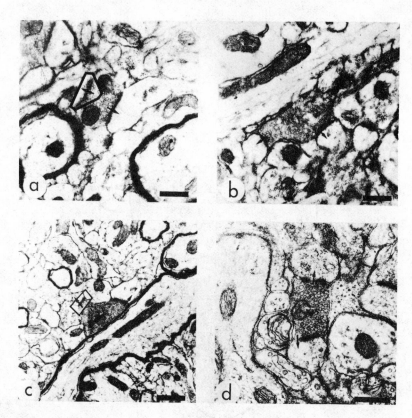

Figure 10.2. Electron micrographs showing four examples of degenerating axodendritic and axospinous terminals in the walls of 'barrels' in layer IV of the primary somatosensory cortex of the mouse 4–5 days after section of the corpus callosum. Scales: a, b, d 0.5 μm; C, 0.8 μm (From Perentes (1977), by courtesy of the author)

1970), has been said to be almost devoid of callosal terminals (Wise and Jones, 1976; York and Caviness, 1975), but recently Perentes (1977) has produced electron microscopic evidence of degenerating terminals in the 'walls' of barrels after callosal lesions in mice (figure 10.2).

Some of the differences in the extent of callosal projections in various studies may be due to alternative techniques, such as axonal degeneration investigated with light or electron microscopy at different survival times, axonal transport or physiology. However, different mutations may be implicated, for Shatz (1977) has recently shown that Siamese cats have much more of their area 17 in receipt of callosal axons than 'gutter' cats. Jones, Burton and Porter (1975) and Künzle (1976) have shown that callosal axons end in columns or bands in the cortex rather than in areas of even density, and this adds another complicating factor (figure 10.3).

Commissural fibres terminate widely through the cortical layers. Many authors

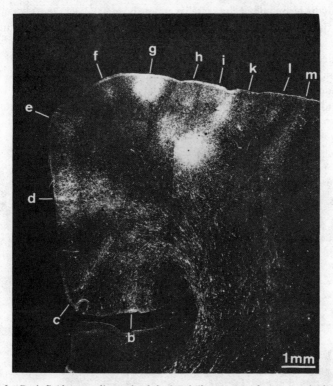

Figure 10.3. Dark-field autoradiograph of the band-like pattern of axon terminals in the motor cortex of the monkey after injection of tritiated proline in the contralateral motor cortex. The letters refer to distinct bands of high grain density traceable in serial sections. (From Künzle (1976), by courtesy of the author and *Brain Research*)

claim that most end in the middle and deep layers, but it has also been shown that more superficial layers may receive a proportion of the commissural fibres (see Garey, 1976 for detailed references). Sloper (1973) has reported relatively more commissural terminals in the deep layers (V and VI) of the primate motor cortex than the somatosensory, and Fisken *et al.* (1975) found them in all layers of area 18, but mainly in layers III and IV of area 17 of the monkey. Several reasons can be postulated for these differences. The laminar pattern of corticocortical fibres is less distinct than that of thalamocortical, and there are variations between different animals and different cortical areas within a single species. Technical difficulties with the silver impregnation technique used in many studies may confuse the interpretation. For example, differences in survival time after the making of the lesion have been shown to emphasise degeneration in certain layers (Zeki, 1970). Also, deep layers contain degenerating fibres passing to their termination more superficially, making the differentiation of terminal degeneration difficult.

Grafstein (1959) suggested that callosal fibres which originate from superficial cortical layers terminate in the same layers of the contralateral cortex, and that similarly the deep cells project to the deep layers of the opposite side, and Ribak (1977) has made similar observations in rat visual cortex.

Evidence as to the identity of structures postsynaptic to commissural axons has come from two main sources. First, the number of spines on the oblique branches of apical dendrites of pyramidal cells impregnated by the Golgi method was reduced after section of the corpus callosum (Globus and Scheibel, 1967). Secondly, elec-

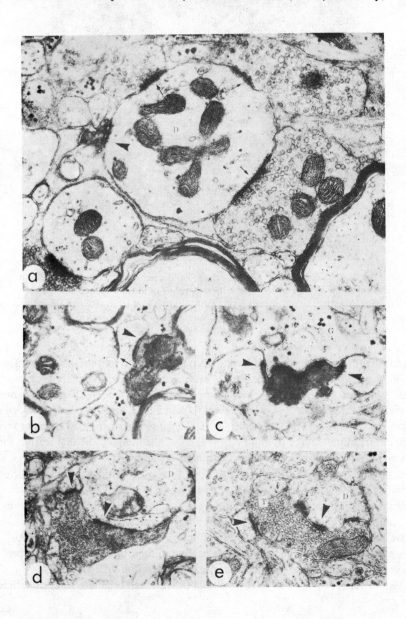

tron microscopy has shown that callosal fibres terminate mainly on dendritic spines, but also on the dendritic shafts of pyramidal and stellate cells on the stellate somata, and have asymmetrical membrane thickenings (Fisken *et al.*, 1975; Jones and Powell, 1970; Lund and Lund, 1970; Sloper, 1973; Szentágothai, 1973)—see figure 10.4.

From the results of many of the degeneration studies quoted above, in which small lesions were made, it can be stated that, in general, areas which do not receive callosal connections do not send any. The cells of origin of callosal fibres have been studied recently in several species using the technique of retrograde transport of horseradish peroxidase (Jacobson and Trojanowski, 1974). The majority of the cells seem to be pyramidal neurons in layer III, but some deeper pyramids are involved and also some stellates in layer IV. In the visual areas of the cat the extent of cortex from which callosal axons originate seems wider than that in which callosal terminals are usually described, extending further into area 17 (Innocenti and Fiore, 1976).

The presence of a group of large pyramidal cells in layer III at the border of areas 17 and 18 of the cat was noted by Shoumura (1974). They may correspond to the cells of the OBγ region of Von Economo (1927) in the primate, which degenerate when the corpus callosum is cut (Glickstein and Whitteridge, 1976) and which can be filled with horseradish peroxidase from an injection in the contralateral area 17/18 boundary (Winfield, Gatter and Powell, 1975; Wong-Riley, 1974). These neurons are much larger than the other pyramids in the vicinity in the monkey (figure 10.5), less so in the cat, and in rodents they are not larger (Dürsteler *et al.*, 1979). Callosal axons terminate near these cells in the primate (figure 10.5).

Although the corpus callosum is the main neocortical commissural pathway in placental mammals, there is also the anterior commissure. Indeed, in marsupials, which have no corpus callosum, the anterior commissure takes over its role (Ebner, 1967). The anterior commissure connects parts of the neocortex, especially the temporal lobes (Fox *et al.*, 1948; Pandya *et al.*, 1973; Whitlock and Nauta, 1956) and the olfactory system. Downer (1962) found that in the monkey visual discriminatory transfer was still possible after cutting the optic chiasma and corpus callosum, so long as the anterior commissure was intact. This was not, however, true in the

Figure 10.4   (a) A large dendrite (D) in layer III of the visual cortex of the cat which receives a degenerating asymmetrical synapse (arrowhead) following a lesion of the visual cortex of the opposite side. The dendrite receives three other synapses (arrows) from normal axon terminals. The dendrite is presumed to be one of a stellate cell. (b) A degenerating commissural terminal in layer III of the visual cortex of the cat forming an asymmetrical synapse upon a small spine (arrowhead): the spine also receives a normal, symmetrical terminal (arrow). (c) A degenerating commissural terminal in layer V of the cat's visual cortex making asymmetical contacts (arrowheads) upon two spines, one of which (S) has a spine apparatus. (d) An axon terminal at a relatively early stage of degeneration in layer VI of the visual cortex of the monkey after a lesion of the opposite visual cortex. The terminal makes asymmetrical synaptic contacts (arrowheads) with a dendrite (D) and a small spine. (e) An axonal terminal (T) in layer II of the cat's visual cortex, at an early stage of degeneration after a lesion of the opposite visual cortex. The terminal makes asymmetical synapses (arrowheads) upon a small spine and a small dendrite (D).

(From Fisken *et al.* (1975), by courtesy of the Royal Society)

cat (Myers and Sperry, 1953). Do, then, primates have direct access to the anterior commissure from the visual cortex, or is the pathway indirect? Further discussion of the other commissural pathways is beyond the scope of the present text, and the reader is referred to Doty and Negrão (1973) for a fuller treatment of the subject.

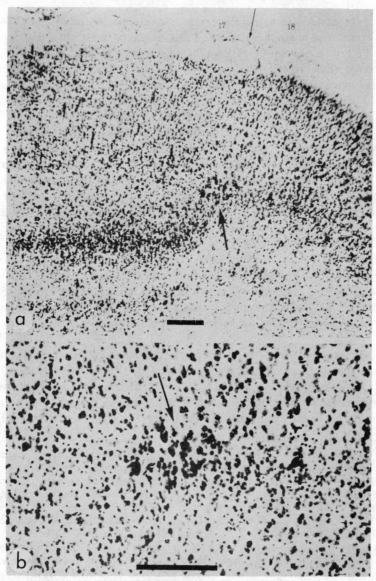

Figure 10.5. (a) The cortex at the boundary of areas 17 and 18 of the monkey (OBγ) to show the large pyramidal cells in the deep part of layer III (large arrow). Scale: 250 μm. (b) High power of the large pyramidal cells (arrow). Scale: 250 μm. (From Fisken *et al.* (1975), by courtesy of the Royal Society)

In conclusion, one may try to summarise some of the problems in present studies on commissural connections. The corpus callosum is very large, especially in primates, and contains very many fine fibres. It seems to be the main transfer channel for cortical learned activity and higher functions, and yet clinical and experimental psychological deficits after its loss seem, proportionately, relatively difficult to determine precisely. Cortical areas connected through the callosum are fairly symmetrical; there is a good degree of somatotopia in the connections, and 'acallosal' or 'weakly callosal' regions neither send nor receive dense projections. These unfavoured areas are often described as being away from the representation of midline structures, such as hands, feet and peripheral visual field. Yet there is new anatomical and physiological evidence that this may not be strictly accurate. The laminae of termination of callosal fibres within the cortex are still uncertain, and the significance of the band-like organisation of these terminals remains to be investigated. We know little about the ontogenetic aspects of the corpus callosum, and its relationship with other commissures is still not fully elucidated.

REFERENCES

Berlucchi, G. (1972). Anatomical and physiological aspects of visual functions of corpus callosum. *Brain Res.,* **37**, 371–92

Bridgman, C. S. and Smith, K. U. (1945). Bilateral neural integration in visual perception after section of the corpus callosum. *J. comp. Neurol.,* **83**, 57–68

Choudhury, B. P., Whitteridge, D. and Wilson, M. E. (1965). The function of the callosal connections of the visual cortex. *Q. Jl exp. Physiol.,* **50**, 214–19

Cowan, W. M., Gottlieb, D. I., Hendrickson, A. E., Price, J. L. and Woolsey, T. A. (1972). The autoradiographic demonstration of axonal connections in the central nervous system. *Brain Res.,* **37**, 21–51

Diamond, I. T., Jones, E. G. and Powell, T. P. S. (1968). Interhemispheric fiber connections of the auditory cortex of the cat. *Brain Res.,* **11**, 177–93

Doty, R. W. and Negrão, N. (1973). Forebrain commissures and vision. In *Handbook of Sensory Physiology,* vol. VII/3B (R. Jung, ed.), Springer, Berlin, pp. 543–82

Downer, J. L. de C. (1959). Changes in visually guided behaviour following midsagittal division of optic chiasm and corpus callosum in monkey (*Macaca mulatta*). *Brain,* **82**, 251–59

Downer, J. L. de C. (1962). Interhemispheric integration in the visual system. In *Interhemispheric Relations and Cerebral Dominance* (V. B. Mountcastle, ed.), Johns Hopkins Press, Baltimore, pp. 87–100

Dürsteler, M. R., Blakemore, C. and Garey, L. J. (1979). Projections to the visual cortex in the golden hamster. *J. comp. Neurol.,* in press

Ebner, F. F. (1967). Afferent connections to neocortex in the opossum (*Didelphis virginiana*). *J. comp. Neurol.,* **129**, 241–68

Ebner, F. F. and Myers, R. E. (1965). Distribution of the corpus callosum and anterior commissure in cat and raccoon. *J. comp. Neurol.,* **124**, 353–66

Fisken, R. A., Garey, L. J. and Powell, T. P. S. (1975). The intrinsic, association and commissural connections of area 17 of the visual cortex. *Phil. Trans. R. Soc. B,* **272**, 487–536

Fleischhauer, K. and Wartenberg, H. (1967). Elektronmikroskopische Untersuchungen über das Wachstum der Nervenfasern und über das Auftreten von Markscheiden im Corpus callosum der Katze. *Z. Zellforsch.*, **83**, 568-81

Fox, C. A., Fisher, R. R. and Delsalva, S. J. (1948). The distribution of the anterior commissures in the monkey (*Macaca mulatta*). *J. comp. Neurol.*, **89**, 245-78

Garey, L. J. (1976). Synaptic organization of afferent fibres and intrinsic circuits in the neocortex. In *Handbook of Electroencephalography and Clinical Neurophysiology*, vol. 2A (A. Rémond, ed.), Elsevier, Amsterdam, pp. 57-85

Garey, L. J., Jones, E. G. and Powell, T. P. S. (1968). Interrelationships of striate and extrastriate cortex with the primary relay sites of the visual pathway. *J. Neurol. Neurosurg. Psychiat.*, **31**, 135-57

Gazzaniga, M. S. (1970). *The Bisected Brain*. Appleton-Century-Crofts, New York, p. 172

Gazzaniga, M. S. and Sperry, R. W. (1967). Language after section of the cerebral commissures. *Brain*, **90**, 131-48

Glickstein, M. and Whitteridge, D. (1976). Degeneration of layer III pyramidal cells in area 18 following destruction of callosal input. *Brain Res.*, **104**, 148-51

Globus, A. and Scheibel, A. B. (1967). Synaptic loci on parietal cortical neurons: terminations of corpus callosum fibers. *Science*, **156**, 1127-29

Grafstein, B. (1959). Organization of callosal connections in suprasylvian gyrus of cat. *J. Neurophysiol.*, **22**, 504-15

Hubel, D. H. and Wiesel, T. N. (1967). Cortical and callosal connections concerned with the vertical meridian of visual fields in the cat. *J. Neurophysiol.*, **30**, 1561-73

Innocenti, G. M. and Fiore, L. (1976). Morphological correlates of visual field transformation in the corpus callosum. *Neurosci. Lett.*, **2**, 245-52

Innocenti, G. M., Manzoni, T. and Spidalieri, G. (1974). Patterns of the somesthetic messages transferred through the corpus callosum. *Expl. Brain Res.*, **19**, 447-66

Jacobson, S. and Trojanowski, J. Q. (1974). The cells of origin of the corpus callosum in rat, cat and rhesus monkey. *Brain Res.*, **74**, 149-55

Jones, E. G. and Powell, T. P. S. (1968). The commissural connexions of the somatic sensory cortex in the cat. *J. Anat.*, **103**, 433-55

Jones, E. G. and Powell, T. P. S. (1969). Connexions of the somatic sensory cortex of the rhesus monkey. II—Contralateral cortical connexions. *Brain*, **92**, 717-30

Jones, E. G. and Powell, T. P. S. (1970). An electron microscopic study of the laminar pattern and mode of termination of afferent fibre pathways in the somatic sensory cortex of the cat. *Phil. Trans. R. Soc. B*, **257**, 45-62

Jones, E. G., Burton, H. and Porter, R. (1975). Commissural and cortico-cortical 'columns' in the somatic sensory cortex of primates. *Science*, **190**, 572-74

Kristensson, K. and Olsson, Y. (1971). Retrograde axonal transport of protein. *Brain Res.*, **29**, 363-65

Künzle, H. (1976). Alternating afferent zones of high and low axon terminal density within the macaque motor cortex. *Brain. Res.*, **106**, 365-70

LaVail, J. H. and LaVail, M. M. (1972). Retrograde axonal transport in the central nervous system. *Science*, **176**, 1416-17

Leicester, J. (1968). Projection of the visual vertical meridian to cerebral cortex of the cat. *J. Neurophysiol.*, **31**, 371-82

Lund, J. S. and Lund, R. D. (1970). The termination of callosal fibres in the paravisual cortex of the rat. *Brain Res.,* **17**, 25–45

Mitchell, D. E. and Blakemore, C. (1970). Binocular depth perception and the corpus callosum. *Vision Res.,* **10**, 49–54

Myers, R. E. (1956). Function of corpus callosum in interocular transfer. *Brain,* **79**, 358–63

Myers, R. E. (1959). Localization of function in the corpus callosum. *Archs Neurol.,* **1**, 74–77

Myers, R. E. (1962). Commissural connections between occipital lobes of the monkey. *J. comp. Neurol.,* **118**, 1–16

Myers, R. E. and Henson, C. O. (1960). Role of corpus callosum in transfer of tactuokinesthetic learning in chimpanzee. *Archs Neurol.,* **3**, 404–409

Myers, R. E. and Sperry, R. W. (1953). Interocular transfer of a visual form discrimination in cats after section of the optic chiasma and corpus callosum. *Anat. Rec.,* **115**, 351–52

Pandya, D. N., Karol, E. A. and Heilbronn, D. (1971). The topographical distribution of interhemispheric projections in the corpus callosum of the rhesus monkey. *Brain Res.,* **32**, 31–43

Pandya, D. N., Karol, E. A. and Lele, P. (1973). The distribution of the anterior commissure in the squirrel monkey. *Brain Res.,* **49**, 177–180

Perentes, E. (1977). Analyse du cortex somatosensoriel (PMBSF) de la souris: ultrastructure des bords des tonneaux et des septa. *Doctoral thesis,* University of Lausanne

Ribak, C. E. (1977). A note on the laminar organization of rat visual cortical projections. *Expl Brain Res.,* **27**, 413–18

Shatz, C. (1977). A comparison of visual pathways in Boston and Midwestern Siamese cats. *J. comp. Neurol.,* **171**, 205–28

Shoumura, K. (1974). An attempt to relate the origin and distribution of commissural fibers to the presence of large and medium pyramids in layer III in the cat's visual cortex, *Brain Res.,* **67**, 13–25

Sloper, J. J. (1973). An electron microscope study of the termination of afferent connections to the primate motor cortex. *J. Neurocytol.,* **2**, 361–68

Sperry, R. W. (1966). Brain bisection and mechanisms of consciousness. In *Brain and Conscious Experience* (J. C. Eccles, ed.), Springer, Berlin, pp. 298–308

Stone, J. (1965). A quantitative analysis of the distribution of ganglion cells in the cat's retina. *J. comp. Neurol.,* **124**, 337–52

Szentágothai, J. (1973). Synaptology of the visual cortex. In *Handbook of Sensory Physiology,* vol. VII/3 (R. Jung, ed.), Springer, Berlin, pp. 269–324

Tomasch, J. (1954). Size, distribution and number of fibers in the human corpus callosum. *Anat. Rec.,* **119**, 119–35

Tomasch, J. and MacMillan, A. (1957). The number of fibres in the corpus callosum of the white mouse. *J. comp. Neurol.,* **107**, 165–68

Von Economo, C. (1927). *Zellaufbau der Grosshirnrinde des Menschen,* Springer, Berlin, p. 145

Whitlock, D. G. and Nauta, W. J. H. (1956). Subcortical projections from the temporal neocortex in *Macaca mulatta. J. comp. Neurol.,* **106**, 183–212

Wilson, M. E. (1967). Cortico-cortical connexions of the cat visual areas. *J. Anat.,* **102**, 375–86

Winfield, D. A., Gatter, K. C. and Powell, T. P. S. (1975). Certain connections of the visual cortex of the monkey shown by the use of horseradish peroxidase. *Brain Res.*, **92**, 456–61

Wise, S. P. and Jones, E. G. (1976). The organization and postnatal development of the commissural projection of the rat somatic sensory cortex. *J. comp. Neurol.*, **168**, 313–44

Wong-Riley, M. T. T. (1974). Demonstration of geniculocortical and callosal projection neurons in the squirrel monkey by means of retrograde axonal transport of horseradish peroxidase. *Brain Res.*, **79**, 267–72

Woolsey, T. A. and Van der Loos, H. (1970). The structural organization of layer IV in the somatosensory region (SI) of mouse cerebral cortex. *Brain Res.*, **17**, 205–42

Yorke, C. H. and Caviness, V. S. (1975). Interhemispheric neocortical connections of the corpus callosum in the normal mouse: a study based on anterograde and retrograde methods. *J. comp. Neurol.*, **164**, 233–46

Zeki, S. M. (1970). Interhemispheric connections of prestriate cortex in monkey. *Brain Res.*, **19**, 63–75

11

ON THE NORMAL ARRANGEMENT OF FIBRES AND TERMINALS AND LIMITS OF PLASTICITY IN THE CALLOSAL SYSTEM OF THE RAT

J. R. WOLFF and L. ZÁBORSZKY

INTRODUCTION

It is well established that callosal connections are distributed unevenly in the neocortex. For instance, those parts of the primary sensory areas which are related to the midline of the body or the vertical meridian of the visual field are strongly interconnected, while other parts of the same areas appear 'acallosal' (Berlucchi, 1972, Wise and Jones, 1976). Recently, evidence has been presented in favour of a much higher specificity indicating that certain neurons in a particular lamina of homotopic parts of the hemispheres seem to be interconnected, while other cells of the same part of the cortex are not (Caviness and Yorke, 1976; Wise and Jones, 1976). If this were to be a general arrangement, then callosal terminals should be aggregated in irregular clusters corresponding to those of the cells of origin (Innocenti et al., 1977; Jacobson and Trojanowski, 1974). In the cortex, neurons of origin and preterminal branches of callosal fibres are more diffusely spread during early postnatal stages (Innocenti et al., 1977; Wise and Jones, 1976). It is unknown whether the misplaced axons are withdrawn or survive as non-myelinated axons. These two possibilities could be discriminated, when the distribution of terminals and fibres is compared in the same adult brains.

In the present chapter we report on results which were obtained with two sensitive methods which stain, consistently and selectively, degenerating fibres and lysosomes, respectively (Gallyas et al., 1979). After short survival times the latter method mainly demonstrates terminal degeneration. The two methods being applied to consecutive frozen sections of the same brains allow comparison of the distribution of fibres and terminals. The chronology of degeneration of both components was followed in a series of callosotomies made 0.5 to 30 days before the albino rats were killed. The atlas of Krieg (1946) was used throughout this study, although several parts of the map have been found to be incorrect.

147

TOPOGRAPHIC ARRANGEMENT

No area seems to be homogeneously filled with callosal fibres or terminals. In a number of areas the terminals are concentrated along the borders (areas 1, 6, 39, 40), while in others they form patches and clusters (areas 2, 41, 10). Terminals are more regularly aggregated along the borders between the frontal, motor, somato-sensory, acoustic, visual, retrohippocampal and limbic regions of the cortex. The highest density of terminals has been found at corners between three and more areas. The lowest terminal density occurs in the primary sensory areas. A small number of terminals is diffusely distributed in area 17, but forms more or less distinct patches in areas 2 and 41.

COLUMNAR ARRANGEMENT

Many zones, bands and patches, all of which are rich in callosal terminals, are composed of more or less fusing, vertically oriented columnar subunits. These columns can often be separated by two properties:

(1) Columns are often delimited from each other by narrow rims containing fewer callosal terminals than the centres (figure 11.1a). This delimitation is most obvious in tangential sections and has been observed in most parts of the cortex (occipital: areas 18, 18a; temporal: 39, 40, parts of 41; parietal: 1, 2, 3). A delimitation is hardly visible where the overall density is too high (thick sections, areas 29c/18; parts of 10, etc.), or too low (areas 17, parts of 2 and 41, etc.).

(2) Within columns the highly variable laminar distribution pattern of callosal terminals (see below) is uniform, but may change from one column to another. This has become a good criterion for delimiting columns in coronal and parasagittal sections (figure 11.1b).

Using these criteria the columns form cylinders with an average diameter of 150–250 μm extending through the whole thickness of the cortex. They often, but not always, contain a centrally located radial blood vessel and tend to aggregate in rows (bands) or bundles (patches). Wider columns (diameter: 350–500 μm) can be identified mostly by one of the above-mentioned criteria as complex columns being composed of several fused columnar units.

Beside the columns which are filled with callosal terminals, there are more or less empty columns with similar diameters forming holes, gaps and zones of low density (figure 11.1a and 11.1b). At the border between filled and empty columns some callosal terminals seem to spread into the neighbouring column (lamina Ib > VI > III > V; figures 11.1b and 11.2). This differential spread causes the well-known sandglass-like arrangement of callosal terminals, as seen in many areas (Heimer *et al.*, 1967).

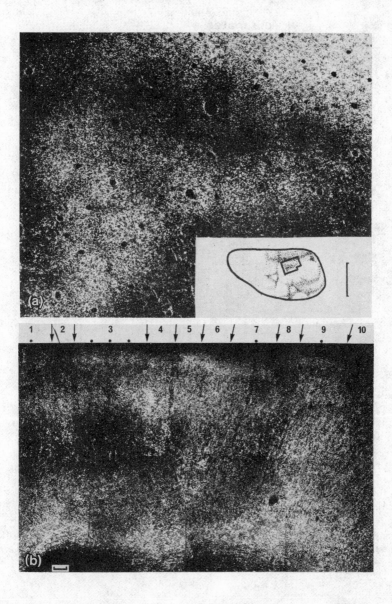

Figure 11.1.   Columnar arrangement of callosal connections (bars = 100 μm) 5 days after a complete callosotomy. (a) Horizontal section through the indicated zone at the border between areas 17/18/7. Note the more or less filled and empty appearing columns. (b) Coronal section through the anterior border of areas 29c and 18. The numbers mark columns with different laminar patterns. Note the lack of terminals in lamina Ib in 1, 2, 8 and in lamina IV in 1, 3, 5, 8; filled columns in 6 and 9 and 'empty' column in 8

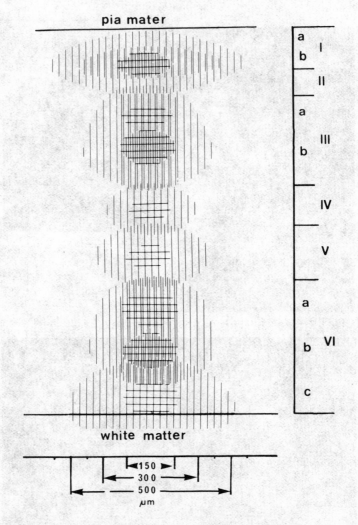

Figure 11.2. Schematic summary of all observed laminar patterns. Horizontal lines mark centres of callosal terminals, vertical lines represent the horizontal and vertical spread or scatter

LAMINAR ARRANGEMENT

The laminar distribution pattern of callosal terminals varies greatly not only within the same cortical area, but also between neighbouring columns. Laminas IIIb and VIb are most frequently filled with terminals, but also laminas Ib, IIIa, V and VIa may be populated. In the neocortex, only laminas Ia and II do not seem to form their own centre of callosal connections, but they may be reached by diffusely spreading terminals from the neighbouring laminae (see figure 11.2). Thus, callosal terminals are arranged in laminar patterns which are characteristic neither for the neocortex nor for any cortical area, but vary between smaller yet undefined units and often between single columns. The limbic cortex and areas 13 and 14 ('insular' cortex of Krieg (1946)) show some peculiarities.

RELATION BETWEEN DISTRIBUTION OF FIBRES AND TERMINALS

Like the terminals, the callosal fibres are unevenly distributed even in the deep layers of the neocortex. There is, for instance, a dense accumulation of fibres along the border between limbic and neocortical areas (e.g. 29c/18, figure 11.3b) which

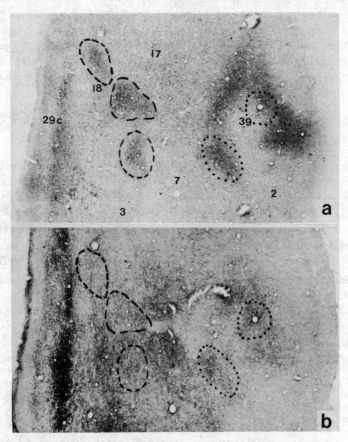

Figure 11.3. Comparison of the distribution of terminal degeneration (a) and degenerating fibres (b) in horizontal sections through the same rat brain 7 days after a complete callosotomy. The numbers represent area numbers according to Krieg (1946). For further explanation see text

corresponds to some extent to the distribution of terminals. This is also true for some other borders between areas, such as 39/7 and 39/41, as indicated by dotted lines in figure 11.3. However, there are also zones which contain many terminals but only few fibres (broken lines in figure 11.3), irrespective of the survival time after callosotomy, indicating that this is not due to differences in the progress of degeneration.

Although the staining method for lysosomes might reveal some unmyelinated fibres, it is difficult to estimate how many of these very thin axons remain invisible. Therefore, it is probably more significant to demonstrate that regions exist which contain many callosal fibres and only few terminals. This is, for instance, the case in the anterior part of area 17, and areas 7 and 3 (see figure 11.3). Correspondingly, in coronal sections the columnar and laminar arrangement of terminals is not strictly related to the location of ascending fibres, preterminal and terminal branches. Thus, there are columns and laminae in many areas in which the number of terminals is not related to the distribution of fibres, in spite of some rough correspondence between the number of fibres and terminals in some other regions. Golgi preparations confirmed that the intracortical course and the preterminal arborisation of many callosal fibres do not correspond to the width of columns.

LIMITS OF PLASTICITY

In a series of experiments, lesions of varying size were made in the occipital cortex, all of which penetrated the subcortical white matter. The persisting callosal connections were demonstrated by a complete callosotomy following 1–3 months of survival. The main result of these experiments was that a lesion had to surpass a length of 2 mm in the mediolateral direction to produce a detectable defect in callosal connections along the posterior border of the visual cortex. Even with lesions of that size there was a considerable number of terminals degenerating after callosotomy, although a short time after the first lesion a heavy terminal degeneration had taken place. Obviously, a reorganisation of callosal terminals must have occurred, the origin of which is obscure. One possibility would be that new terminals arise from persisting fibres terminating in the occipital cortex, but taking an unusual course through the anterior corpus callosum. An argument in favour of this possibility is that defects are more complete when the lesions are situated more laterally.

DISCUSSION

The present results confirm many aspects of earlier observations on the areal and laminar distribution of callosal connections in rodent brains (see Jacobson, 1970, Wise and Jones, 1976, Yorke and Caviness, 1975). This suggests that the new staining methods, as used in the present study, produce results which are comparable to other methods of tracing interneuronal connections.

Until now, little attention has been paid to the columnar arrangement of callosal terminals. Recently, corticocortical connections in monkeys were found to be organised in columns (Goldman and Nauta, 1977; Jones *et al.*, 1975). The smallest columns of these much larger brains show a similar width to the callosal columnar units in rats, i.e. about 200 μm. The similar diameter in monkeys and rats, the common tendency to fuse, forming complex columns, patches, bands, etc., as well as the presence of 'empty columns', might indicate that columns represent a more general unit of space organisation in the cortex.

The extension and distribution of callosal columns resemble very much those of the smallest vascular modules which develop as a result of the tangential growth of the cortex during the first and the second postnatal week (Wolff, 1976, 1978), i.e. when callosal fibres enter the cortex (Wise and Jones, 1976). The corresponding blood vessels supply mainly lamina III, which contains many callosal terminals and the majority of neurons giving rise to callosal fibres (Jacobson and Trojanowski, 1974).

Nevertheless, as shown in the present study, the callosal axon terminals often do not follow the distribution of preterminal fibres. This suggests that the callosal afferents, although influencing the formation of callosal connections, do not determine precisely the intracortical arrangement of the latter. Nor are the callosal terminals aggregated in the same irregular clusters as the cells of origin (see Innocenti *et al.*, 1977). Hence, the distribution of the neurons producing the callosal fibre system is also similar to, but not identical with, the distribution of callosal terminals. Consequently, a rather complicated spatial relationship seems to exist between callosal axons and the cells of origin in the contralateral hemisphere. The latter seem to attract a local accumulation of callosal terminals in certain columns and even laminae (Caviness and Yorke, 1976) without being the only postsynaptic element.

Our experiments on plastic changes of callosal connections are still much too prelimary to allow for any definite statement. Nevertheless, they suggest that destroyed callosal connections can be replaced by an unknown mechanism (axon sprouting, augmentation of terminals from persisting fibres with an unusual course). However, this capacity seems to be limited with respect to the size of the lesion.

REFERENCES

Berlucchi, G. (1972). *Brain Res.*, **37**, 371-92
Caviness, V. S. Jr. and Yorke, C. H., Jr. (1976). *J. comp. Neurol.*, **170**, 449-60
Gallyas, F., Böttcher, H. and Wolff, J. R. (1979). In press
Goldman, P. S. and Nauta, W. J. H. (1977). *Brain Res.*, **122**, 393-415
Heimer, L., Ebner, F. F. and Nauta, W. J. H. (1967). *Brain Res.*, **5**, 171-77
Innocenti, G. M., Fiore, L. and Caminiti, R. (1977). *Neurosci. Lett.*, **4**, 237-42

Jacobson, S. (1970). *Exp. Neurol.,* **28**, 193–205
Jacobson, S. and Trojanowski, J. Q. (1974). *Brain Res.,* **74**, 149–55
Jones, E. G., Burton, H. and Porter, R. (1975). *Science,* **190**, 572–74
Krieg, W. J. S. (1946). *J. comp. Neurol.,* **84**, 277–323
Wise, S. P. and Jones, B. G. (1976). *J. comp. Neurol.,* **168**, 313–44
Wolff, J. R. (1976). *Drug Res.,* **26**, 6, 12
Wolff, J. R. (1978). In *Architectonics of the Cerebral Cortex* (M. A. B. Brazier and
    H. Petsche, eds.), Raven Press, New York
Yorke, C. H. and Caviness, V. S., Jr. (1975). *J. comp. Neurol.,* **164**, 233–46

12
COBALT-INDUCED EPILEPSY IN THE RAT: SOME STUDIES ON THE MIRROR FOCUS

JUDITH K. McQUEEN and R. C. DOW

INTRODUCTION

The corpus callosum is known to be of primary importance in the propagation of focal epileptic activity from one hemisphere to a contralateral homotopic point. Various workers (Morrell, 1960; Mutani et al., 1973; Woodruff, 1975) have established that section of the corpus callosum prevents the spread of focal seizures produced by agents like penicillin or ethyl chloride. However, Isaacson et al. (1971) and Nie et al. (1974) have described, in addition, the possibility of descendant propagation into subcortical structures and subsequent spread into cortical areas as an alternative route.

It has also been suggested that the normal hemisphere may exert an inhibitory effect on the 'epileptic' one via the corpus callosum (Kopeloff et al., 1950; Mutani et al., 1973). Such an effect might explain why complete forebrain commissurotomy in cats apparently accelerated the development of kindled seizures (Wada and Sato, 1975). However, Racine et al. (1972) reported that commissurotomy retarded the kindling process in rats.

With the exception of studies on alumina lesions in monkeys, where secondary foci can develop in spite of complete commissurotomy, other studies have concentrated on acute foci and on observation periods of only hours. The present study was designed to examine the part played by the corpus callosum in both the development and maintenance of a secondary focus following implantation of cobalt into the sensorimotor cortex of the rat. Because the foci persist for several weeks in this model the long-term effects of sectioning the corpus callosum, on both the primary and the secondary foci, could be evaluated.

METHODS

Cobalt implantation

For this study, adult male Piebald Virol Glaxo (PVG) rats, weighing 180–220 g, were used. The operative technique for the implantation of cobalt and for the inser-

155

tion of stainless steel recording electrodes is described in detail by Dow *et al.* (1972). In these experiments a cobalt–gelatine pellet, 1 mm in diameter, was implanted into the cortex at a position 3 mm anterior to the coronal suture and 3 mm lateral to the midline. One recording electrode was inserted into the skull immediately above the implant and another was placed over the corresponding position in the cortex of the contralateral hemisphere. Two further electrodes were inserted 4 mm posterior to the coronal suture and 3 mm either side of the sagittal suture. The animals were allowed 48 h to recover from the operative procedure. Bipolar recordings of the electrocorticogram (ECoG) were made from the conscious, unrestrained rat at frequent intervals thereafter in order to monitor the development of both primary and secondary foci. Ten-minute ECoG recordings were made on magnetic tape and analysed for epileptiform spikes by the automated method of Hill and Townsend (1973). Monitoring the focal discharges in this way showed that spikes took several days to develop but they then continued for 30 days or more. Epileptiform spikes were recorded not only from the implant side but also from the homotopic point on the contralateral cortex. There was incomplete synchrony between the two hemispheres and many more spikes arose from the secondary focus.

Section of the corpus callosum

The operative procedure for sectioning the corpus callosum is a modification of the technique described by Bures *et al.* (1964) and is described in detail by Ashcroft *et al.* (1972).

Two bur holes (1.5 mm in diameter) were drilled in the skull: one 1 mm anterior to the coronal suture and 1 mm left of the midline; one 1 mm anterior to the lambdoid suture and 1 mm right of the midline. Using a No. 21 curved triangular suture needle a catgut suture was then passed in the anterior bur hole and out the posterior one passing under the dura and the medial sagittal sinus, thus avoiding major haemorrhage. Each end of the suture was then passed through the eyes of two needles fixed 10 mm apart on a steel holder. The needles were inserted vertically into the bur holes to a depth of 4 mm anteriorly and 3 mm posteriorly. The suture was then pulled tight at both ends. The resultant central section cuts through the corpus callosum from splenium to genu and through the commissures of the fornix and hippocampus. However, the anterior and posterior commissures and the habenula remain intact. This was confirmed at *post mortem* in most rats.

This operative procedure will henceforth be referred to as 'callosotomy'. Control animals with cobalt implants were subjected to 'sham callosotomy', in which the entire procedure was carried out except that the ends of the suture were not pulled tight. These surgical procedures were carried out either immediately before cobalt implantation, i.e. in the same operation, or at 2, 4 or 7 days thereafter. All animals were recorded regularly to monitor the development of primary and secondary focal discharges.

RESULTS AND DISCUSSION

Electrocorticogram records from two rats eight days after cobalt implantation into the right frontal cortex are shown in figure 12.1. In the sham-operated animal epileptiform spikes are seen in the ECoG both from the site of the implant and from the contralateral cortex. A secondary focus, as evidenced by asynchrony of discharge together with greater amplitude on the contralateral side, is clearly present.

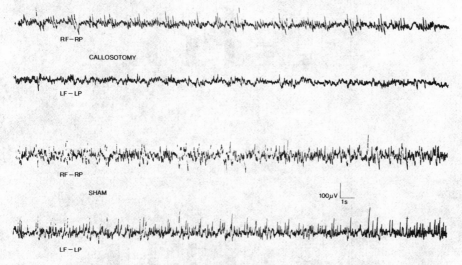

Figure 12.1. Electrocorticogram records obtained eight days after cobalt implantation into the right frontal cortex. Upper two channels from rat subjected to callosotomy procedure. Lower two channels from rat subjected to sham operation. RF–RP bipolar recording between right frontal (primary focus) and right parietal electrodes; LF–LP, bipolar recording between left frontal (secondary focus) and left parietal electrodes

In the rat which had the corpus callosum cut at the time of implantation, although a primary focus has apparently developed normally, there are no epileptiform spike discharges from the secondary focus. This observation was confirmed by objective spike counts.

To demonstrate the effects of callosotomy at various times after implantation the spike counts from groups of at least four animals were averaged. The effects on the development of the primary focus are shown in figure 12.2 which has been simplified by incorporating only some of the recording times for which we have data. However, the general picture would not be altered by that additional data. In both groups of animals, epileptiform spikes first appear at two days, develop over the next week and then persist for several weeks. Callosotomy, either at the time of cobalt implantation or at two or four days thereafter had no significant effect on the level of spiking of the primary focus. Thus there is no evidence from these experiments that the contralateral cortex in cobalt rats exerts an inhibitory influ-

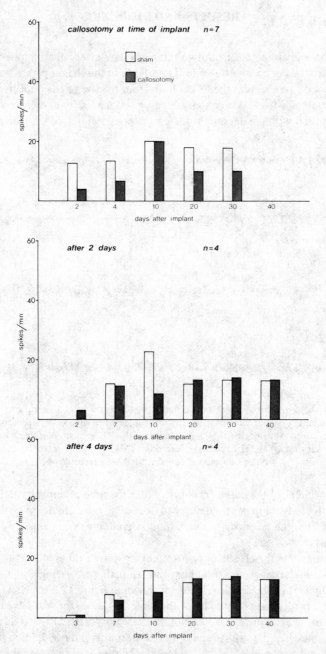

Figure 12.2. Effects of callosotomy on epileptiform spike discharges from the site of cobalt implantation (the primary focus). Ordinate, spikes per min in the ECoG; abscissa, days after cobalt implantation. 'After 2 days' and 'after 4 days' refers to timing of callosotomy or sham operation

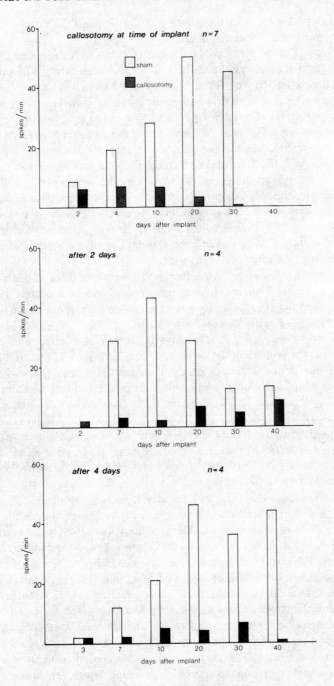

Figure 12.3. Effects of callosotomy on epileptiform spike discharges from the homotopic point on the contralateral cortex (the secondary focus). Details as in figure 12.2

ence on the primary focus via the corpus callosum. Perhaps the anterior commissure might mediate this function in rats.

The effects of callosotomy on the number of spikes arising from the area of the secondary focus are shown in figure 12.3. In the sham-operated group spikes first appear in the contralateral cortex at two days and then persist for several weeks. This time course is similar to that of the primary focus. However, when callosotomy was carried out either at the time of cobalt implantation or at two or four days thereafter, very few spikes were recorded from the area of the secondary focus. In some cases spike counts of five per minute were recorded, contrasting with counts of 40 per minute in the sham-operated group. Even 40 days after implantation a secondary focus had not developed. This is despite the presence of an actively discharging primary focus and despite the presence of other commissural connections between the hemispheres. This suggests that the corpus callosum, or possibly the commissures of the fornix and hippocampus, is the only pathway by which secondary foci are set up following cobalt implantation. Even in the absence of these pathways alternatives do not appear to be used.

Several months after cobalt implantation subconvulsant doses of pentylentetrazole (5 mg/kg i.p.) will produce both primary and secondary discharges. However, in rats subjected to the callosotomy procedure only a primary focus could be elicited confirming the absence of a secondary focus.

If callosotomy is withheld to seven days, it has little or no effect on the development of either the primary or the secondary focus, as is shown in figure 12.4. Similar spike counts are found in both groups of animals. Thus there is no evidence that callosotomy significantly suppresses or enhances established foci. This implies that the secondary focus is no longer dependent on transcallosal connections with the primary. Indeed if the primary lesions/area is removed after seven days the secondary focus persists, although not for as long as usual. As we have shown that callosotomy at seven days does not shorten the life of either the primary or secondary focus, this would suggest that other commissural connections between the hemispheres may be responsible for this effect.

As cobalt salts have been used to trace axonal pathways (Pitman et al., 1972) it seemed possible that cobalt could be transported from the implant via the corpus callosum to the contralateral cortex. The secondary focus itself might even result from the presence of cobalt. Sectioning the corpus callosum would interrupt this transport and this might be why the secondary focus failed to develop. Certainly, Clayton and Emson (1976) found signs of degenerating cells, terminals and axons in the contralateral cortex of cobalt rats. However, using Timm's histochemical method for demonstrating heavy metals, they could not detect increased concentrations of cobalt in the contralateral cortex. We used the more sensitive technique of atomic absorptiometry to measure levels of cobalt in discrete areas of rat brain. Weighed pieces of brain (10-20 mg) were digested in concentrated nitric acid and 20 μl of the digest (equivalent to approximately 1 mg tissue) were injected into the furnace of a Perkin-Elmer HGA 360 atomic absorptiometer. The cobalt peak was measured at 241.5 nm and a standard curve of cobalt prepared over the range 1-50

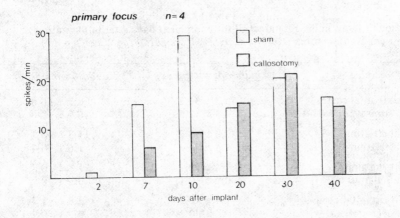

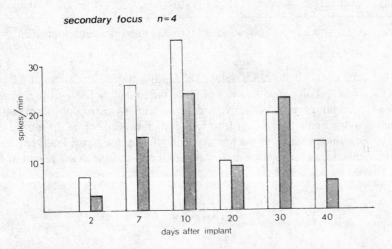

Figure 12.4. Effects of callosotomy at seven days on the number of epileptiform spikes in recordings from the primary focus (upper diagram) and secondary focus (lower diagram)

ppm. The quenching effects of nitric acid were corrected for by analysing control tissues to which known amounts of cobalt were added.

Table 12.1 shows the cobalt distribution, eight days after implantation, in some of the brain areas we have examined. Although the highest concentrations are found round the area of the implant, cobalt is found throughout the right hemisphere extending to the cerebellum and thalamus. Although concentrations in the left side are much lower, significant quantities are found in the region of the secondary focus. However, it does not appear that the cobalt is transported by transcallosal fibres, as callosotomy has no effect on the distribution. Although similar cobalt concentrations are found in the area of the secondary focus in both groups of rats,

Table 12.1

Cobalt levels in discrete areas of rat brain eight days after implantation to right frontal cortex (*Results as μg/g wet weight; mean ± s.e., n = 10*)

Area	Sham-operated group	Callosotomy group
Right frontal cortex	66.2 ± 31.2	58.7 ± 16.8
Left frontal cortex	4.3 ± 1.5	6.0 ± 2.6
Right striatum	7.8 ± 2.0	11.3 ± 3.1
Left striatum	1.6 ± 0.4	1.6 ± 0.4
Right thalamus	1.2 ± 0.1	1.8 ± 0.3
Left thalamus	0.9 ± 0.1	0.9 ± 0.2
Right occipital cortex	1.4 ± 0.3	2.8 ± 1.3
Left occipital cortex	0.8 ± 0.1	0.8 ± 0.1
Right cerebellum	2.1 ± 0.7	1.1 ± 0.3

Callosotomy or sham operation carried out at the same time as cobalt implantation

only the sham-operated animals developed epileptiform spike discharges in this area. Therefore, cobalt *per se* does not produce the secondary focus—it presumably develops as a result of spread of activity from the primary focus probably across the corpus callosum. Some time, i.e. at least four days, is needed before the secondary focus becomes independent of the primary, and interruption of the interhemispheric connections at any time during this period prevents the development of the secondary focus.

SUMMARY

(1) Adult male rats have been rendered epileptic by the implantation of cobalt into the sensorimotor cortex of one hemisphere. The effects of cutting the corpus callosum and the commissures of the fornix and hippocampus on the development of a secondary focus in the contralateral cortex have been examined.

(2) Callosotomy either before or after cobalt implantation had no effect on spike discharges from the primary focus.

(3) Callosotomy up to four days after implantation prevented the usual development of a secondary focus. Other commissural connections do not appear to be used even in the absence of transcallosal fibres.

(4) Callosotomy at seven days had no effect on either the primary or the secondary foci, suggesting that callosotomy had no effect on established foci in the rat.

(5) Cobalt was found in significant concentrations in the contralateral cortex. Callosotomy did not affect cobalt distribution, suggesting that the presence of a secondary focus is unrelated to cobalt concentration.

REFERENCES

Ashcroft, G. W., Dow, R. C., Harris, P., Hill, A. G., Ingleby, J., McQueen, J. K. and Townsend, H. R. A. (1972). Effects of surgical lesions on cobalt-induced epileptic foci in the rat. *Proc. Fifth European Symposium on Epilepsy* (M. J. Parsonage, ed.), pp. 109-15

Bures, J., Buresova, O. and Fifkova, E. (1964). Interhemispheric transfer of a passive avoidance reaction. *J. comp. physiol. Psychol.,* **57**, 326-30

Clayton, P. R. and Emson, P. C. (1976). Spread of cobalt from a cortical epileptic lesion induced by a cobalt–gelatine implant into the frontal cortex of the rat. *Experientia,* **32**, 1303-1305

Dow, R. C., McQueen, J. K. and Townsend, H. R. A. (1972). The production and detection of epileptogenic lesions in rat cerebral cortex. *Epilepsia,* **13**, 459-65

Hill, A. G. and Townsend, H. R. A. (1973). The automatic estimation of epileptic spike activity. *Int. J. Bio-Med. Computing,* **4**, 149-56

Isaacson, R. L., Schwartz, H., Persoff, N. and Pinson, L. (1971). The role of the corpus callosum in the establishment of areas of secondary epileptiform activity. *Epilepsia,* **12**, 133-46

Kopeloff, N., Kennard, M. A., Pacella, B. L., Kopeloff, L. M. and Chusid, J. G. (1950). Section of corpus callosum in experimental epilepsy in the monkey. *Archs Neurol. Psychiat.,* **63**, 719-27

Morrell, F. (1960). Secondary epileptogenic lesions. *Epilepsia,* **1**, 538-60

Mutani, R., Bergamini, L., Fariello, R. and Quattrocolo, G. (1973). An experimental investigation of the mechanisms of interaction of asymmetrical acute epileptic foci. *Epilepsia,* **13**, 597-608

Nie, V., MacCabe, J. J., Ettlinger, G. and Driver, M. V. (1974). The development of secondary epileptic discharges in the rhesus monkey after commissure section. *Electroenceph. clin. Neurophysiol.,* **37**, 473-81

Pitman, R. M., Tweedle, C. D. and Cohen, M. J. (1972). Branching of central neurons: intracellular cobalt injection for light and electron microscopy. *Science* **176**, 412-14

Racine, R., Okujava, V. and Chipashvili (1972). Modification of seizure activity by electrical stimulation. III Mechanisms. *Electroenceph. clin. Neurophysiol.,* **32**, 295-99

Wada, J. A. and Sato, M. (1975). The generalized convulsive seizure state induced by daily electrical stimulation of the amygdala in split brain cats. *Epilepsia,* **16**, 417-30

Woodruff, M. L. (1975). Midbrain and callosal influences on the spread of focal cortical epileptic activity. *Brain Res.,* **85**, 53-8

13
INTEROCULAR TRANSFER OF VISUAL LEARNING IN THE RAT

I. STEELE RUSSELL, J. F. BOOKMAN and G. MOHN

'It is an excellent scientific maxim not to appeal to central processes as long as there remains the possibility of explaining the given phenomenon in peripheral terms.' (Hunter, 1930.)

INTRODUCTION

A basic assumption in the studies of cerebral disconnection is that interocular transfer is perfect in the intact animal. By this we mean that when a normal animal is trained monocularly on a visual discrimination and when the untrained eye is tested on the same task it will show perfect retention of the learned information. Failure of interocular transfer in the split-brain animal is usually taken as evidence of disruption of commissural integration of cerebral unity.

It is the purpose of this chapter to present a series of experiments which cast doubt on that assumption, because they show that normal non-operated rats often show complete failure of interocular transfer (IOT). In accounting for the impairment of IOT in the split-brain animal little attention has been given to the role of peripheral factors. Hunter's maxim that central explanations should defer to the exclusion of peripheral artefacts is as relevant to commissure research as it was to Lashley's work on mass action. Failure to observe this advice has on occasion had disastrous consequences in neurophysiology, e.g. Hernandez-Peon's neglect of peripheral factors that occur during attentional shifts. The necessity to transect the optic chiasm in addition to division of the commissures in order to disrupt interocular transfer in higher mammals is a potential source of considerable artefact. Severe distortions of normal vision occur owing to the loss of visual field resulting from the bitemporal hemianopia. In addition, in cat and monkey there will be considerable defocusing of objects in the proximal field because of the chronic pupillary dilation (Behr's pupil sign) resulting from chiasm section.

Using the rat with its almost completely crossed fibres in the optic chiasm, lateralisation of the visual input can be obtained by monocular eye occlusion. This was done by using a textile patch which was attached by surgical adhesive cement to one side of the animal's head. Not only did this ensure a lightproof coverage of one eye, but it did so in a completely benign and atraumatic fashion. The training appa-

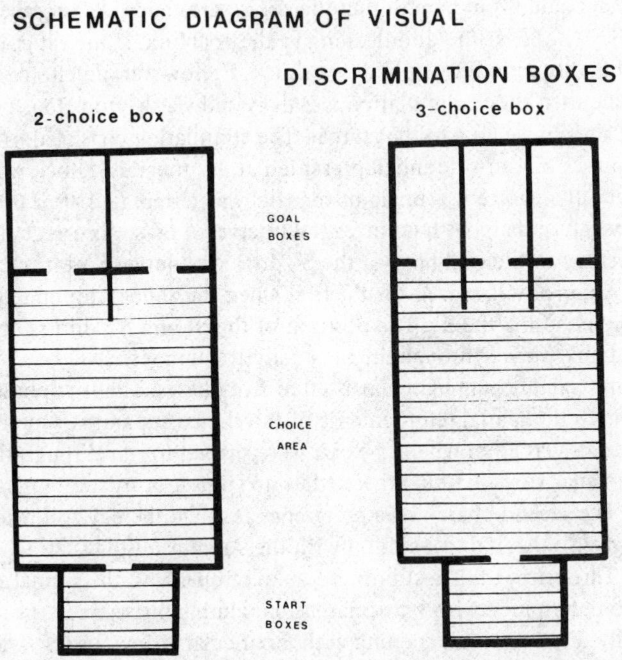

SCHEMATIC DIAGRAM OF VISUAL

DISCRIMINATION BOXES

2-choice box   3-choice box

GOAL
BOXES

CHOICE
AREA

START
BOXES

Figure 13.1. The ground floor plan for both two- and three-door Malet boxes. The shock grid does not continue into the goal box areas, which had hardboard flooring. For clarity no attempt is made to represent the start or goal box doors

ratuses used are shown schematically in figure 13.1. Essentially each consists of a start box (30 × 25 cm) connected via a choice area (60 × 45 cm) to the separate goal boxes (each 30 × 25 cm). The 20 cm high walls of each compartment and the floor of the goal boxes were painted a uniform orange colour which to the rat's monochromatic vision appears as neutral grey. The grid floor of the start box and choice area was composed of 1 cm stainless steel rods spaced at 2.5 cm intervals. The 20 cm high walls of the apparatus were covered by a clear Perspex ceiling. A double-door system separated the start box from the choice area. A vertical guillotine door, which was used to start the trial sequence, gave access to the choice area via a second flap door. This door was hinged from the ceiling and only opened in the forward direction to prevent retracing. The door to each goal box was similarly flap-hinged, with cardboard visual stimulus displays attached to the front of each door. A 15 cm long divider panel was inserted between each pair of doors to facilitate the scoring of errors.

The animals were trained on the visual discrimination tasks using shock motivation. A correction procedure was always used, whereby each trial was continued until the animal made a correct choice and entered the goal box. A trial sequence began when the animal was placed in the start box with the guillotine door closed. After 10 s the door was raised and a 5 s avoidance period was started. During this time the animal could avoid by entering the choice area and selecting the correct stimulus display (S^+) over the door leading to the goal box. If the rat entered the goal box during this period it would avoid shock. If, however, no choice was made within this time then shock stimulation was delivered via the grid floor of both the start box and the choice area to the animal. The stimulation consisted of 0.5 s square wave pulses of 1 mA dc shock presented at 2 s intervals. Shock was continued either until a choice was made or the trial was terminated after 60 s. Thirty such trials were given daily with an intertrial interval of 60 s. A correct choice was defined as an entry to the goal box via the S^+ door without any prior response to the S^- door. An error was scored for the trial when the animal responded to the S^- door before choosing the S^+. The position of the S^+ and S^- doors for each trial were randomly varied throughout each daily training session.

The standard training paradigm consisted of five phases. The first phase pretrained the rats to the spatial requirements of the choice apparatus. One training session of 30 trials was given where the rats were shaped to run through the apparatus with binocular vision. During these trials no stimulus cards were placed on the choice doors. The second phase was a preference test. On the day following shaping the rats were given a 20-trial test session with the stimulus displays attached to the choice doors. Throughout this test both doors were open and the animal's stimulus preference was determined with binocular vision. During phase three the animals were given daily discrimination training with monocular vision. The S^+ was the non-preferred stimulus and the S^- was the preferred stimulus. Training was continued until a criterion of 18 consecutively correct responses was made within one daily session. Following completion of discrimination training the rats were tested for interocular transfer. In phase four the rats were tested for retention of the discrimination, with each eye, on separate days. In each group of rats the order of testing with either the trained or naive eye was counterbalanced. Each test consisted of 20 trials where the stimuli were randomly presented. In phase five the rats were monocularly retrained with the naive eye to the original learning criterion to obtain a relearning measure in addition to the retention scores. The combination of measures was used because the use of savings scores derived from relearning measures can have certain weaknesses. Non-specific factors, such as learning set and test sophistication, can all produce as great a facilitory effect on savings scores as can the effect of specific transfer of training. The contribution of these non-visual components of the discrimination could well facilitate acquisition with the naive eye and thus bias the results in the direction of overestimating the amount of interocular transfer.

ROLE OF NON-VISUAL FACTORS IN INTEROCULAR TRANSFER

From several points of view it would appear that many of the standard conventions of discrimination training are geared to encourage non-visual strategies in the solution of the visual problems. An example is the use of the pseudo-random Gellerman sequences which although effective in suppressing position preferences nevertheless do encourage such sequential behaviours as Win–Stay or Lose–Shift patterns of responding. Indeed in every experiment it is a common occurrence to observe an animal make a correct response without any demonstrable visual inspection of the choice alternatives. Furthermore the almost invariable use of a two-choice comparison test method can additionally favour switching strategies where, after making a false choice, the animal simply selects the other alternative. To do this, visual guidance is neither necessary nor indeed is it appropriate as there is no other possibility. Obviously, then, in standard tests of visual performance such confounding of both visual and non-visual elements could well lead to the danger of a serious overestimation of the amount of interocular transfer in a commissure-sectioned or normal animal.

The present experiment undertook therefore to examine interocular transfer both where the participation of non-visual components in the discrimination performance was allowed and where such non-visual strategies were excluded. A group of 32 normal hooded rats were trained to make a two-choice black-white discrimination using the standard avoidance training procedure described previously. A second group of 32 rats were trained using the same procedure on the same task in a three-choice situation. The three-choice situation gives greater randomisation of the position of the visual display cards, such that simple sequential strategies are ineffective in finding the correct door. Furthermore switching responses are made ineffective by virtue of the fact that an incorrect response no longer reduces uncertainty, as an animal is still faced with two remaining alternatives.

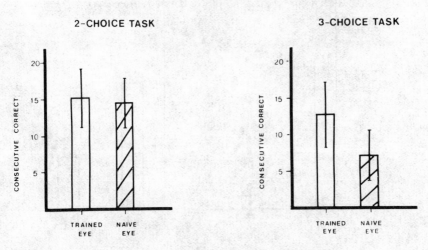

RETENTION OF BRIGHTNESS DISCRIMINATION

Figure 13.2. Retention scores for each eye following monocular training on either a two-choice or three-choice brightness discrimination. The average number of consecutive correct choices made in each 20 trial retention test

When both groups were tested for interocular transfer considerable differences were found between them. The animals that had learned a two-choice discrimination showed no difference in retention scores between the performance with the trained eye and that with the untrained eye. Overall retention was above 95% and as can be seen in figure 13.2 run lengths of 15 consecutively correct choices were made with either eye. Furthermore the retraining scores showed 92% savings, as only a few trials were required to reach criterion with the naive eye. Thus both measures were in agreement in establishing that there was perfect interocular transfer following two-choice discrimination training.

The contribution of non-visual factors to this performance is clearly considerable when the results of the three-choice discrimination task are considered. A comparison of the naive eye with the trained eye reveals a severe impairment of interocular transfer. As can be seen in figure 13.2 the trained eye had a retention of 13 consecutively correct responses, with the overall retention being 91% correct. Retention by the untrained eye was markedly inferior, with a retention score of 75% and a run of seven consecutively correct responses. Following retention testing the animals were divided into two sub-groups and retrained on the same problem. One group was retrained with the original eye and the other with the untrained eye (i.e. the eye that showed poor IOT). The original learning and relearning scores are given in figure 13.3. It can be seen that virtually no relearning trials are required if the same eye is used. When, however, the untrained eye is retrained almost 60 trials are required to learn. This represents a saving of only 58%, which together with

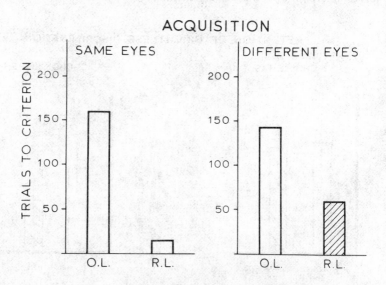

Figure 13.3. Acquisition scores for the three-choice monocular brightness discrimination. Trials to criterion are plotted for relearning (RL) the problem either with the same eye or different eye from that used during original learning (OL)

the retention scores shows a severe impairment in IOT. Thus, in so far as the three-choice training excluded sequential strategies and response switching, it would appear clear that these non-visual components of the discrimination played a significant role in the apparently perfect IOT in the two-choice situation.

EFFECT OF DECISION TIME ON INTEROCULAR TRANSFER

In the previous experiments each training trial began with a 5 s avoidance period during which the animal was free to make its choice without shock stimulation. The intention was that this time period would permit the rat to enter the choice area and have adequate time to make visual comparisons of the choice stimuli without any distraction by shock. It is possible that this period could be used by the animals not for visual inspection of the choice stimuli but for sequential learning. The likelihood of this possibility arises from the fact that on those trials where the rat was inspecting the choice stimuli when the avoidance period ended, the onset of shock would act as a punishment for such visual comparisons.

Accordingly an investigation was made of the effect of eliminating the decision time (avoidance) on discrimination learning and IOT. For this two groups of rats were trained on the two-choice discrimination task. A control group of 10 rats was monocularly trained on a black-white discrimination with the standard avoidance procedure. An experimental group of 10 rats was also monocularly trained on the same task using an escape procedure to eliminate the decision time period. In this group, as soon as the guillotine door was raised in the start box there was an immediate presentation of shock to the grid floor. In all other respects the training procedure was identical for both groups.

Both groups learned the discrimination in the same number of trials, suggesting that the variable of decision time was not a powerful determinant of learning. Although it does not significantly affect the rate of acquisition it nevertheless had a clear effect on interocular transfer. As can be seen in figure 13.4 there was perfect IOT of the black-white discrimination when it was learned with the avoidance paradigm. Performance of the trained and the naive eye was 95% and 93%, respectively, with run lengths of 12 and 11 consecutively correct choices. These results are comparable with those obtained for two-choice learning in the previous experiment. When the results of the escape group (i.e. animals trained without any decision time) are examined, a clear impairment of IOT is found. Overall performance during retention testing gave 96% correct for the trained eye with 69% correct for the naive eye. As can be seen in figure 13.4 the trained eye made 14 consecutively correct whereas the naive eye made only seven consecutive. The relearning scores for this group were 38 trials to relearn the original discrimination with the naive eye. This gives 49% savings on the original learning of 78 trials. Thus the decision time available to the animal to make a choice as to which visual target to select directly affects the amount of IOT obtained. This would suggest that the use of the avoid-

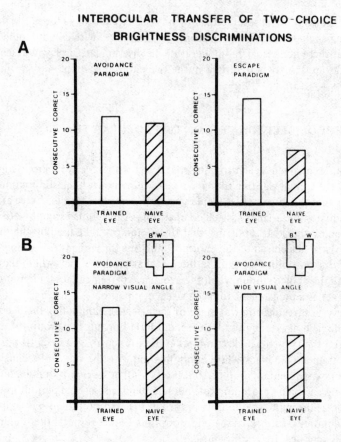

Figure 13.4.   Determinants of interocular transfer. (A) A comparison of the effects of learning with an avoidance versus an escape paradigm. (B) The effect of changes in visual angle in interocular transfer

ance paradigm not only failed to facilitate visual choice behaviour but may well have contributed to the susceptibility of the animal to employ non-visual strategies in its discrimination.

EFFECT OF CHANGES IN VISUAL ANGLE ON INTEROCULAR TRANSFER

The last experiment clearly demonstrated that the use of the two-choice procedure itself is not inherently subject to contamination by non-visual artefacts such as sequencing and switching strategies. Rather it would appear that this occurs when there is no time constraint on the actual choice behaviour itself. Where the animal is given minimal choice time it would appear that the optimal pay-off is to concentrate on visual cues and to ignore non-visual strategies in the solution of the discrimination. Under these circumstances it is possible that the discrimination performance becomes closely linked to the animal's monocular scanning patterns.

It is therefore possible that an additional factor responsible for the impairment of IOT in the three-choice box could be related to this variable of monocular scanning. In this situation the animal, in addition to being confronted with a greater number of visual choices (3 versus 2), has also to contend with a broader visual horizon than it does in the two-choice situation. Obviously the visual angle over which the animal must scan to examine the visual targets is much greater for the three-choice situation. The present experiment was designed to disentangle the relative contributions of the size of visual angle and the number of choices as determinants of IOT. A three-choice box was accordingly modified to provide either a wide angle two-choice situation or a narrow angle two-choice task. For a wide visual angle the apparatus was altered by blocking off the centre choice area with a barrier across the two partitions (see figure 13.4B). The narrow visual angle was obtained by using only two adjacent choice areas by closing off one side of the apparatus on each trial (see figure 13.4B). The position of the closed off side was varied randomly from left to right throughout training to control against the possible genesis of motor patterns specific to the start box centre choice door axis.

Animals were trained monocularly on the black-white discrimination using the avoidance paradigm. No significant differences in acquisition were obtained between groups, although the narrow visual angle group took slightly more trials to reach criterion than did the wide visual angle group. Despite this, IOT for this group was found to be perfect. Retention overall was around 90% and 95% for both eyes with run lengths of 13 and 12 consecutive correct for the trained and naive eye, respectively (see figure 13.4B). With the wide visual angle a marked impairment in IOT was found. Here the naive eye showed a poor overall retention of 73% and only eight consecutively correct responses. The trained eye in contrast showed 95% correct overall with a run length of 15 consecutive correct responses. The relearning scores show 52% savings for the naive eye, which supports the picture of impaired IOT following training with a wide visual angle. These results suggest that where the animal has to scan over the broad visual angle to compare visual targets then in some way discrimination performance becomes dependent upon this monocular condition. It is possible that, during monocular occlusion, the animal develops stereotyped oculomotor scanning strategies to enable it both to compensate for the reduction in visual field and effectively survey the broader horizon required by the wide angle task. The performance of the discrimination could then become state-dependent to such oculomotor habits which would be disrupted by reversal of eye occlusion.

EFFECT OF REPEATED TESTING ON INTEROCULAR TRANSFER

In all of the experiments considered so far, the results have all been obtained from animals tested for IOT after training on a single problem. It is entirely possible that different results would be obtained with animals that had been accustomed to learn-

ing under monocular eye occlusion, i.e. trained to several problems. If for example
an impairment in IOT was found only on the first problem but was then observed
to disappear on subsequent problems, then the most likely explanation would be
that it was an effect of novelty. In particular terms the explanation offered as to
the failure of IOT with a wide visual angle could well be accounted for as an artefact
of novelty. If the apparent failure in IOT derived from a monocular dependency on
oculomotor scanning habits, it would be expected that when the naive eye was
tested there would be a disruption in performance. Further it would also be expected
that repeated exposure to the training situation with each eye should therefore
familiarise the animal such that it is accustomed to visual 'search' routines with
either eye. Experience acquired from learning a series of different visual problems
could then be expected to lead to perfect IOT.

To examine this possibility two groups of 10 rats were monocularly trained with
the same eye on three successive visual problems using the three-choice situation.
In the first group the animals were trained on a brightness problem (black versus
white), then an orientation discrimination (vertical versus horizontal) and finally a
two-dimension form discrimination (diamonds versus squares).

Figure 13.5 gives the results of the retention tests for all three tasks. As expected,
poor IOT was obtained on the brightness problem. The trained eye showed an overall retention of 91% with a run length of 15 consecutive correct responses. The
naive eye, as can be seen in figure 13.5, obtained only eight consecutive correct
choices, with an overall retention score of 68%. The performance on the IOT tests
for the subsequent problems showed a progressive increase in the impairment

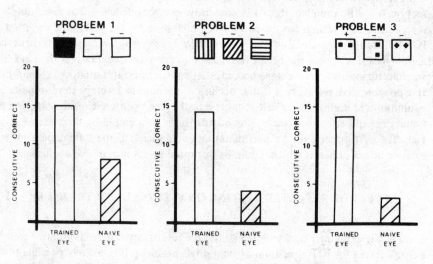

Figure 13.5. The effect of repeated monocular training on interocular transfer

of IOT. As can be seen in figure 13.5, the difference between the trained and naive eyes for the line orientation task is much greater than it was for the previous brightness problem. This trend continues for the pattern discrimination where the naive eye scores only three consecutively correct choices compared with the 15 consecutive of the trained eye. At this point it is interesting to note that the performance by the naive eye is no better than chance or that of an untrained animal. Contrary to expectation, these results show that the impairment in IOT in the normal rat does not dissipate with test sophistication. The fact that impairment was maintained over three different visual problems clearly excludes novelty as a contributing factor.

The results strongly suggest that the amount of IOT is determined by the type of visual input. The three problems used can be graded in complexity level from the brightness task, then the orientation task to the pattern problem being the most demanding. Here complexity would be defined in terms of the type of feature extraction that is required to distinguish between the visual displays. For the brightness problem the requirement is minimal, compared with either of the other tasks. It would appear that where the visual display required detailed feature extraction the amount of IOT diminished. A second group of animals were monocularly trained under the same conditions on these same problems, but in the reverse order. They were given the pattern task first, then the orientation problem and finally the brightness discrimination. The results showed that IOT depended upon the type of visual input and hence an order effect could be excluded. Thus the amount of IOT is determined by the extent to which the animal is involved in detailed visual scanning responses during monocular discrimination learning.

ROLE OF VISUAL SCANNING MECHANISMS IN INTEROCULAR TRANSFER

The finding of the last experiment concerning the potential role of visual scanning mechanisms in IOT may well provide a clue to a unifying theme for the present series of experiments as a whole. A common factor in these situations is that the degree of IOT appears to be related to the extent that the problem encourages the animal to develop patterns of visual scanning responses as part of the solution of the discrimination. Table 13.1 provides a summary of the differing situational variables and their effect on IOT. It can be seen that when visual scanning involving efficient or detailed oculomotor integration is required then IOT deteriorates. It would appear as if the monocular visual guidance system used by the animal in the discrimination performance becomes highly dependent upon or tied to these visuomotor mechanisms. When the monocular occlusion is changed to the opposite eye then there will be a lateral inversion of such oculomotor patterns. Where the animal's performance is tightly coupled to such visuomotor integrations then reversed eye patching will produce a profound disorganisation of its visual guidance system, and block IOT. From this point of view the summary of the experiments on IOT provided by Table 13.1 would now appear more coherent and less arbitrary. For example, the effects of training with either a three-choice or a wide angle two-choice

Table 13.1

Testing conditions	IOT
Number of choices	
two-choice	Perfect
three-choice	Impaired
Decision time	
long	Perfect
short	Impaired
Visual angle	
narrow	Perfect
wide	Impaired
Visual input	
brightness	Perfect
orientation	Impaired
pattern	None

task are the same in terms of impairing IOT. These tasks also required more visual scanning over a wide horizon, and thus increase the animal's susceptibility to being dependent on oculomotor habits. Changes in the amount of decision time have a similar effect. Animals trained with an escape paradigm are forced to adopt highly efficient visual guidance of their behaviour in order to minimise shock.

If in all these cases the observed failure of IOT was due to the blocking of the discrimination record by a misalignment of oculomotor integration, it would follow that if this misalignment could be corrected then the impairment in IOT would disappear. The last experiment was concerned to explore this possibility, by attempting to 'decouple' the visual discrimination from the animal's visual guidance habits in the three-choice box. In order to do this the standard training procedure was

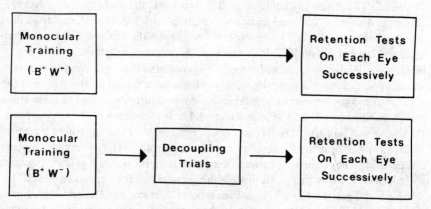

Figure 13.6. Schematic of decoupling procedure

modified slightly by the interpolation of an additional training procedure (figure 13.6). This consisted of a session of 10 'decoupling' trials given the day after mono-cular learning and before testing for IOT. This decoupling procedure was intended to break the animal's dependency on the original monocular visuomotor habits by giving the naive eye visual experience in the test situation, without exposing it to the discrimination. In this manner it was intended that the procedure would realign the animal's visuomotor co-ordination without giving any additional discrimination training.

EFFECT OF DECOUPLING WITH BINOCULAR VISION

A group of eight rats were initially monocularly trained on a brightness discrimina-tion using the avoidance paradigm in the three-choice situation. After reaching criterion the animals were given the decoupling procedure with both eyes open and the display cards removed from the goal box doors, to preclude discrimination learning during this phase. During these trials one door was open and the other was closed. The position of the open door was randomly changed over the 10 trials. On the following days the animals were then tested for IOT with the black and white display cards replaced on the goal box doors. The results are given in figure 13.7(A) and show a clear impairment in IOT. The retention of the trained eye was at 90% with 15 consecutively correct choices, whereas the naive eye showed an overall re-tention of less than 70% correct, scoring only six consecutively correct. It was clear that the decoupling procedure was without any effect.

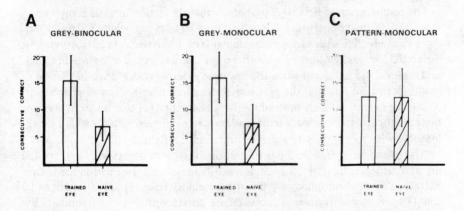

Figure 13.7. The role of oculomotor habits in interocular transfer. All groups were monocular-ly trained on a three-choice brightness discrimination. (A) The effect of 10 binocular decoup-ling trials before IOT testing. (B) Effect on IOT of 10 decoupling trials with the trained eye occluded. (C) The effect of novel visual information during the 10 decoupling trials with the trained eye occluded

EFFECT OF DECOUPLING WITH MONOCULAR VISION

One possible reason for the lack of effect of the decoupling treatment could be that the monocular training produced an ocular dominance. If this were the case then it is possible that the animals only processed visual information with the trained eye and did not use the naive eye. A second group of eight rats were trained on the same three-choice brightness discrimination as before. During the decoupling procedure the trained eye was occluded in order to force visual guidance by the untrained eye. The same stimulus conditions and alternation procedure were used as in the previous group. The results of the IOT tests were negative as can be seen in figure 13.7(B). The trained eye had an overall retention of 95% correct with a run of 16 consecutively correct choices. The retention by the naive eye was impaired with a performance of 74% overall correct where only seven consecutively correct choices were made. There was still a marked impairment in IOT, despite the attempt to familiarise the naive eye visually.

A final group of eight rats were monocularly trained as before on the same brightness discrimination. As the previous groups had been exposed to a visually uniform choice area during the decoupling procedure it is possible that this visually featureless situation acted as a ganzfeldt and served to de-emphasise visual processing even further by the naive eye. In order to safeguard against this possibility the decoupling procedure was slightly modified. During the 10 trials when the animals were trained with the naive eye, vertical–horizontal striated display cards were placed over the goal box doors. Thus the orientation discrimination stimuli provided novel visual material for the animals to inspect during the decoupling procedure. At the same time it was unrelated to the originally trained brightness task and could not therefore serve to contribute to any additional training.

The results, given in figure 13.7(C), show that this procedure was completely successful. Both eyes performed equally during IOT testing, where retention was approximately 90% with each eye making at least 13 consecutive correct responses. Perfect IOT was only obtained when the naive eye was forced to engage in visual guidance and did not occur when there was no external visual 'demand'. These results clearly indicate that the previous observations of either impaired or absent IOT in the normal rat were misleading. They suggest rather that under many conditions monocular training leads to dependence on oculomotor habits which can interfere with accessibility to visual information stored in the brain.

The relevance of these findings to split-brain research is obvious. First, the failure of interocular transfer does not necessarily mean that information has been lateralised to one hemisphere as a unilateral memory trace. The impairment of IOT could be due to an information access failure caused perhaps more frequently by peripheral factors than has been realised. The fact that an impairment in IOT can be induced by oculomotor integration mechanisms implies that much more emphasis should be given to normal control observations than has frequently been the case. It is certainly clear that an impairment in IOT can by itself no longer be attributed to a failure in hemispheric integration.

Conversely, it is also possible that the presence of apparently perfect IOT does not necessarily derive from the presence of a bilateral record of the information. Efficient IOT could equally well be obtained from a unilateral trace that was binocularly accessible. Furthermore, such sensory access could be achieved either by the peripheral pathways of the optic chiasm or such central ones as the corpus callosum or other commissures.

The present report also suggests that failure of IOT need not always be symptomatic of a disconnection syndrome where communication between hemispheres has been disrupted due to some central lesion. On the contrary it would suggest that under certain conditions an absence of interhemispheric communication is a characteristic of the intact brain. Indeed for tactile discriminations with primates (Semmes and Mishkin, 1965) it is well known that intermanual transfer (IMT) is frequently not seen in normal animals whose only experimental experience is unimanual training. Reliable transfer is only seen when animals are given extensive experience with each hand separately prior to IMT testing.

Wall (1970) drew attention to the possibility that animals can adopt different strategies to solve various tactile problems dependent on the type of sensory input that they use, i.e. whether or not they use information from joint or tactile receptors. Joint receptors, particularly those of the fingers of the hand, project entirely contralaterally in the monkey to cortical areas devoid of callosal connections. It is possible therefore that such tactile information would remain confined to the input hemisphere. Support for this conjecture is found in the report (Butler and Francis, 1973) that there is a total lack of IMT in normal monkeys trained on a tactile discrimination requiring the use of joint receptors.

On interhemispheric communication of visual information in the intact brain following monocular input several points need to be made. First, the failure to observe any IOT does not necessarily imply an absence of interhemispheric communication. Test conditions have been reported where information is relayed from one hemisphere to the other, but cannot be initially utilised by the other hemisphere (Butler, 1968; Noble, 1968). On other occasions the failure of IOT may be due to an absence of interhemispheric communication despite the presence of an intact commissural system. Several reports have shown the trained hemisphere to learn normally and then fail to exchange this information across the midline (Berlucchi, 1972; Butler, 1966; Zeki, 1967). Anatomical studies have shown that commissural connections do not arise with equal density from all brain areas—for example, the main connections of the corpus callosum arise from neurons in the cortical area representing the vertical meridian (Berlucchi and Rizzolatti, 1968; Cragg and Ainsworth, 1969). Hence, such disturbances of interhemispheric communication may well be attributable to an absence of callosal connections.

Alternatively, the practice of monocular testing may not only be anomalous but could itself facilitate ocular independence and de-emphasise IOT (van Hof and Steele Russell, 1977; Voneida and Robinson, 1970). The present findings have drawn attention to a wide range of conditions where monocular training leads to a dependency on oculomotor habits which can interfere with IOT. Furthermore, marked ocular asymmetries that totally disrupt IOT have been reported to occur spontaneously in 30% of normal intact rabbits (van Hof and van der Mark, 1976). It would appear unlikely that this ocular dominance derives from any hemispheric asymmetry as its incidence has been found to be independent of neonatal eye patching (van Hof and van der Mark, 1976). It is possible that this phenomenon is an artefact of monocular training, and it could well be another example of discrimination learning becoming state dependent on oculomotor habits.

Considering the role of visuo-oculomotor integration in the split-brain animal, there are two major reasons to suspect that the cerebral bisection procedure in combination with monocular occlusion would result in marked abnormalities of visual function. First, midsaggittal section of the optic chiasm produces clear signs of pupillary dysfunction. The pupils are typically dilated (Behr's pupil) and show abnormalities of constriction during blinking, eye movement and also during flash stimulation (Pasik and Pasik, 1972). The Pasiks (1964) first drew attention to the role of the corpus callosum as a pathway for visuo-oculomotor integration. They found that following chiasm section electro-oculograms were entirely normal. Symmetrical responses were obtained during optokinetic stimulation for both monocular and binocular conditions, e.g. stimulation of the right eye produced normal optokinetic nystagmus (OKN) both to the left and the right. Section of the corpus callosum severely impaired this, and produced a pronounced dissociation of the OKN. Stimulation of the right eye gave a normal response to the left but not to the right, where the nystagmus was profoundly impaired. This deficit was only uncovered with monocular testing, because entirely normal responses were obtained with binocular stimulation. As conjugate gaze mechanisms and OKN are subserved by the same pathways (Bender and Shanzer, 1964; Pasik and Pasik, 1964) it is likely that both are similarly affected by transection of the corpus callosum. Thus it is probable that monocular training in the split-brain animal would produce difficulty in recognising the visual problem which could appear distorted to the untrained eye. For example, Bender and Feldman (1967) have found evidence that impairments in conjugate gaze can lead to aberrations in visual perception. Further, Trevarthen (1965) has suggested that such deficits in conjugate gaze could cause neglect of half of the horizontal stimulus array in the testing of split-brain monkeys and thus disrupt IOT.

A second source of artefact derives from the bisection of the optic chiasm. This will result in a loss of the nasal hemiretinae, producing a bitemporal hemianopia. Under monocular conditions the horizontal visual angle is drastically reduced to $65°$ in the chiasm-sectioned monkey compared with $155°$ in the normal animal. There is no reduction in the visual angle in the vertical meridian. In view of this it is not unreasonable to expect anomalies in IOT as a consequence of the abnormal nature of the compensatory eye movements that are required to restore horizontal panoramic vision during monocular eye closure. Because of the lack of change in the vertical meridian these changes in oculomotor integration would be restricted to the horizontal plane.

Anomalies in IOT in either chiasm-sectioned animals or in species with almost total crossing of the fibres in the optic chiasm have frequently been reported when they were tested with 'mirror-image' pattern orientations (Hamilton *et al.*, 1973; Starr, chapter 28 in this volume). Typically, animals when they are monocularly trained with an oblique striation task would, when tested for IOT with the untrained eye, select the opposite orientation to the one with which they had been originally trained. This mirror-image transfer although widely reported for laterally reversed displays has never been observed for vertical pattern inversions, suggesting the phenomenon is related to the field deficits produced by the bitemporal hemianopia. This would implicate the role of visuo-oculomotor mechanisms where the performance of the discrimination becomes tied to the pattern of compensatory visual scanning movements. Thus, for example, a 45° oblique display could be coded as a feature oriented *nasal-up* and *lateral-down*, *when using the left eye*. Thus when the right eye is tested for IOT such a visuomotor code would match the 135° obliques and mis-match the original 45° striations due to the lateral inversion of the visuomotor co-ordination.

The anatomical explanation (Noble, 1966) of mirror-image IOT in terms of a topographic inversion of sensory information by the commissures between hemispheres, is not only highly speculative but also factually inaccurate.

An overall consideration of the present findings and related studies of IOT make it clear that the role of visuo-oculomotor mechanisms has been seriously neglected. In lower mammals with laterally implanted eyes, it was demonstrated that IOT could be frequently blocked by the state-dependency of the learning on monocular visuomotor habits. In higher mammals the disruption of IOT following chiasm and commissure section is no longer solely explicable in terms of memory confinement to one hemisphere. Alternative explanations, such as deficits in conjugate gaze and anomalies of visual scanning due to visual field impairment, now deserve serious consideration.

REFERENCES

Bender, M. B. and Shanzer, S. (1964). Oculomotor pathways defined by electrical stimulation and lesions in the brain stem of monkey. In *The Oculomotor System* (M. B. Bender, ed.), Harper and Row, New York, pp. 81–140

Bender, M. B. and Feldman, M. (1967). Visual illusions during head movement in lesions of the brain stem. *Archs Neurol.* **17**, 354–64

Berlucchi, G. (1972). Anatomy and physiology aspects of visual functions of the corpus callosum. *Brain Res.*, **37**, 371–92

Berlucchi, G. and Rizzolatti, G. (1968). Binocularly driven neurons in visual cortex of split-chiasm cats. *Science*, **159**, 308–10

Butler, C. R. (1966). Cortical lesions and interhemispheric communication in monkeys. *Nature*, **209**, 59–61

Butler, C. R. (1968). A memory record for visual discrimination habits produced in both cerebral hemispheres of monkey when only one hemisphere has received direct visual information. *Brain Res.*, **10**, 152-67

Butler, C. R. and Francis, A. C. (1973). Split-brain behavior without splitting: tactile discriminations in monkeys. *Israel J. med. Sci.*, **9**, Suppl., 79-84

Cragg, B. G. and Ainsworth, A. (1969). The topography of the afferent projections of the circumstriate visual cortex (CVC) of the monkey studied by the Nauta method. *Vision Res.*, **9**, 733-49

Hamilton, C. R., Tieman, S. B. and Winter, H. L. (1973). Optic chiasm section affects discriminability of asymmetric patterns by monkeys. *Brain Res.*, **49**, 427-31

Hunter, W. S. (1930). A consideration of Lashley's theory of the equipotentiality of cerebral action. *J. gen. Psychol.*, **3**, 455

Noble, J. (1966). Mirror-images and the forebrain commissures in the monkey. *Nature*, **211**, 1263-5

Noble, J. (1968). Paradoxical interocular transfer of mirror-image discriminations in the optic chiasm sectioned monkey. *Brain Res.*, **10**, 127-51

Pasik, T. and Pasik, P. (1964). Optokinetic nystagmus: an unlearned response altered by section of the chiasma and corpus callosum in monkeys. *Nature* **203**, 609-11

Pasik, T. and Pasik, P. (1972). Transmission of 'elementary' visual information through brain commissures as revealed by studies on optokinetic nystagmus in monkeys. In *Cerebral Interhemispheric Relations* (J. Cernacek and F. Podivinsky, eds), Slovak Academy Science, Bratislava, Czechoslovakia, pp. 267-85

Semmes, J. and Mishkin, M. (1965). A search for the cortical substrate of tactile memories. In *Functions of the Corpus Callosum* (G. Ettlinger, ed.), Churchill, London

Trevarthen, C. (1965). Functional interactions between cerebral hemispheres of the split-brain monkey. In *Functions of the Corpus Callosum* (G. Ettlinger, ed.), Churchill, London, pp. 24-41

Van Hof, M. W. and Steele Russell, I. (1977). Binocular vision in the rabbit. *Physiol. Behav.*, **19**, 121-28

Van Hof, M. W. and van der Mark, F. (1976). Monocular pattern discrimination in normal and monocularly light-deprived rabbits. *Physiol. Behav.*, **16**, 775-81

Voneida, T. J. and Robinson, J. S. (1970). Effect of brain bisection on capacity for cross comparison of patterned visual input. *Expl Neurol.*, **26**, 60-71

Wall, P. D. (1970). The sensory and motor role of impulses travelling in the dorsal columns towards cerebral cortex. *Brain*, **93**, 505-24

Zeki, S. M. (1967). Visual deficits related to size of lesion in prestriate cortex of optic chiasma sectioned monkeys. *Life Sci.*, **6**, 1627-38

14
SOME STUDIES OF
INTERHEMISPHERIC INTEGRATION IN
THE RAT

I. STEELE RUSSELL and SARAH C. MORGAN

INTRODUCTION

The most central problem of the study of the commissures and hemispheric integration is the question of whether or not a single or a duplex record of experience is established in the brain. In other words when an animal is trained on a visual problem with binocular vision, is the information stored as two separate and independent records in the two hemispheres, or as a single record across both hemispheres? The interest in the question derives from the early work of Sperry (1961) which established the essential point that monocular visual training in the cat with both chiasm and commissures sectioned resulted in memory lateralisation to one hemisphere. By contrast, monocular training in either the chiasm-sectioned or the callosum-sectioned animal did not produce memory lateralisation. These findings were interpreted to imply that in the normal intact brain the visual information is integrated during binocular vision by both the chiasm and the commissural system to result in two separate records, one in each cerebral hemisphere. This is what is known as the bureaucratic theory of the brain, where everything is stored in duplicate form at least at a cortical level. If we consider the colliculi, it may even be necessary to think in terms of quadruplicate storage.

A number of papers have drawn attention to the fact that in fish (Savage—see chapter 3), pigeon (Graves and Goodale—see chapter 6), and rat (Cowey and Parkinson, 1973; Levinson and Sheridan, 1969; Russell and Safferstone, 1974; Russell et al.—see chapter 13), monocular training per se has a number of anomalous features in many testing situations. Furthermore, in higher mammals, such as cat and monkey, the bisection of the optic chiasm results in a profoundly altered visual preparation from several points of view. The division of chiasm produces both a permanent pupil dilation (Behr's pupil sign) and a bitemporal hemianopia. In such an animal one would expect neither normal visual learning under monocular training conditions nor a memory record similar to that in normal animals. Instead of arguing from the findings of split-brain experiments as to whether or not learning in normal animals entails a single record or dual records, it is believed that a different approach is required. A more appropriate model for normal brain organisation during visual learning is obtained from animals with intact commissures that have been trained with binocular vision. If a duplex memory system normally subserves learning, then retention of learning should be perfect following hemidecortication. This in the rat is relatively simple to do and the animal sustains it easily with no motor side effects such as circling or unilateral hemiplegia. Furthermore the rat has the additional advantage that due to the almost complete crossover of optic fibres, division of the chiasm is not necessary for routing of the visual input to one hemisphere.

EFFECT OF HEMIDECORTICATION UPON RETENTION OF A BRIGHTNESS DISCRIMINATION

The first experiment undertook to examine the nature of the cortical engram established for a simple brightness discrimination. The animals were given successive discrimination training using an operant go/no-go procedure. All animals were given identical pretraining in a Skinner box to establish a stable pattern of bar pressing prior to visual learning. This entailed 10 days of bar training where every bar press was rewarded by a pellet of food (FR1). Following this they were shaped by successive approximations to an intermittent reward schedule of one food pellet for every 15 responses (FR15). After five days of stabilisation at FR15, discrimination training was started. The visual stimuli used for the brightness discrimination consisted of the presence or absence of the ambient illumination provided by an overhead light in the ceiling of the test chamber. For half the animals the positive stimulus (S^+) was the presence of light, and for the remainder it was the absence of light (S^-). Throughout training an asymmetrical reward procedure was used. During each daily 60-min training session the presentation of S^+ and S^- periods was alternated at 2-min intervals, with FR15 reinforcement during S^+ and no reward given during S^- periods. During each session 30 such alternations of S^+ and S^- stimuli were given. Each group of six rats received at least 75 days' binocular training to ensure reliable asymptotic performance of the discrimination.

Following this, one group of animals was hemidecorticated by surgically removing the pial vascular bed from the surface of one hemisphere and asphyxiating the underlying cortex. Care was taken to avoid any damage to the sagittal and transverse sinuses, as well as the olfactory bulb. This procedure results in a relatively atraumatic and uniform decortication in the rat and avoids damage to subcortical structures such as the dorsal hippocampus. The completeness of the removal varied from 80% to 95% in the animals studied. Following the operation all animals were given six weeks to recover, after which they were retrained on the discrimination. The results showed a clear memory deficit, where all signs of retention of the originally learned discrimination appeared to be lost following the removal of one cortical hemisphere. Figure 14.1 gives a comparison of the first 10 days of the original acquisition with the first 10 days of the relearning of the task following hemidecortication by the same animals.

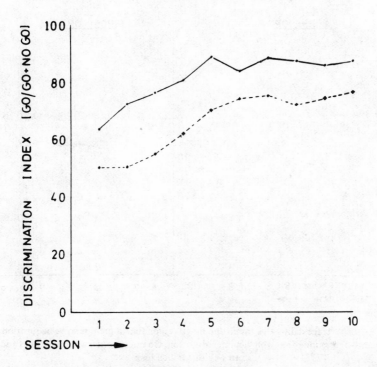

Figure 14.1. The average daily discrimination index (go/go + no-go), throughout the first 10 days of acquisition for normals (solid line) and the first 10 days of retraining after hemidecortication (dashed line)

The learning curve for both was obtained from the percentage of correct responses out of each daily response total. Looking at the initial acquisition curve, when the rats learned the task with both hemispheres intact, it can be seen that within the first session the animals had already significantly departed from the chance level of 50%, and by the tenth session had attained an 80% correct discrimination level. With subsequent training the discrimination level approached an asymptote of 95% correct responding. Examining the relearning curve there is no indication of any retention of the former learning during the first 10 days of retraining. Performance during the first two days stayed at chance and thereafter the acquisition curve more or less parallels the original learning curve. Control animals that had received a sham operation followed by a six-week recovery period showed perfect retention when exposed to the retraining.

An examination of the separate response rates for the go and no-go periods revealed that the animals learned the discrimination by suppressing responding during the no-go periods. Figure 14.2 shows that, during original learning, response rates to both S^+ and S^- started at equal levels and during training the rate remained constant to S^+ but declined systematically to S^-. Looking at the retraining phase it is immediately apparent that the animals relearned the discrimination in a totally

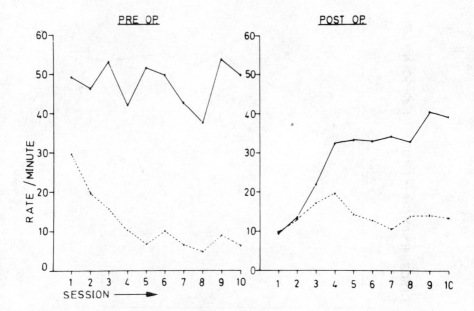

Figure 14.2. Average daily rates for go and no-go responding in pre-operative acquisition and postoperative retraining following hemidecortication. Go rates are given by solid lines and no-go rates by the dashed lines

different way from that during original acquisition. The effect of hemidecortication appeared to produce a total disruption of the memory record, as can be seen by the loss of all bar pressing both to the S^+ and the S^- stimuli. Both the go and no-go responding build up over the first few sessions with a subsequent fall in the no-go responding as the discrimination is relearned. However, it should be noted that the level of S^- responding declines more slowly than it did during original learning. In fact the level of errors remains high over the next 30 or 40 days of retraining.

An alternative interpretation of these results could be that the effect of hemidecortication was not an interference with memory, but rather a reduction in motivation level which would lead to a loss of responding. Two sources of evidence however make this unlikely. First, the disruptive effect of hemidecortication on memory was solely restricted to the discrimination problem. Animals which had only learned an FR15 bar press task without any discrimination requirement were not affected by hemidecortication. Following recovery from the operation these animals had perfect retention of the bar press task, which showed not only that there was no motivational deficit but also that this simple learning was represented in duplex form in the brain. Secondly, not all discrimination trained animals showed such a massive postoperative lowering of the overall response rate. One example can be seen in figure 14.3. Looking at the pre-operative discrimination performance it can be seen that the animal was responding at approximately 95% correct. Six weeks after hemidecortication the first retraining session shows an initial reduction in responding

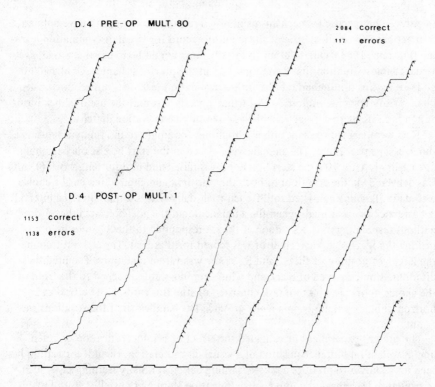

Figure 14.3. Cumulative response records for an individual pre-operative go/no-go discrimination and also the first postoperative retention test on the same animal. The sequence of S^+ and S^- periods in the 60-min training period is indicated by the event marker at the bottom of the lower tracing

followed by a rapid recovery of responding. There is a complete absence of the discrimination, which is relearned without savings during the subsequent 30 days of retraining. This loss of the discrimination without any motivational deficit suggests that there is a unitary memory record for the brightness task.

EFFECT OF HEMIDECORTICATION ON RETENTION OF VISUAL DISCRIMINATION MOTIVATED BY SHOCK

The previous experiment presented evidence that argued strongly against a dual memory record. However, it was noted from control observations that the interdependency or unity of the two hemispheres appeared to be dependent upon the presence of a learned visual discrimination. Nevertheless these results could be peculiar to the use of a go/no-go procedure. It could be argued that the loss of cortex, and in particular the damage to frontal cortex, resulted in the animals having difficulty in inhibiting a learned response. Thus the effect of hemidecortication might well be specific to mechanisms of no-go response control, and have only an indirect bearing on the nature of the memory record for visual discrimination learning (Pribram, 1961). One solution to this dilemma would be to use the two-choice visual training situation that we reported on in the previous chapter. Unlike go/no-go learning this simultaneous either/or discrimination task does not require or depend on any response inhibition. A further advantage is that the use of shock motivation is a safeguard against possible lesion-induced motivation deficits.

Rats were trained to make either a brightness or a pattern discrimination using a shock escape procedure. The animals were placed in the start box at the beginning of each trial. After 10 s the start box door was raised and intermittent shock (1 mA) was delivered via the grid floor of both the start box and choice area until a choice was made. Training consisted for 30 such trials daily with a 1 min intertrial interval. A correct choice was made when the animal entered the goal box with the S^+ door without responding to the S^- door. If the rat responded to the S^- door before making the S^+ choice, then an error was scored for that trial. Throughout training the left-right position of the S^+ and S^- doors was varied randomly. The brightness discrimination consisted of black and white stimulus cards attached to the front of the choice doors. The pattern task consisted of stimulus cards with vertical and horizontal black striations on a white ground. The bandwidth of the striations was 5 mm.

The present experiment investigated the effect of hemidecortication on retention as well as on initial acquisition of a visual discrimination. Hemidecortication has been long known to produce a severe learning deficit for many learning tasks such as avoidance learning and go/no-go discrimination learning (Russell, 1969). Dependent on the particular details of the situation, this deficit can be either marginal or considerable (Russell and Plotkin, 1972). No such deficit has, however, been reported for either simple Pavlovian tasks or Pavlovian discriminations (Oakley and Russell, 1975, 1976). It would appear that one factor in common with tasks that show a hemidecorticate learning deficit is that they readily lateralise in the split-brain animal. It would further suggest that during normal learning both cortical hemispheres operate as a unitary whole; hence the learning deficit that results from the disconnection of one hemisphere from another.

Effect of hemidecortication on binocular visual learning

The first experiment therefore examined the effect of hemidecortication on the learning of both brightness and pattern discriminations. A group of normal and a group of hemidecorticate rats were first trained on the brightness task and then the pattern problem. A further group of normal and a group of hemidecorticate animals learned the same tasks in a counterbalanced order, i.e. the pattern problem first and the brightness second. There were eight rats in each group. The hemidecorticated animals were surgically prepared 6–8 weeks before the beginning of the experiment in the same manner as was earlier described. All animals in each group were binocularly trained to the same criterion of 18 consecutive correct choices for each problem.

Looking at the results, we can see in figure 14.4 the learning curves for both normal and hemidecorticate groups for first the brightness and then the pattern problem. The learning curves are here presented in terms of the number of trials required to attain each criterion out of an ensemble of training criteria arranged from high to low. Thus the number of trials are given to reach 3 consecutively correct choices, followed by 6, 9, 12, 15 and 18 consecutive. Thus a learning profile can be examined across an entire range of criterion levels.

The performance of the normal animals on the first problem showed a clear inflection point in the number of trials required for the different criterion levels. An asymptote in difficulty level was approached between the nine and 12 consecutive correct criteria. The hemidecorticates showed a marked learning deficit which increases as a direct function of the criterion level. At the 18 consecutive correct level

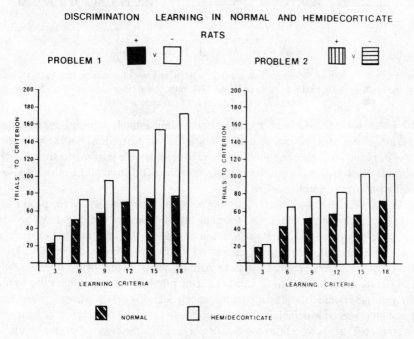

Figure 14.4. Average number of trials to successive criterion levels of consecutive correct choices for both normal and hemidecorticated rats. Both groups were exposed to the brightness task first, and were then given the pattern problem. The stipled columns represent the trials to criterion (exclusive of criterion trials) for the normal animals' performance. Similarly the plain columns represent the performance by the hemidecorticate animals

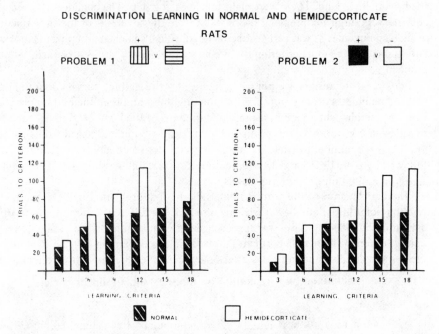

Figure 14.5. Learning by normal and hemidecorticate animals of a pattern task first, followed
by the brightness discrimination. As in figure 14.4, only the average number of trials to reach
criterion were plotted for each criterion level

the deficit was maximal, with the hemidecorticated animals requiring approximately
100 more trials than normal animals to reach the same criterion. For the single hemisphere animal on the second problem there is considerable learning-to-learn effect,
which is much less in the normal animal. Nevertheless there is still a substantial and
highly significant learning deficit.

Figure 14.5 gives the results for the two groups of animals where the problems
were learned in reverse order, i.e. striations first followed by the brightness problem.
On the first problem the normals took approximately the same number of trials to
reach criterion as did the normal animals on the first problem in the previous groups.
The hemidecorticates showed the same learning deficit as that of the previous hemidecorticate animals and also required the same number of trials as those did to reach
criterion (see figure 14.4). The hemidecorticate learning deficit was still present
although it was considerably reduced in comparison to the normal performance.
From these results two principal points emerge. First, the removal of one hemisphere produces a generalised deterioration in the learning of both visual discriminations. Secondly, there is no apparent difference in difficulty level of either the pattern or brightness tasks for both normal and hemidecorticate animals. Independent
of the task material the first problem was always more difficult to learn than the
second. The fact that both the brightness and pattern problems were learned with
equal ease is of great significance when retention results are considered.

Retention of binocular visual learning after hemidecortication

The main experiment is concerned with the effect of hemidecortication on retention of previous learning. Three separate groups, each of eight normal animals, were
trained on the black-white discrimination with binocular vision. Following acquisition of this discrimination, two groups were hemidecorticated, and a sham operative
procedure was given to the control group. All three groups were allowed six weeks to
recover from surgery during which time no training was given. After this period they
were then retrained with binocular vision. In each group of eight hemidecorticated
animals half of the animals had the right hemisphere and half had the left hemisphere removed.

As can be seen in figure 14.6 there were no differences between any of the groups
when their initial acquisition was examined. Considering retention first in the normal

NORMAL ACQUISITION AND RETENTION OF A
BRIGHTNESS DISCRIMINATION AFTER
HEMIDECORTICATION

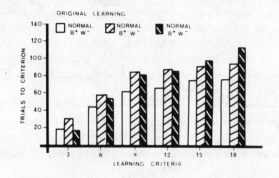

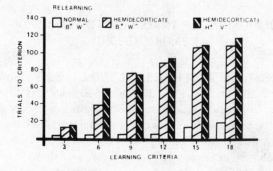

Figure 14.6. Normal acquisition and retention of a brightness discrimination after hemidecortication. The average scores of each group are plotted for each criterion level during original
learning and subsequent retention

control animals, it is clear that there was no spontaneous loss of the training due to forgetting during the six-week recovery period. Performance at all criterion levels was virtually perfect, requiring no more than a few trials to regain the highest criterion. In the hemidecorticate groups a totally different picture was seen. Both required as many trials to relearn the task as they did in the beginning. The most obvious interpretation of these results would be that they reflect a total loss of the visual memory. However, this conclusion should not be accepted without reservation, when it is recalled that naive hemidecorticates take approximately twice as long as normal animals to learn a visual task (see figures 14.4 and 14.5). The present results (figure 14.6) gave no evidence of any hemidecorticate learning deficit, as the relearning following hemidecortication is identical to original learning, i.e. it is characteristic of normal learning. This comparison clearly suggests that there is some preservation of the memory record.

It is for that reason that the control hemidecorticate group is crucial. They were initially trained on the brightness problem, and following recovery from hemidecortication they were then retrained on the pattern discrimination. This task has previously been shown (figure 14.4 and 14.5) to be indistinguishable in difficulty level from the brightness problem. The results showed that whether or not the animals received postoperative training on the same or on a different problem, none the less the outcome was the same. There were no savings for the animals, when they were retrained on the same or a new problem. Therefore these results argue very strongly that hemidecortication resulted in a complete loss of the visual memory record. The absence of a hemidecorticate learning deficit is explicable in terms of the fact that the relearning is equivalent to acquiring a second and a different problem where such a deficit is minimal.

Thus, considering both the go/no-go and the either/or discrimination results, it would appear that this type of visual learning has a single representation in the brain where the memory trace encompasses both hemispheres as a unitary whole. There is no evidence to suggest that separate and independent records exist in each hemisphere.

EFFECT OF MONOCULAR TRAINING ON DISTRIBUTION OF THE MEMORY RECORD

A number of papers (van Hof and Russell, 1977; Voneida and Robinson, 1970) have drawn attention to the possibility that monocular training is different from binocular in terms of its de-emphasis of interhemispheric integration mechanisms. Accordingly the last experiment was concerned to evaluate the effect of hemidecortication upon retention of visual learning following monocular training, to see if this affected the distribution of the memory trace. Figure 14.7 shows schematically the general experimental procedure. The animals, after initial monocular training, were divided into two sub-groups each of eight rats, which were hemidecorticated by using cortical spreading depression (CSD) and then tested for retention. This experi-

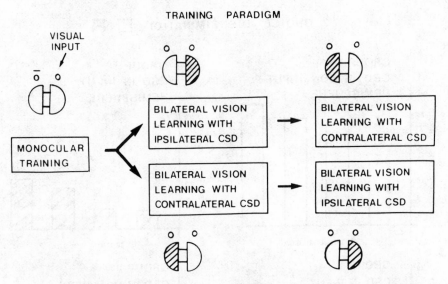

Figure 14.7. Schematic of the experimental procedure. Following monocular training on a brightness discrimination, the animals were tested for binocular retention of the task with either the primary-input or the secondary hemisphere functionally decorticated

mental procedure has the main advantage that results are obtained from animals uncontaminated by any possible contribution of neural compensation. A further benefit is that the use of CSD also permits repeated testing of the same animals where each hemisphere can be functionally ablated on successive occasions.

Two groups were compared. One group, after the monocular training, was first tested with binocular vision with the secondary hemisphere depressed, i.e. the hemisphere that did *not* receive the primary visual projection during learning. Following this they were then tested with the primary hemisphere depressed, i.e. the hemisphere that received visual information via the primary crossed projections in the optic chiasm during original training. The other group was exposed to the same procedure but in counterbalanced order. Each testing phase consisted of four 30-trial sessions of training where two sessions were given on each of two consecutive days. On each day, there was a 30-min rest interval between training sessions. The longest run of consecutive correct responses was plotted for each session.

Looking at the results in figure 14.8, for the first group, we see that when the non-input hemisphere is depressed there is perfect retention. There was no effect of hemidecortication in terms of interfering with the discrimination performance. All animals retained the task perfectly well, with a 90% overall level of correct responding. On the first session the longest run of consecutive correct responses was 15, followed by 28, 28 and 29 on the subsequent sessions. The finding of perfect retention following hemidecortication of the non-input hemisphere has two main implications. First, it establishes the point that hemidecortication by itself was atraumatic. As such the memory loss produced by hemidecortication after binocular training

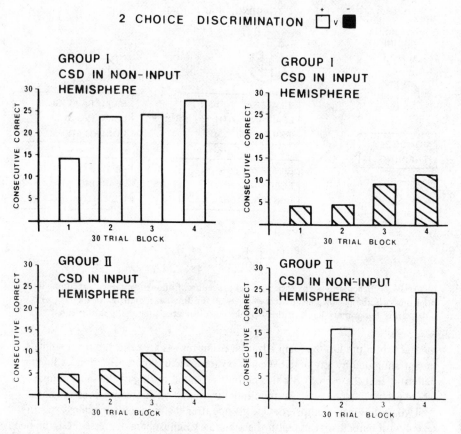

Figure 14.8. Retention scores following hemidecortication of either the primary or secondary hemisphere. The longest run of consecutive correct responses is given for each 30-trial retention test

cannot then be attributed to non-specific effects of the surgical procedure. Secondly, these results suggest that the non-input hemisphere contained no elements of the memory record. In marked contrast to this, when the primary input hemisphere was depressed, there appeared to be a complete obliteration of the memory trace. This was indicated by the presence of a *de novo* acquisition curve, where the animals performed identically to naive surgical hemidecorticates (see figure 14.4). The results for the second group (see figure 14.8, lower row) gave the same outcomes when the testing was given in counterbalanced order, thus excluding any dependence on order effects.

To conclude, it would appear that under normal conditions of training an animal establishes a single memory record with both hemispheres highly unified. Interference with either hemisphere surprisingly results in a substantial if not a total impairment of the memory record. Whether or not the memory loss is total remains to be seen.

What is beyond question is that any notions of a duplex memory record seem highly unlikely for complex visual learning as opposed to such simpler problems as non-discriminative bar press tasks.

Following monocular training a remarkably different picture emerged. Under these conditions animals appeared to have also established a single memory record, but one which was clearly localised to one hemisphere. The other hemisphere contained no information in store of the monocular learning. This finding does not seem to be restricted to rats but has also been found in primates. Both Myers (1962) and Downer (1962) reported that, in the chiasm-sectioned monkey, after monocular training it was possible to show interocular transfer. However, if these trials were kept to a minimum and the callosum was cut, then interocular transfer was abolished. The untrained eye no longer has access to the lateralised information. If this is true for both simple and advanced mammals it would suggest that in the split-brain rat and also the split-brain monkey the severance of the callosum does not lateralise memory and confine it to one hemisphere. What does occur instead is that the monocular training *alone* results in memory being stored in a lateralised form. Cutting the corpus callosum then denies the animal the opportunity to access that record from the naive or non-input hemisphere. Thus information retrieval from the unilateral record is interfered with by callosal section, and memory lateralisation occurs due to monocular training.

REFERENCES

Cowey, A. and Parkinson, A. M. (1973). Effects of sectioning the corpus callosum on interocular transfer in rat. *Expl Brain Res.*, **18**, 433–45

Downer, J. L. de C. (1962). Interhemispheric integration in the visual system. In *Cerebral Dominance and Interhemispheric Relations* (V. B. Mountcastle, ed.), Johns Hopkins Press, Baltimore

Levinson, D. M. and Sheridan, C. L. (1969). Monocular acquisition and interocular transfer of two types of pattern discrimination in hooded rats. *J. comp. physiol. Psychol.*, **67** (4), 468–72

Myers, R. E. (1962). Transmission of visual information within and between the hemispheres: A behavioral study. In *Cerebral Dominance and Interhemispheric Relations* (V. B. Mountcastle, ed.), Johns Hopkins Press, Baltimore

Oakley, D. A. and Russell, I. S. (1975). Role of cortex in Pavlovian discrimination learning. *Physiol. Behav.*, **15**, 315–21

Oakley, D. A. and Russell, I. S. (1976). Subcortical nature of Pavlovian differentiation in the rabbit. *Physiol. Behav.*, **17**, 947–54

Pribram, K. H. (1961). A further experimental analysis of the behavioral deficit that follows injury to the primate frontal cortex. *Expl Neurol.*, **3**, 432

Russell, I. S. (1969). Cortical mechanisms and learning. In *Animal Discrimination Learning* (N. S. Sutherland and R. Gilbert, eds.), Academic Press, London, pp. 335–56

Russell, I. S. Plotkin, H. C. (1972). Interhemispheric relations and learning in the split-brain rat. In *Cerebral Interhemispheric Relations* (J. Cernacek, ed.), Slovak Academy of Science, Czechoslovakia, pp. 299-317

Russell, I. S. and Safferstone, J. F. (1974). Interocular transfer and stimulus control of visual discriminations in the rat. *Brain Res., 66*, 355-56

Sperry, R. W. (1961). Cerebral organization and behavior. *Science, 133*, 1749

van Hof, M. W. and Russell, I. S. (1977). Binocular vision in the rabbit. *Physiol. Behav.,* **19** 121-29

Voneida, T. J. and Robinson, J. S. (1970). Effect of brain bisection on capacity for cross comparison of visual input. *Expl Neurol., 26*, 60-71

15
ULTRASTRUCTURE AND CONDUCTION PROPERTIES OF VISUAL CALLOSAL AXONS OF THE RABBIT

HARVEY A. SWADLOW and STEPHEN G. WAXMAN

INTRODUCTION

The corpus callosum of most mammals is comprised of both myelinated and non-myelinated axons, most of which are less then 1 μm in diameter (Fleischhauer and Wartenberg, 1967; Seggie and Berry, 1972; Tomasch, 1954; Tomasch and MacMillan, 1957; Waxman and Swadlow, 1976a). Characteristics of impulse conduction along such axons in the central nervous system are relatively unstudied. In the present chapter we review our work on the ultrastructure and conduction properties of visual callosal axons of the rabbit and also present preliminary data on the conduction properties of callosal axons of the macaque monkey.

For ultrastructural studies, adult Dutch rabbits (12–24 months) were perfused through the left ventricle with physiological saline followed by 5% gluteraldehyde in 1/15 M Sorensen's phosphate buffer (pH 7.4). Subsequent specimen preparation methods have been previously described (Waxman and Swadlow, 1976b). In physiological studies, extracellular single-unit recordings were obtained from visual areas I and II (Swadlow, 1977; see also chapter 16) of chronically prepared unanaesthetised, unparalysed adult Dutch rabbits. Recordings were obtained from the cell bodies of neurons which sent an axon across the corpus callosum (callosal efferent neurons). Recording techniques have been described previously (Swadlow, 1974a; Swadlow and Waxman, 1976). Banks of stimulating electrodes were implanted near the midline of the corpus callosum, and in some cases at other locations along the course of the callosal axons. Electrical stimuli were presented singly or, in order to determine the dependence of conduction properties on prior activity, in pairs (a conditioning stimulus followed by a test stimulus). In some cases the conditioning stimulus consisted of a train of pulses. In other experiments, stimuli were triggered at various intervals following a spontaneous spike. Callosal efferent neurons were identified by their antidromic activation following electrical stimulation of the callosal axon. Antidromic activation was differentiated from synaptic activation by means of collision tests (Bishop et al., 1962; Swadlow, 1974a), and by examination of refractory periods and spike waveform (Bishop et al., 1962; Phillips, 1959; Phillips et al., 1963).

For units which were shown to be antidromically activated by stimulation of the corpus callosum, latency to a single test pulse was determined at various intervals following either a single conditioning pulse or a train of conditioning pulses. Conditioning and test pulses in most cases were delivered via the same electrode. Since variations in both threshold and latency to a test volley follow conditioning volleys, the stimulus threshold was determined at each conditioning stimulus-test stimulus interval and the test stimulus intensity was adjusted to 1.2× threshold value at that particular conditioning stimulus-test stimulus interval.

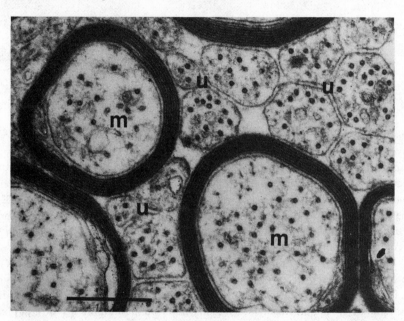

Figure 15.1. Electron micrograph showing a transverse section through the splenium of the rabbit corpus callosum. Both myelinated (m) and non-myelinated axons (u) are present. Calibration bar indicates 0.5 μm

ULTRASTRUCTURE OF CALLOSAL AXONS

Figure 15.1 presents an electron micrograph of the rabbit splenium. Both myelinated (m) and non-myelinated (u) fibres are present. Non-myelinated axons generally are found in small clusters of at least 3–4 axons. Most myelinated axons are less than 1 μm in diameter. Figure 15.2 presents a fibre diameter spectrum of 872 axons in the rabbit splenium. Non-myelinated axons comprise 45% of this sample and ranged from 0.08 to 0.6 μm ($\overline{X}$ = 0.20, s.d. = 0.08). Myelinated axons ranged from 0.3 to 1.85 μm ($\overline{X}$ = 0.74, s.d. = 0.24). In low power fields containing thousands of axons, occasional axons larger than 2 μm were seen, but these were very rare. Both myelinated and non-myelinated axons have a morphology typical of that of central axons (Hirano and Dembitzer, 1967).

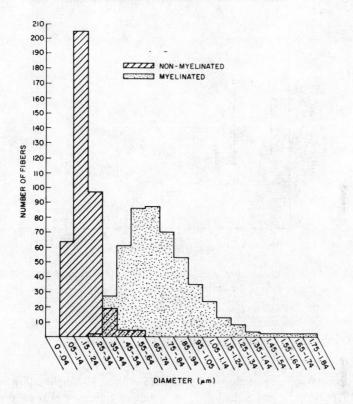

Figure 15.2. Diameter spectra for myelinated (stippling) and non-myelinated axons (oblique lines) in the splenium of the rabbit corpus callosum. (From Waxman and Swadlow, 1976b)

CONDUCTION VELOCITY AND REFRACTORY PERIODS

Figure 15.3 shows the estimated conduction velocity of 75 visual callosal axons. Conduction velocities range from 0.3 to 12.9 m/s and have a median value of 2.8 m/s. These values are similar to those which would be expected on the basis of the diameter spectrum, assuming that the relationship between conduction velocity and diameter is similar to that for peripheral nerve (Gasser, 1950; Hursh, 1939; Rushton, 1951). On the basis of the above morphological data, we can conservatively estimate (Swadlow and Waxman, 1976) that axons with a conduction velocity of less than 0.8 m/s are non-myelinated and that axons with conduction velocities of more than 3.4 m/s are myelinated.

The refractory period of most callosal axons studied was determined using double-volley antidromic stimulation at 2× threshold intensity. Refractory periods ranged from 0.6 to 2.0 ms (Swadlow and Waxman, 1976) and as in peripheral nerve (Paintal, 1967), the faster axons generally had shorter refractory periods than did the slower axons.

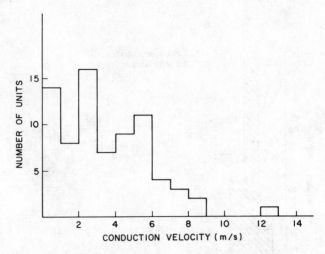

Figure 15.3.   Estimated conduction velocity of 75 visual callosal axons in the rabbit (From Swadlow and Waxman, 1976)

THE SUPERNORMAL PERIOD

All but two axons of more than 100 studied (Swadlow, 1974b; Swadlow and Wax-man, 1976; Waxman and Swadlow, 1976a), showed a decrease in latency and thres-hold to an antidromic test stimulus that followed an antidromic conditioning stim-ulus at appropriate intervals. At conditioning stimulus-test stimulus intervals of 1–2 ms (during the relative refractory period) an increase in latency and threshold to

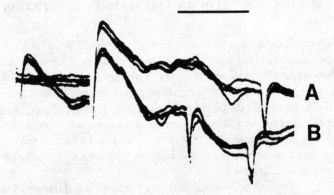

Figure 15.4.   (A) Oscilloscope tracing showing antidromic latency to a test stimulus presented in the absence of a conditioning stimulus. The latency is 12.1 ms. (B) The test stimulus is pre-sented 5.2 ms following a conditioning stimulus and the latency to the test stimulus is reduced to approximately 11.2 ms. The calibration bar equals 5 ms. Positivity is downward.

the test stimulus was usually observed. At intervals of 2–4 ms, latency and threshold decreased below control values to reach a low value at intervals of 3–17 ms.

In figure 15.4(A), an antidromic test stimulus is presented in the absence of an antecedent conditioning stimulus. Control latency is 12.1 ms. In figure 15.4(B), an antidromic test stimulus is presented 5.2 ms. following an antidromic conditioning stimulus. Threshold to the test stimulus at this conditioning stimulus-test stimulus interval was 21% lower than the control value. To minimise the possibility of activating the axon further from the stimulating electrode, the intensity of the test stimulus was reduced by 21%. Latency to the test stimulus at this interval was approximately 11.2 ms.

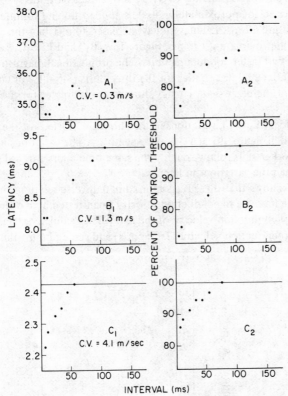

Figure 15.5. (A_1–C_1) Variations in latency to antidromic activation for three neurons with axon conduction velocities of 0.3, 1.3 and 4.1 m/s. Latency to antidromic activation to a test stimulus, as a function of conditioning stimulus-test stimulus interval, is shown. The antidromic latency at each conditioning stimulus-test stimulus interval is represented by closed circles. Pairs of stimuli were delivered at a rate of 1/3.3 s. Each conditioning stimulus is presented at 1.5× threshold intensity. The test stimulus is presented at a fixed multiple (1.2×) of threshold at each conditioning stimulus-test stimulus interval. (A_2–C_2) Variations in threshold to antidromic test volley following a single antidromic conditioning volley for the same three units which were presented in A_1–C_1. The changes in threshold follow a similar time course to the changes in latency. (From Swadlow and Waxman, 1976)

Note that the decrease in latency is due to a decrease in the latency of the 'A' or axon hillock component of the spike.

In figure 15.5(A_1–C_1), the antidromic latency to a test stimulus is shown as a function of conditioning stimulus-test stimulus interval for three units of different conduction velocities (control conduction velocities of 0.3, 1.3 and 4.1 m/s, respectively). The conditioning stimulus is presented at 1.5× threshold in all cases. The test stimulus is presented at 1.2× threshold at each conditioning stimulus-test stimulus interval. Latency at each conditioning stimulus-test stimulus interval is represented by the closed circles. Figure 15.5(A_1) shows a very slow callosal axon, with a control antidromic latency of 37.5 ms (conduction velocity = 0.3 m/s). Latency decreased to approximately 34.7 ms at conditioning stimulus-test stimulus intervals of 10 and 17 ms. Latency slowly increased to re-attain the control value at an interval of approximately 170 ms. Figure 15.5(B_1) and 15.5(C_1) show decreases in latency for two faster conducting units. The proportional magnitude of the maximal decrease in latency was similar for the three units (7.5–11% of control values). The duration of the decrease in latency, however, was greater for the slower conducting axons.

In figures 15.5(A_2–C_2), variations in threshold are plotted for the same three units presented in figures 15.5(A_1–C_1), respectively. The variations in threshold for these and for other cells follow roughly the same time course, or a slightly longer time course than the variations in latency.

Figure 15.6 shows that there is an approximate inverse relationship between the duration of the increase in conduction velocity (manifested by a decrease in latency) and the control conduction velocity of the axon. The sample contains many myelinated axons (conduction velocities > 3.4 m/s) and some non-myelinated axons

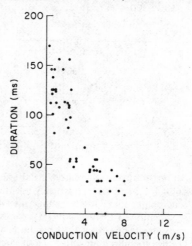

Figure 15.6. Relationship between conduction velocity and the duration of the decrease in latency for the callosal axons. Each point represents a single unit (From Swadlow and Waxman, 1976)

(conduction velocities < 0.8 m/sec). The duration of the increase in conduction velocity appears to vary continuously with conduction velocity, and there is no discrete change which might suggest a qualitative difference between myelinated and non-myelinated axons.

As noted above, the refractory period also appears to vary continuously with the conduction velocity of the axon. These findings on central axons are similar to those of Paintal (1967), who observed that although rise time, fall time and spike duration of peripheral myelinated and non-myelinated axons vary systematically with conduction velocity, there is no obvious qualitative difference between the two types of fibres.

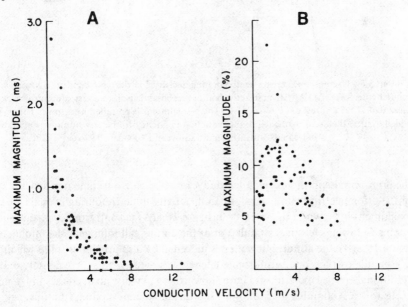

Figure 15.7. Relationship between conduction velocity and magnitude of the decrease in latency. (A) The maximum absolute magnitude of the decrease in latency; (B) the relative magnitude (percent decrease) of the decrease in latency. (From Swadlow and Waxman, 1976)

Figure 15.7(A) shows the maximal *absolute* magnitude of the decrease in latency for the units in which this variable was studied. The maximal *absolute* magnitude of the decrease in latency is much smaller for fast units than for slow units.

Figure 15.7(B) shows, for the same units, the relationship between *proportional* magnitude of the maximal latency decrease and conduction velocity. The magnitude of the decrease in latency ranged from 3% to 22% of the control latency. No consistent relationship between the proportional magnitude of the decrease in latency and the conduction velocity was observed.

Various control experiments indicate that the reduction in latency resulted from

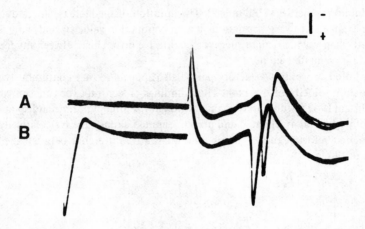

Figure 15.8. Oscilloscope tracing demonstrating decreased antidromic latency following a spontaneous spike. (A) Antidromic activation of a callosal neuron to a test stimulus (arrow) presented at 1.2× threshold intensity. (B) The test stimulus is preceded by a spontaneous spike which triggers the oscilloscope. Note the reduction in latency to the test stimulus. Calibration bar equals 5 ms. (From Swadlow and Waxman, 1976)

the prior impulse in the axon under study, rather than from some non-specific effect of the prior electrical stimulation, or from activity in neighbouring axons. One such experiment is shown in figure 15.8. In figure 15.8(A), an antidromic spike is elicited 4.9 ms following electrical stimulation of the corpus callosum near the midline. In figure 15.8(B), the antidromic volley is preceded by a spontaneous spike which triggers the oscilloscope. Antidromic latency was reduced to approximately 4.4 ms. Additional control experiments have shown that (1) while no decreases in latency occur to a test stimulus that follows a sub-threshold conditioning stimulus, decreases in latency of a similar magnitude and time course occur to a test stimulus that follows a conditioning stimulus which is presented at either 1.1 or 1.5× threshold; and (2) when the intensity of conditioning stimulus is just at threshold, a decrease in latency occurs to the test stimulus only when the conditioning stimulus results in a spike (Swadlow and Waxman, 1976).

The physiological studies also show that the activity dependent variations in conduction velocity occur along the main axonal trunk within the corpus callosum. For these experiments, two pairs of stimulating electrodes activate the axon at different distances from the cell body. In figure 15.9(A), for example, latency to antidromic activation to a test stimulus is shown as a function of conditioning stimulus-test stimulus interval for a unit stimulated via electrodes 2 mm to the right of the midline (contralateral to the recording microelectrode). In figure 15.9(B) the same neuron is activated by stimulation 2 mm to the left of the midline. Although durations of the decrease in latency in the two experiments are approximately equal, the magnitudes of the decrease in latency following stimulation at the two sites are

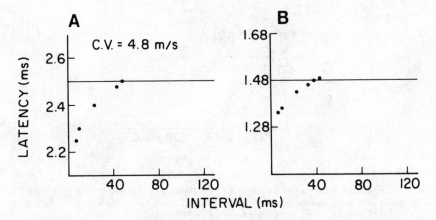

Figure 15.9. Experiment showing that the magnitude of the decrease in latency is proportional to conduction path length. The changes in conduction velocity therefore occur along the axonal trunk within the corpus callosum. (A) Both conditioning and test stimuli are delivered through a stimulating electrode located approximately 2 mm to the right of midline. (B) Both stimuli are delivered via a stimulating electrode located approximately 2 mm to the left of the midline. The latency to the test stimulus is represented by closed circles. The conditioning stimulus was delivered at 1.2X threshold at each conditioning stimulus-test stimulus interval. Antidromic control latency at 1.2X threshold is represented by the horizontal line

not equal, and in fact are approximately proportional to the control latency at each stimulation site. Observations of this type indicate that the latency decrease occurs along the callosal axonal trunk, and is not dependent on changes which occur only in the non-myelinated terminals and/or non-myelinated segments near the cell body.

THE SUBNORMAL PERIOD

For some units, following a single antidromic conditioning volley, a slight *increase* in latency to a test stimulus follows the initial decrease in latency. This increase in latency is augmented both in magnitude and duration by an increase in the number of conditioning pulses. Even those units showing no increase in latency to a test stimulus after a single conditioning volley show a clear increase in latency after a conditioning stimulus consisting of a train of pulses (Swadlow and Waxman, 1976). In figure 15.10, the response to a test stimulus is shown for a unit which received a conditioning stimulus consisting of 1, 20 or 54 pulses (330 pulses/s). As shown in this figure, the magnitude of the increase in latency was related to the number of conditioning pulses. In some units, the duration of the increase in latency following a conditioning stimulus consisting of 20 pulses was as long as 1.5 s. Two lines of evidence indicate that the increases in latency are a result of previous impulse activity along the axon: (1) increases in latency occur during and following periods of heightened 'spontaneous' or orthodromically driven activity, and (2) no increases

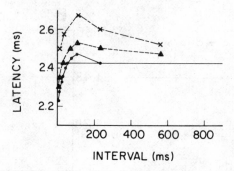

Figure 15.10. Graph showing the time course of the increase in latency for one unit when the conditioning stimulus consisted of a single pulse (•—•), 20 pulses (▲---▲---▲) or 54 pulses (X—X—X) delivered at 330 pulses/s

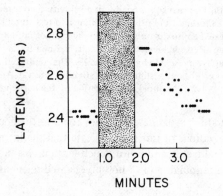

Figure 15.11. Long-lasting increase in antidromic latency for a single unit (control conduction velocity of 5.3 m/s). To the left of the solid bar closed circles represent a period during which baseline latency was obtained. Antidromic volleys were presented at 1 pulse/3.3 s. The width of the solid bar represents the duration of a period of tetanic stimulation (33 pulses/s). Latency was not measured during this period of tetanic stimulation. To the right of the bar, closed circles represent antidromic latency at various intervals following the tetanic stimulation. During this period a single test pulse was presented every 3.3 s. In this experiment, all stimuli were presented at 1.5X the control threshold

in latency are noted following a conditioning train which is just sub-threshold (Swadlow and Waxman, 1976).

For some units, changes in conduction velocity persist for more than a minute following tetanic stimulation. Figure 15.11 shows a unit with a control conduction velocity of 5.3 m/s. Points to the left of the solid bar represent a control period during which baseline latency was obtained. During this control period, antidromic volleys were presented at 1 pulse/3.3 s. The solid bar represents a period of tetanic stimulation (33 pulses/s). Latency was not measured during this period of stimulation. The points to the right of the bar represent antidromic latency at various intervals following the tetanic stimulation. During this period a single test pulse was presented every 3.3 s. All stimuli were presented at 1.5× the control threshold. Following a 60 s train, the latency increased from just over 2.4 ms to approximately 2.7 ms and did not return to control levels for more than 90 s.

CONDUCTION PROPERTIES OF MACAQUE CALLOSAL AXONS

More recently we have looked at the conduction properties of visual callosal axons of the macaque monkey (Swadlow *et al.*, 1979). Of the 61 axons studied thus far, 60 have demonstrated activity dependent variations in conduction properties very similar to those seen in the rabbit. Figure 15.12 illustrates variations in latency to a test stimulus following a single conditioning volley (closed circles) and following a conditioning volley consisting of 20 antidromic pulses (open circles). This cell was located in prelunate gyrus and was antidromically activated by a stimulating electrode located in the contralateral prelunate gyrus.

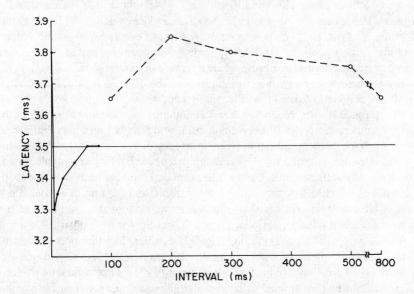

Figure 15.12. Activity dependent variation in the conduction velocity of a macaque callosal axon. Time course of latency variation to an antidromic test stimulus at various intervals following a conditioning stimulus. The conditioning stimulus consists of either a single pulse (•—•) or a train of 20 pulses (o--o) presented at 330/s

CONCLUSIONS AND IMPLICATIONS

The results of these experiments show that the conduction velocity and excitability of visual callosal axons are not constant, but on the contrary vary dynamically with the history of impulse conduction along the individual axon. Increases and decreases in conduction velocity and excitability occur. Moreover, they occur along the length of the callosal axon. The total range (increase and decrease) of the variations in conduction velocity for an axon may exceed 25% of the conduction velocity of that axon in its resting state. Activity dependent variations in conduction properties may last for more than 1 min. These variations occur in both myelinated and non-myelinated axons, but are more readily observed in the slowly conducting axons. An important question concerns the generality of these observations. Several lines of evidence indicate that activity dependent variations in conduction properties are not unique to visual callosal axons of the rabbit. (1) The morphology of these axons is unremarkable. (2) We have observed very similar after-effects in somatosensory callosal axons of the rabbit (Swadlow and Waxman, 1976) and visual callosal axons of the monkey (Swadlow *et al.,* 1979). After-effects of shorter duration and lesser magnitude were observed in some corticotectal axons of the rabbit (Swadlow and Waxman, 1976). (3) Similar after-effects have been observed in axons in other regions of both peripheral (Bliss and Rosenberg, 1974; Bullock, 1951; Gilliatt and Willison, 1963; Lass and Abeles, 1975; Newman and Raymond, 1971) and central (Gardner-Medwin, 1972) nervous systems. A series of events following the action potential (action potential → refractory period → supernormal period → subnormal period) may thus represent a rather general feature of axonal physiology.

Since the absolute magnitude and duration of the decrease in latency is greater for slowly conducting axons than for rapidly conducting axons one would expect that antidromic latency variability in fast conducting axons would be small. In the present studies, neurons with axon conduction velocities of more than 7 m/s, see figure 15.7(A), had a maximum decrease in latency of 0.1 ms or less, a figure which is often cited as a criterion for the maximum latency variability acceptable for an antidromically activated unit. On the other hand, all but four units with conduction velocities of less than 6 m/s exhibited latency decreases of 0.1 ms or greater. On the basis of latency measurements alone, these units would probably have been inappropriately classified as synaptically activated (Swadlow and Waxman, 1975).

The above results are thus methodologically significant with respect to the criteria for the identification of antidromically and synaptically actived neurons. As we have noted previously (Swadlow and Waxman, 1975), since conduction velocity varies with the history of impulse activity along the axon, an invariant latency does not constitute a necessary condition for the identification of antidromically activated neurons. Conversely, a variable latency does not constitute a sufficient condition for the identification of synaptically activated neurons. Impulse collision tests, examination of refractory periods and observations of waveform changes following the second of two closely spaced volleys, together with systematic exploration of latency and threshold variability, provide in our opinion the most appropriate criteria for differentiating antidromic from synaptic activation.

Activity dependent variation in conduction velocity may be significant with respect to mechanisms of coding and temporal summation of neural information (Swadlow and Waxman, 1975). For some axons in the splenium of the rabbit corpus callosum, the total range of activity dependent increases and decreases in antidromic latency is more than 3 ms. Although some postsynaptic neurons may not discriminate temporal variation of this magnitude in the timing of the incoming spikes, other neurons are exquisitely sensitive to small differences in the timing of presynaptic (see Hall, 1965 and Yasargil and Diamond, 1968) impulses. For axons in a system requiring preservation of temporal relationships between impulses, the interval between spike initiation near the cell body and the time of arrival of the impulse at the axon terminal might be expected to be nearly constant. We would expect impulse conduction along most visual callosal axons to fulfil this requirement only if no prior impulse had occurred for at least several hundred milliseconds. It may be relevant, with regard to this point, that the great majority of visual callosal neurons in the rabbit have spontaneous firing rates of less than one spike/s (Swadlow, 1974a). In addition to the possible effects of activity dependent variations in conduction velocity, activity dependent variations in threshold could modulate the spatial distribution of impulses along the terminal arbors which are invaded via branch points of low safety factor. This idea has been fully explored previously (Chung et al., 1970). Moreover, transmitter dynamics might also be expected to vary with variations in terminal excitability (Hubbard and Willis, 1962; Takeuchi and Takeuchi 1959).

The diameter is of the largest axons in the splenium of the rabbit corpus callosum is more than 20 times that of the smallest axons, and the volume is thus greater by a factor of more than 400. As we have noted previously (Swadlow and Waxman, 1976), the above considerations may be relevant to the evolutionary constraints which have determined the diameter of axons within a tract of fibres. For a tract of fixed cross-sectional area, increases in axonal diameter will necessitate a decreased number of independent axonal channels. On the other hand, increased diameter will result in a number of changes in conduction properties. One of these is an increase in conduction velocity. This may be of functional significance not only with regard to decreasing the absolute conduction time, but may in addition provide a mechanism for mediating synchrony (Bennett, 1968; Waxman and Melker, 1971). As described above for central axons, and as demonstrated by Paintal (1967) in peripheral nerve, the refractory period is briefer for more rapidly conducting axons. The maximum possible impulse frequency will therefore be higher for larger diameter axons. Finally, let us consider systems in which a constant axonal conduction time may be critical (as in the superior accessory olive, where cells are sensitive to interaural differences as small as 100 μs; Hall, 1965). The demonstration that the magnitude and duration of activity dependent variation in conduction velocity are smaller for fast, than for slowly conducting axons suggests that large axons may provide the most appropriate channels for such systems.

With regard to interhemispheric communication, the functional significance of the large range of fibre diameters and resultant conduction velocities (in the rabbit we have observed a range of 40-1 in the conduction velocities of callosal axons) is unclear. Berlucchi and Rizzolatti (1968) have shown that one function of the visual callosal system of the cat is to fill in the ipsilateral component of the receptive fields of cells which have their receptive field centres very near the vertical meridian. One might expect fast myelinated axons to mediate such a function, so that ipsilateral thalamic and contralateral cortical input would activate the cell receiving this information nearly simultaneously. In the human, simple reaction time experiments that require interhemispheric integration may be subject to an interhemispheric delay of 5 ms or less (see, for example, Berlucchi et al., 1971). Such integration would also be mediated by the larger myelinated axons.

The function of small myelinated and non-myelinated axons is more problematical. The corpus callosum of the rat (Seggie and Berry, 1972), rabbit (Waxman and Swadlow, 1976b), cat (Fleischhauer and Wartenberg, 1967; see Bishop and Smith, 1964 and Naito et al., 1971 for different findings), and human (Tomasch, 1954) reportedly contain 40-50% non-myelinated axons. In the rabbit, the slower visual callosal axons conduct impulses at 0.3-0.5 m/s. In the human, where conduction distance may exceed 100 mm, such conduction velocities would yield interhemispheric conduction times of 200-400 ms. If callosal axons of the human demonstrate activity dependent variations in conduction velocity which are similar to those of monkey and rabbit, the conduction time along such axons would be subject to variations of tens of milliseconds. The function of such slow and possibly history dependent channels of interhemispheric communication is a matter of considerable interest.

ACKNOWLEDGEMENTS

This work was supported in part by grants from the National Institutes of Health (NS-12307, NS-00010), the Bell Telephone Laboratories Inc. and the Health Sciences Fund (78-10). We thank Ms E. Hartwieg for excellent technical assistance.

REFERENCES

Bennett, M. V. L. (1968). Neural control of electric organs. In *The Central Nervous System and Fish Behavior* (D. Ingle, ed.), University of Chicago Press, pp. 147-69

Bergmans, J. (1973). Physiological observations on single human nerve fibres. In *New Developments in Electromyography and Clinical Neurophysiology*, vol. 2 (J. E. Desmedt, ed.), Karger, Basel, pp. 89-127

Berlucchi, G. and Rizzolatti, G. (1968). Binocularly driven neurons in visual cortex of split-chiasm cats. *Science*, **159**, 308-10

Berlucchi, G., Heron, W., Hyman, R., Rizzolatti, G. and Umilta, C. (1971). Simple reactions times of ipsilateral and contralateral hand to lateralized visual stimuli. *Brain*, **94**, 419-30

Bishop, G. H. and Smith, J. M. (1964). The size of nerve fibers supplying the cerebral cortex. *Expl Neurol.*, **9**, 483-501

Bishop, P. O., Burke, W., and Davis, R. (1962). Single-unit recording from anti-dromically activated optic radiation neurons. *J. Physiol., Lond.*, **162**, 432-50

Bliss, T. V. P. and Rosenberg, M. E. (1974). Supernormal conduction velocity in the olfactory nerve of the tortoise. *J. Physiol., Lond.*, **239**, 60-61P

Bullock, T. H. (1951). Facilitation of conduction rate in nerve fibers. *J. Physiol., Lond.*, **114**, 89-97

Chung, S., Raymond, S. A. and Lettvin, J. (1970). Multiple meaning in single visual units. *Brain, Behav. Evol.*, **3**, 72-101

Fleischhauer, K. and Wartenberg, H. (1967). Elektronenmikroskopische Unter-suchungen über das Wachstum der Nervenfasern und über das Auftreten Von Markscheiden im Corpus Callosum der Katze. *Z. Zellforsch.*, **83**, 568-81

Gardner-Medwin, A. R. (1972). An extreme supernormal period in cerebellar paral-lel fibers. *J. Physiol., Lond.*, **22**, 357-71

Gasser, H. S. (1950). Unmedullated fibers originating in dorsal root ganglia. *J. gen. Physiol.*, **33**, 651-90

Gilliatt, R. W. and Willison, R. G. (1963). The refractory and supernormal periods of the human median nerve. *J. Neurol. Neurosurg. Psychiat.*, **26**, 136-43

Hall, J. L. (1965). Binaural interaction in the accessory superior olivary nucleus of the cat. *J. Acoust. Soc. Am.*, **37**, 814-23

Hirano, A. and Dembitzer (1967). A structural analysis of the myelin sheath in the central nervous system. *J. Cell. Biol.*, **34**, 555-67

Hubbard, J. I. and Willis, W. D. (1962). Hyperpolarization of mammalian motor nerve terminals. *J. Physiol., Lond.*, **163**, 115-37

Hursh, J. B. (1939). Conduction velocity and diameter of nerve fibers. *Am. J. Physiol.*, **127**, 131-39

Lass, Y. and Abeles, M. (1975). Transmission of information by the axon: I. Noise and memory in the myelinated nerve fiber of the frog. *Biol. Cyb.*, **19**, 61-67

Naito, H., Miyakawa, F. and Ito, N. Diameters of callosal fibers interconnect-ing cat sensorimotor cortex (1971). *Brain Res.*, **27**, 369-72

Newman, E. A. and Raymond, S. A. (1971). Activity dependent shifts in excitability of frog peripheral nerve axons. *Q. Prog. Rep., M.I.T. Res. Lab. Electronics*, **102**, 165-87

Paintal, A. S. (1967). A comparison of the nerve impulses of mammalian non-medul-lated nerve fibres with those of the smallest diameter medullated fibres. *J. Physiol., Lond.*, **193**, 523-33

Phillips, C. G. (1959). Actions of antidromic pyramidal volleys on single Betz cells in the cat. *Q. Jl exp. Physiol.*, **44**, 1-25

Phillips, C. G., Powell, T. P. S. and Shepherd, G. M. (1963). Responses of mitral cells to stimulation of the lateral olfactory tract in the rabbit. *J. Physiol., Lond.*, **168**, 65-88

Rushton, W. A. H. (1951). A theory of the effects of fibre size in medullated nerve. *J. Physiol., Lond.,* **115**, 101-22

Seggie, J. and Berry, M. (1972). Ontogeny of interhemispheric evoked potentials in the rat: significance of myelination of the corpus callosum. *Expl Neurol.,* **35**, 215-32

Swadlow, H. A. (1974a). Properties of antidromically activated callosal neurons and neurons responsive to callosal input in rabbit binocular cortex. *Expl Neurol.,* **43**, 424-44

Swadlow, H. A. (1974b). Systematic variations in the conduction velocity of slowly conducting axons in the rabbit corpus callosum. *Expl Neurol.,* **43**, 445-51

Swadlow, H. A. (1977). Relationship of the corpus callosum to visual areas I and II of the rabbit. *Expl Neurol.,* **57**, 516-31

Swadlow, H. A. and Waxman, S. G. (1975). Observations on impulse conduction along central axons. *Proc. natn Acad. Sci. U.S.A.,* **72**, 5156-59

Swadlow, H. A. and Waxman, S. G. (1976). Variations in conduction velocity and excitability following single and multiple impulses of visual callosal axons in the rabbit. *Expl Neurol.,* **53**, 128-50

Swadlow, H. A., Rosene, D. and Waxman, S. G. (1979). Characteristics of inter-hemispheric impulse conduction between prelumate gyri of the Rhesus monkey. *Expl Brain Res.,* in press

Takeuchi, A. and Takeuchi, N. K. (1962). Electrical changes in the pre- and post-synaptic axons of the giant synapse of *Loligo. J. gen. Physiol.,* **45**, 1181-93

Tomasch, J. (1954). Size, distribution and number of fibers in the human corpus callosum. *Anat. Rec.,* **119**, 119-35

Tomasch, J. and MacMillan (1957). The number of fibers in the corpus callosum of the white mouse (1957). *J. comp. Neurol.,* **107**, 165-68

Waxman, S. G. and Bennett, M. V. L. (1972). Relative conduction velocities of small myelinated and nonmyelinated fibres in the central nervous system. *Nature New Biol.,* **238**, 217-19

Waxman, S. G. and Melker, R. J. (1971). Closely spaced nodes of Ranvier in the mammalian brain. *Brain Res.,* **32**, 445-48

Waxman, S. G. and Swadlow, H. A. (1976a). Morphology and physiology of visual callosal axons: evidence for a supernormal period in central myelinated axons. *Brain Res.,* **113**, 179-87

Waxman, S. G. and Swadlow, H. A. (1976b). Ultrastructure of visual callosal axons in the rabbit. *Expl Neurol.,* **53**, 115-27

Yasargil, G. M. and Diamond, J. (1968). Startle-response in Teleost fish: an element-ary circuit for neural discrimination. *Nature (Lond.),* **230**, 241-43

16
INTERHEMISPHERIC COMMUNICATION BETWEEN NEURONS IN VISUAL CORTEX OF THE RABBIT

HARVEY A. SWADLOW

INTRODUCTION

Whereas the physiological properties of the callosal system of the cat have been subjected to extensive investigation (see, for example, Berlucchi *et al.*, 1967; Choudhury *et al.*, 1965; Hubel and Weisel, 1967; Innocenti *et al.*, 1974), those of other species have remained relatively unstudied. This chapter will review recent investigations of the visual callosal system of the rabbit. The physiological properties and the distribution of cells of origin of the corpus callosum (callosal efferent neurons) and cells which are synaptically activated by callosal input will be examined.

The optical axis of the rabbit's eyes are directed about $2°$ anterior of laterally and approximately $13°$ above the horizontal plane (Hughes, 1971). This situation yields a nearly panoramic view of the world, most of which is monocular. Approximately $24-30°$ of visual space directly in front of the rabbit is, however, accessible to either eye (Hughes, 1971) and about 10% of optic nerve fibres of pigmented rabbits pass ipsilaterally (Giolli and Guthrie, 1969). Thompson *et al.* (1950) first showed that, in the rabbit, a strip of cortex which straddles the border of visual areas I and II receives input from the ipsilateral as well as the contralateral eye and that the border of V–I and V–II is the cortical representation of the nasotemporal division of the retina. The region of visual space represented by the border of visual areas I and II was called the line of decussation, which is thus analogous to the vertical meridian of carnivores and primates.

One might therefore expect that, as in the cat (see, for example, Berlucchi, *et al.*, 1967; Berlucchi and Rizzolatti, 1968; Choudhury *et al.*, 1965; Hubel and Weisel, 1967; Toyama *et al.*, 1974), the border of visual areas I and II would be maximally involved in interhemispheric communication. In fact, this border has been shown to receive extensive callosal terminals (Hughes and Wilson, 1969; Towns *et al.*, 1977). As will be shown below, however, the cells of origin of the corpus callosum (callosal efferent neurons) and the effects of synaptic input via callosal terminals are not limited to this border region but, on the contrary, are more widely distributed in both visual areas I and II.

211

METHODS

In the physiological experiments, extracellular recordings were obtained from the cell bodies of callosal efferent neurons in adult, unanaesthetised, unparalysed, Dutch rabbits. Recording procedures (Swadlow, 1974; Swadlow and Waxman, 1976) and techniques for tracking the eye of the awake rabbit during the determination of receptive field position (Swadlow, 1977) have been thoroughly described. The use of the awake rabbit was considered important for several reasons. First, the callosal system is very sensitive to both barbiturate (Bremer, 1958; Purpura and Girado, 1959; Sypert et al., 1970) and chloralose (Robinson, 1973) anaesthesia. Synaptic transmission via callosal terminals is dramatically reduced by as little as 8 mg/kg of pentobarbital (Purpura and Girado, 1959). Secondly, the use of the unanaesthetised but paralysed preparation also poses problems, for the animal is often in a sleep-like state from which it cannot be aroused (Mountcastle, et al., 1969). Berlucchi and Rizzolatti (1968) have pointed out the importance of an 'aroused' preparation in their studies of interhemispheric transfer of visual information.

In physiological studies, callosal efferent neurons were identified by their antidromic activation following electrical stimulation via electrodes chronically implanted at one or several sites along the course of the callosal axon. Banks of stimulating electrodes were implanted in the contralateral hemisphere (Swadlow, 1974, 1977) and/or in the corpus callosum near the midline (approximately 2 mm from the midline, contralateral to the recording microelectrode). Antidromic activation was differentiated from synaptic activation by collision tests (Bishop et al., 1962; Swadlow, 1974) in conjunction with examination of refractory periods and spike waveforms (Bishop et al., 1962; Phillips, 1959; Phillips et al., 1963).

In anatomical studies (Swadlow et al., 1978) the horseradish peroxidase (HRP) 'dark' reaction (Mesulum, 1976) was used to identify callosal efferent neurons. The border between visual areas I and II was determined by physiologically observing the reversal in receptive field position as successive microelectrode penetrations were made in a medial–lateral direction. This procedure has an accuracy of ± 0.3 mm (Swadlow, 1977). A microlesion was made at the border of visual areas I and II by passing 20–40 μA (cathodal) through the microelectrode for 10–15 s. Injections of 0.15–0.40 μl of 20% HRP (Sigma) were placed in the contralateral hemisphere. Injections were made at intervals of 1.0–1.5 mm and extended 4–5 mm medial and at least 3 mm lateral of the point which was homotopic to the microlesion. For technical reasons, all microlesions were made at points on the border of V-I and V-II representing the lower and middle visual field. Following survival times of 40–52 h, rabbits were perfused with a solution consisting of 1% paraformaldehyde and 1.25% gluteraldehyde in 0.1 M phosphate buffer (pH 7.4). Brains were post-fixed for 1 h in the perfusate and stored overnight in buffer. The next day, 40 μm frozen sections were cut and reacted (Mesulum, 1976).

RESULTS

Figure 16.1 illustrates the distribution of callosal efferent neurons in a frontal section (40 μm thick) through the left visual cortex after multiple injections of HRP in
the right visual cortex. Each closed circle represents an HRP filled cell. The arrow
marks the physiologically defined border of visual areas I and II. In V-I, callosal
efferent neurons are found in high concentrations as far as 2.0–2.5 mm medial of

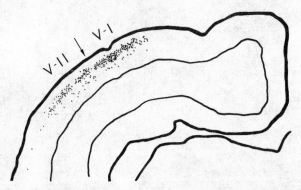

Figure 16.1.   Distribution of callosal efferent neurons in left visual cortex (40 μm section).
Arrow marks the physiologically defined border of visual areas I and II. The figure is a frontal
section through the left hemisphere. Heavy lines outline the surface of the brain, while lighter
lines outline the white matter

the border of V-I and V-II. An occasional callosal efferent neuron was found in
more medial regions of V-I, even as far as 1 mm from the medial border of striate
cortex. In V-II, many callosal efferent neurons were found as far as 2–4 mm lateral
of the border with V-I. In both V-I and V-II, the majority of HRP-labelled cells were
located in layer II-III which, in the rabbit, is fused (Rose, 1931). HRP filled cells
were found to a lesser extent in layers IV and V, whereas none were found in layers
I and VI. Most callosal efferent neurons were pyramidal cells. Figure 16.2 shows a
micrograph of callosal efferent neurons in the lateral portion of visual area I.
  Physiological experiments (Swadlow, 1977) enabled a more precise determination of the distribution of callosal efferent neurons in defined regions of V-I and
V-II. The distribution of cells which were activated synaptically following callosal
input was also studied. In these experiments the border between visual areas I and
II and the corresponding line of decussation in the visual field was defined by observing the reversal in receptive field position with anterior–lateral movements of
the microelectrode. A map of V-I and V-II of individual rabbits was thereby constructed. Control procedures (Swadlow, 1977) determined the reliability of these
methods to be ± 3°. Small regions of cortex in V-I and V-II were characterised with
respect to (a) the region of visual space which was represented and (b) the number

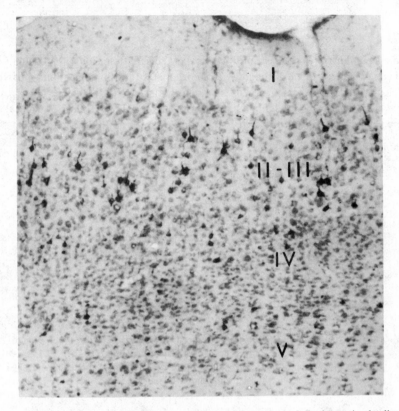

Figure 16.2.   Photomicrograph of the lateral portion of visual area I. Darkly stained cells are HRP filled callosal efferent neurons

of cells which were antidromically and synaptically activated following electrical stimulation near the midline of the corpus callosum.

The distribution of callosal efferent neurons in cortex with visual field positions of various angular distances from the line of decussation in V-I and V-II is shown. in figure 16.3(A). This figure represents all callosal efferent neurons found in a total of 99 penetrations into identified regions of V-I and V-II. Each penetration yielded recordings from at least three neurons ($\overline{X}$ = 5.8) and was through the full depth of the cortex. Cortical sites which had a field representation of less than 3° from the line of decussation were classified as being on the border of V-I and V-II. In V-I, a mean of one callosal efferent neuron per penetration or more was found up to 23° from the line of decussation. The concentration of callosal efferent neurons dropped markedly at greater angular distances. The most distant callosal efferent neuron in V-I was found 41° from the line of decussation at a distance of 3.3 mm from the V-I–V-II border. The distribution of callosal efferent neurons in V-I encompassed an area somewhat larger than the region of binocular representation.

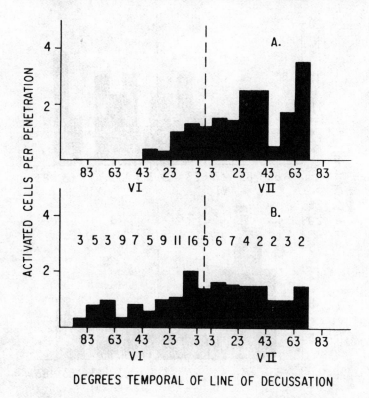

DEGREES TEMPORAL OF LINE OF DECUSSATION

Figure 16.3. In visual areas I and II, the mean number per penetration of callosal efferent neurons (A) and neurons synaptically activated by callosal input (B) which were found in cortical sites with visual field positions of various distances from the line of decussation. Regions of cortex with a visual field representation of less than 3° from the line of decussation were classified as being on the border of V-I and V-II (dashed line). The number above each bin of the histogram in B refers to the number of penetrations (in both A and B) represented by that bin.
(From Swadlow, 1977)

In contrast to V-I, callosal efferent neurons were found at a high concentration throughout the studied region of V-II.

The distribution of synaptically activated units in V-I and V-II is shown in figure 16.3(B). Whereas the concentration of these cells was greater near the line of decussation, synaptically activated units were also found up to 90° from the line of decussation. Units in V-I which were closer to the V-I-V-II border generally responded to each callosal stimulus with a greater number of spikes, at a lower threshold and at a shorter latency. The median antidromic latency of callosal efferent neurons in V-I and V-II which were found in cortical sites with various field positions is shown in figure 16.4(A). Only those field positions in which at least three callosal neurons were found are presented. Although there is a suggestion of a slightly greater latency in V-II, conduction velocity spectra for callosal axons with

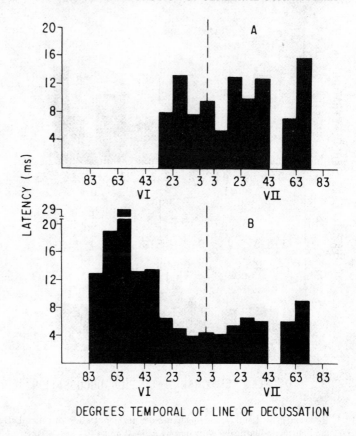

Figure 16.4. Median latency to activation following electrical stimulation of the corpus callosum for callosal efferent neurons (A) and neurons synaptically activated by callosal input (B), found in regions of V-I and V-II with visual field representations of various distances from the line of decussation. (From Swadlow, 1977)

cells of origin in V-I and V-II were roughly equivalent. The corresponding data for units which were synaptically activated by callosal stimulation is shown in figure 16.4(B). Note, in V-I, the abrupt increase in median latency at field positions of greater than 33° from the line of decussation.

In the above experiments, weak ipsilateral input could be found in some cells with receptive field centres as far as 25° and 30° from the line of decussation in V-I and V-II, respectively. Strong binocular input was found in regions of V-I and V-II which represented 0–12° from the line of decussation.

The behaviour of callosal efferent neurons and neurons synaptically activated by callosal input differed significantly in several respects. Figure 16.5 illustrates spontaneous firing rates of (A) all cells, (B) callosal efferent neurons and (C) neurons synaptically activated by callosal input found in a sample of 211 cells in binocular visual cortex (Swadlow, 1974). In this experiment it was not determined which

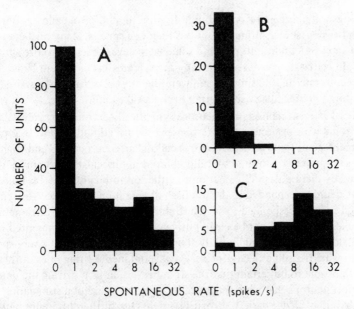

Figure 16.5. Spontaneous firing rates of (A) all cells, (B) callosal efferent neurons and (C) neurons synaptically activated by callosal input found in a sample of 211 cells in binocular visual cortex. (From Swadlow, 1974)

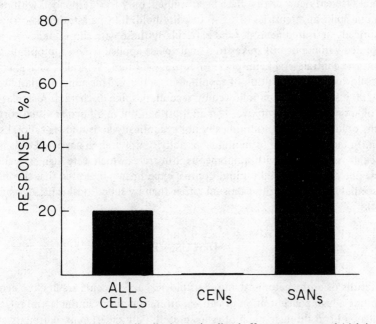

Figure 16.6. Percentage of (left) all cells, (centre) callosal efferent neurons and (right) neurons synaptically activated by callosal input that were activated by diffuse flash illumination to either or both eyes

recordings were obtained from V-I or V-II. More than 85% of callosal efferent neurons had a spontaneous firing rate of less than one spike/s. Many of these cells fired at rates of less than 10/min and some were never observed to fire spontaneously. In contrast, neurons synaptically activated by callosal input had a median spontaneous rate of 10.2 spikes/s and were the most spontaneously active neurons encountered in binocular visual cortex of the awake rabbit.

Callosal efferent neurons and neurons synaptically activated by callosal input also differed with respect to their responses to visual stimuli. Figure 16.6 presents the percentage of (left) all cells, (centre) callosal efferent neurons and (right) neurons synaptically activated by callosal input in binocular visual cortex that were activated by diffuse flash illumination to either or both eyes. Whereas no callosal efferent neurons responded to diffuse flash illumination, nearly 65% of synaptically activated neurons responded to such a stimulus. Many callosal efferent neurons in the awake rabbit could not be clearly driven by discrete stimuli presented in the visual field. Those that could be driven usually responded only to a very specific stimulus with 1-3 spikes. Only the very low spontaneous firing rates of these units made it possible to be certain that the stimulus was, in fact, driving the unit. In contrast, most neurons that were synaptically activated by callosal stimulation were easily driven by a wide variety of visual stimuli. One further difference between callosal efferent neurons and neurons synaptically activated by callosal input was in the number of spikes elicited by a single electrical stimulus. Of more than 150 callosal efferent neurons that have been studied, only four responded with more than one spike at intensities of 1.5-3.0× threshold. In contrast, the majority of synaptically activated neurons (and particularly those with short latency responses) responded with a burst of spikes to a single pulse applied to the appropriate location in the contralateral hemisphere or corpus callosum. Typically, such excitation was followed by an inhibition of spontaneous activity. This inhibition lasted for 100-200 ms and was often followed by secondary spike discharges. A similar inhibition of spontaneous activity was seen in most neurons in binocular visual cortex which could be neither antidromically nor synaptically activated via callosal stimulation. In fact, inhibition of spontaneous activity was seen in nearly all cells in binocular visual cortex with spontaneous firing rates which were high enough to enable detection of this inhibition. Control experiments indicated that the inhibition was mediated by the corpus callosum rather than by subcortical routes (Swadlow, 1974).

DISCUSSION

The results of both anatomical and physiological experiments are in close agreement in finding a high concentration of callosal efferent neurons in the lateral regions of visual area I and through much of visual area II. Callosal efferent neurons were physiologically identified in high concentration in regions of visual area I with visual field representations of 0-23° from the line of decussation and at a lesser concentration at 23–41°. No callosal efferent neurons were physiologically identified in more medial regions of V-I, though a few were anatomically identified in this area. Callosal efferent neurons in V-II were physiologically identified in high concentrations in regions of cortex with visual field representations of 0–66° from the line of decussation. More lateral regions of V-II were not studied physiologically.

Many neurons in both monocular and binocular V-I and V-II were synaptically activated by callosal stimulation. The interpretation of these findings, however, should be made with caution since orthodromic synaptic effects cannot be distinguished from synaptic effects which are mediated by antidromically activated recurrent collaterals of callosal efferent neurons. Furthermore, sub-threshold excitatory synaptic effects cannot usually be detected in extracellular recordings. Neurons in binocular V-I were synaptically activated at a shorter and less variable latency and responded with more spikes at a lower threshold than did those cells that were in monocular regions of V-I. This finding is of interest in light of anatomical studies (Hughes and Wilson, 1969; Towns *et al.*, 1977) which indicate that callosal terminals in V-I are only found near the border with V-II. Whereas the long and variable orthodromic latencies observed in the medial regions of V-I may be due to a number of factors, they are suggestive of a polysynaptic input of this region. The existence of polysynaptic interhemispheric communication between areas 17 is also suggested in the monkey by the behavioural experiments of Doty (1965, 1966), who found that an appetitive response to electrical stimulation of area 17 of one hemisphere is also made to a stimulus which is applied to contralateral area 17. This effect was shown to be mediated by either the anterior commissure or the corpus callosum.

Callosal efferent neurons and neurons synaptically activated by callosal input demonstrate dramatically different patterns of both spontaneous and visually elicited behaviour. Callosal efferent neurons have very low spontaneous firing rates, never respond to diffuse flash illumination and are very difficult to drive from the visual field. In contrast, neurons synaptically activated by callosal input have high spontaneous firing rates and generally respond to a wide range of visual stimuli, including diffuse flash illumination. Similarly, callosal efferent neurons in the somatosensory system of the cat have small and specific receptive fields (Innocenti *et al.*, 1974), whereas cells driven by transcallosal volleys have receptive fields which are wide and bilateral (Fadiga *et al.*, 1972; Robinson, 1973). The divergent characteristics of callosal efferent neurons and neurons that are driven synaptically by callosal input suggest that these classes of neural elements may be all but mutually exclusive. This view is supported by the finding in the rabbit that only four of more than 150 callosal efferent neurons were synaptically as well as antidromically activated by callosal or contralateral cortical stimulation. Furthermore, the intracellular studies of Toyama *et al.* (1974) have indicated that callosal efferent neurons were the only cells near the border of V-I and V-II of the cat which did not generally respond with EPSPs to callosal stimulation.

In binocular cortex, inhibition of spontaneous activity is the most prevalent effect elicited by callosal or contralateral cortical stimulation. Inhibitory phenomena were not studied in monocular cortex. As has been discussed by Doty and Negrão (1972) the lack of inhibitory type synapses formed by callosal terminals in rat para-visual cortex (Lund and Lund, 1970) suggest that such inhibition may be mediated by inhibitory interneurons. Similarly, the results of Toyama *et al.* (1974) strongly suggest that the inhibition mediated by callosal afferents in cat visual cortex is disynaptic.

In the above mapping experiments (Swadlow, 1977) the receptive field proper-ties of callosal efferent neurons were not systematically studied. Rather, for each rabbit, a map of V-I and V-II was constructed and the distribution of callosal effer-ent neurons within identified regions of the mapped area of cortex was then deter-mined. There are, therefore, important methodological differences between the above physiological experiments and studies of the receptive field properties of visual callosal axons of the cat (Berlucchi *et al.*, 1967; Hubel and Weisel, 1967; Shatz, 1977). A comparison of the results from cat and rabbit, however, suggests significant differences in the distribution of callosal efferent neurons in V-I and V-II of these species. The receptive field centres of all but four of the 75 visual cal-losal axons studied by Hubel and Weisel (1967), Berlucchi *et al.* (1967) and Shatz (1977) were less than $10°$ from the vertical meridian. Thus, the great majority of visual callosal efferent neurons in the cat are presumably located in cortical regions with visual field representations of $0–10°$ from the vertical meridian.

These physiological findings in the cat are generally confirmed by recent anatom-ical studies using horseradish peroxidase (Innocenti and Fiore, 1976; see also chap-ters 18 and 19). It thus appears that, in the rabbit, callosal efferent neurons may be more widespread in both V-I and V-II than is the case in the cat. In the primate, the distribution of callosal efferent neurons is apparently even more restricted than in the cat, for anatomical studies in both squirrel monkey (Wong-Riley, 1974) and macaque (Lund *et al.*, 1975) suggest that area 17 is nearly devoid of callosal effer-ent neurons. Whether the progressive restriction of callosal efferent neurons in V-I towards the cortical representation of the vertical meridian represents a phylogene-tic trend or other factors (e.g. species differences in visual acuity or receptive field size) is a matter of some interest.

The axons of visual callosal efferent neurons in the rabbit are both myelinated and non-myelinated (Waxman and Swadlow, 1976) and conduct at velocities of 0.3–12.9 m/s (Swadlow, 1974; Swadlow and Waxman, 1976). Antidromic latencies following stimulation of the callosal axon via electrodes located approximately 2 mm contralateral of the midline ranged from 1.0–37.5 ms, whereas the estimated interhemispheric conduction times for these axons were 1.3–62.0 ms. At present, the functional significance of such a wide range of conduction velocities and result-ant interhemispheric conduction times is unknown. An analysis of the receptive field properties of callosal efferent neurons with various axonal conduction velo-cities would be interesting in this regard.

The cortical representation of the line of decussation (or vertical meridian) of the rabbit interacts extensively with the contralateral hemisphere via the corpus cal-losum. Although the functions of these callosal connections are unknown, they are presumably similar to those proposed for the visual callosal system of the cat (see, for example, Berlucchi *et al.,* 1967; Berlucchi and Rizzolatti, 1968; Choudhury *et al.,* 1965; Hubel and Weisel, 1967). In the rabbit, however, visual cortical areas representing more temporal visual space also give rise to callosal efferent neurons and receive synaptic input via callosal terminals. In this regard it is somewhat surprising that behavioural experiments (Van Hof, 1970; Van Hof and Van Der Mark, 1976) have demonstrated little interocular transfer of learned pattern discriminations.

The widespread distribution of callosal elements in the visual cortex implies that each hemisphere receives substantial information from the contralateral hemisphere regarding a large portion of the ipsilateral visual hemifield. The functional significance of such widespread interhemispheric interaction is unknown. A systematic analysis, under conditions of reversible callosal blockade, of the receptive field properties of neurons located at various distances from the border of V-I and V-II might yield some insight in this direction.

ACKNOWLEDGEMENTS

This work was supported in part by grants from the National Institutes of Health (NS-03606, NS-12307) and the Bell Telephone Laboratories Inc. I thank Ms E. Hartwieg for excellent technical assistance.

REFERENCES

Berlucchi, G. and Rizzolatti, G. (1968). Binocularly driven neurons in visual cortex of split-chiasm cats. *Science,* **159**, 308–10

Berlucchi, G., Gazzaniga, M. S. and Rizzolatti, G. (1967). Microelectrode analysis of transfer of visual information by the corpus callosum. *Arch. Ital. Biol.,* **105**, 583–96

Bishop, P. O., Burke, W. and Davis, R. (1962). Single-unit recording from antidromically activated optic radiation neurons. *J. Physiol., Lond.* **162**, 432–50

Bremer, F. (1958). Physiology of the corpus callosum. In *The Brain and Human Behavior,* vol. 36, Proc. Ass. Res. Nerv. Ment. Dis., Williams and Wilkins, Baltimore, pp. 424–48

Choudhury, P. B., Whitteridge, D. and Wilson, M. E. (1965). The function of the callosal connections of the visual cortex. *Q. Jl exp. Physiol.,* **50**, 214–19

Doty, R. W. (1965). Conditioned reflexes elicited by electrical stimulation of the brain in macaques. *J. Neurophysiol.,* **28**, 623–40

Doty, R. W. (1966). Interhemispheric transfer of conditioned reflexes established to electrical stimulation of neocortex. *The Physiologist,* **9**, 170

Doty, R. W. and Negrão, N. (1972). Forebrain commissures and vision. In *Handbook of Sensory Physiology,* vol. VII/s, Springer-Verlag, Heidelberg

Fadiga, E., Innocenti, G. M., Manzoni, T. and Spidaliere, G. (1972). Transcallosal reactivity of cat trigeminal I neurons. *Brain Res.,* **37**, 368–69

Giolli, R. A. and Guthrie, M. D. (1969). The primary optic projections in the rabbit. An experimental study. *J. comp Neurol.*, **136**, 99-126

Hubel, D. H. and Weisel, T. N. (1967). Cortical and callosal connections concerned with the vertical meridian of visual fields in the cat. *J. Neurophysiol*, **30**, 1561-73

Hughes, A. (1971). Topographical relationships between the anatomy and physiology of the rabbit visual system. *Docum. Opthal. (Den Hagg)*, **30**, 33-159

Hughes, A. and Wilson, M. E. (1969). Callosal terminations along the boundary between visual areas I and II in the rabbit. *Brain Res.*, **12**, 19-25

Innocenti, G. M. and Fiore, L. (1976). Morphological correlates of visual field transformation in the corpus callosum. *Neurosci. Lett.*, **2**, 245-52

Innocenti, G. M., Manzoni, T. and Spidalieri, G. (1974). Patterns of somesthetic messages transfered through the corpus callosum. *Expl Brain Res.*, **19**, 447-66

Lund, J. S. and Lund, R. D. (1970). The termination of callosal fibers in the paravisual cortex of the rat. *Brain Res.*, **17**, 25-45

Lund, J. S., Lund, R. S., Hendrickson, A. E., Bunt, A. H. and Fuchs, A. F. (1975). The origin of efferent pathways from the primary visual cortex, area 17 of the Macaque monkey as shown by retrograde transport of horseradish peroxidase. *J. comp. Neurol.*, **164**, 287-304

Mesulum, M. (1976). The blue reaction product in horseradish peroxidase neurohistochemistry: incubation parameters and visibility. *J. Histochem. Cytochem.*, **24**, 1273-80

Mountcastle, V. B., Talbot, W. H. and Sakata, H. (1969). Cortical neuronal mechanisms in flutter-vibration studies in unanesthetized monkeys. Neuronal periodicity and frequency discrimination. *J. Neurophysiol.*, **32**, 452-84

Phillips, C. G. (1959). Actions of antidromic pyramidal volleys on single Betz cells in the cat. *Q. Jl exp. Physiol.*, **44**, 1-25

Phillips, C. G., Powell, T. P. S. and Sheperd, G. M. (1963). Responses of mitral cells to stimulation of the lateral olfactory tract in the rabbit. *J. Physiol. Lond.*, **168**, 65-88

Purpura, D. P. and Girado, M. (1959). Synaptic mechanisms involved in transcallosal activation of corticospinal neurons. *Arch. Ital. Biol.*, **97**, 95-110

Robinson, D. L. (1973). Electrophysiological analysis of interhemispheric relations in the second somatosensory cortex of the cat. *Expl Brain Res.*, **18**, 131-44

Rose, M. (1931). Cytoarchitektonischer Atlas der Grosshirnrinde des Kaninchens. *J. Psychol. Neurol.*, **43**, 353-440

Shatz, C. (1977). Abnormal interhemispheric connections in the visual system of Boston Siamese cats: A physiological study. *J. comp. Neurol.*, **171**, 229-46

Swadlow, H. A. (1974). Properties of antidromically activated callosal neurons and neurons responsive to callosal input in rabbit binocular cortex. *Expl. Neurol.*, **43**, 424-44

Swadlow, H. A. (1977). Relationship of the corpus callosum to visual areas I and II of the awake rabbit. *Expl Neurol.*, **57**, 516-31

Swadlow, H. A. and Waxman, S. G. (1976). Variations in conduction velocity and excitability following single and multiple impulses of visual callosal axons in the rabbit. *Expl Neurol.*, **53**, 128-50

Swadlow, H. A., Weyand, T. G. and Waxman, S. G. (1978). The cells of origin of the corpus callosum in rabbit visual cortex. *Brain Res.*, in press

Sypert, G. W., Oakley, J. and Ward, Jr. A. A. (1970). Single-unit analysis of propagated seizures in neocortex. *Expl Neurol.*, **28**, 308–25

Thompson, J. M., Woolsey, C. B. and Talbot, S. A. (1950). Visual areas I and II of cerebral cortex of rabbit. *J. Neurophysiol.*, **13**, 277–88

Towns, L. C., Giolli, R. A. and Haste, D. A. (1977). Corticocortico fiber connections of the rabbit visual cortex: a fiber degeneration study. *J. comp. Neurol.*, **173**, 537–60

Toyama, D., Matsunami, K. and Ohno, T. (1969). Antidromic identification of association, commissural and corticofugal efferent cells in cat visual cortex. *Brain Res.*, **14**, 513–17

Toyama, K., Matsunami, K. Ohno, T. and Tokashiki, S. (1974). An intracellular study of neuronal organization in the visual cortex. *Expl Brain Res.*, **21**, 45–66

Van Hof, M. W. (1970). Interocular transfer in the rabbit. *Expl Neurol.*, **26**, 103–108

Van Hof, M. W. and Van Der Mark, F. (1976). A quantitative study on interocular transfer in the rabbit. *Physiol. Behav.*, **17**, 715–17

Waxman, S. G. and Swadlow, H. A. (1976). Ultrastructure of visual callosal axons in the rabbit. *Expl Neurol.*, **53**, 115–27

Wong-Riley, M. T. T. (1974). Demonstration of geniculocortical and callosal projection neurons in the squirrel monkey by means of retrograde axonal transport of horseradish peroxidase. *Brain Res.*, **79**, 267–72

17

INTEROCULAR TRANSFER AND INTERHEMISPHERIC COMMUNICATION IN THE RABBIT

M. W. VAN HOF

INTRODUCTION

Several years ago we investigated interocular transfer in the rabbit (van Hof, 1970). Dutch-belted rabbits were trained to discriminate patterns monocularly. In the training box used in those experiments (van Hof, 1966) the rabbit was exposed to two patterns simultaneously, where the animal was required to choose one pattern by touching it with its nose. If the 'rewarded' pattern was selected a food pellet was given; if the 'unrewarded' pattern was chosen the stimuli were removed and the trial ended without any reward. The animals were trained monocularly by patching one eye with a textile mask. Each eye was exposed daily to a series of 100 discrimination trials. One eye was given a vertical versus horizontal striation problem and the other eye was trained on a 45° versus 135° striation task (figure 17.1). Vertical and 45° striations were rewarded, with the rewarded pattern positioned randomly either left or right.

After the 90% correct choice level was reached interocular transfer was tested. The left eye was exposed to the training problem of the right eye and vice versa. Of 16 rabbits studied only one reached the 90% level with both eyes during the first 100 trials. Three other animals reached this level with the vertical versus horizontal striations and not with the oblique ones. In all cases the performance was close to chance level. In other words, in most cases each eye had access to only one memory trace.

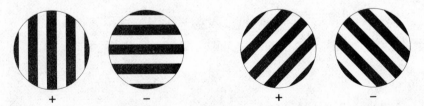

Figure 17.1. Striated patterns as seen by the animal. Vertical versus horizontal striations were offered to one eye and 45° and 135° to the other. Each eye received 100 exposures per day. Vertical and 45° striations were rewarded. Stripe width 1.25 cm

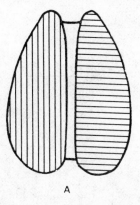 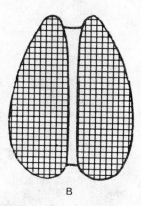

A   B

Figure 17.2. Scheme of the hemispheres of the rabbit seen from above. Memory traces formed by way of the right and left eye are indicated by vertical and horizontal lines, respectively. Two possibilities are discussed: one memory trace in each hemisphere (A) and two memory traces each distributed over both hemispheres (B)

The present chapter deals with the question of whether or not the rabbit is a 'natural split-brain preparation', as suggested by our first experiment (figure 17.2A). However, for this interpretation to be true it would mean that the ipsilateral fibres in the chiasm (some 10% of the total number) do not contribute substantially to memory trace formation during monocular training and that in some way interhemispheric communication via the intercerebral commissures is either absent or actively blocked. If these two assumptions are not valid it is more likely that the two traces are separated but distributed over both hemispheres (figure 17.2B). In that case the low level of interocular transfer would be due to a lack of intrahemispheric rather than interhemispheric communication.

THE ROLE OF IPSILATERAL FIBRES IN MONOCULAR PATTERN DISCRIMINATION

Rabbits have almost laterally implanted eyes and the 10% of the optic fibres which do not cross in the chiasm originate from the posterior part of the retina (Hughes, 1971). Covering different parts of the visual field by means of clear plexiglass caps it was found that during pattern discrimination the rabbit has a tendency to look forward (van Hof and Lagers-van Haselen, 1973) and expose the posterior part of the retina to the patterns. In other words, during pattern discrimination the rabbit has a tendency to use that part of the retina which has a relatively large cortical representation (Hughes, 1971), which is optically adapted to proximal vision (De Graauw and van Hof, 1978) and from which the binocular units arise (van Sluyters and Stewart, 1974). In unpublished experiments by Lagers-van Haselen and van Hof it was found that monocularly trained rabbits also have a tendency to look forward.

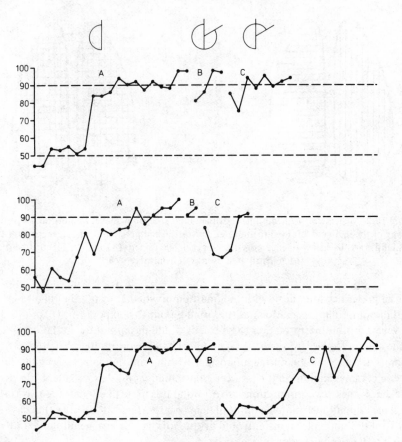

Figure 17.3. Monocular pattern discrimination in three different animals (45° versus 135° striations, 100 trials per day). In each graph, A represents the learning curve with the right eye. The left eye was covered with a textile mask. On the ordinate is the percentage of correct choices, and on the abcissa the sequence of the days. Each dot represents the number of correct choices in a series of 100 trials. In B, in addition to the left eye, the posterior 120° of the visual field of the right eye is occluded. In C, the left eye and the anterior 60° of the right visual field are covered

Three rabbits were trained to discriminate patterns monocularly (figure 17.3). In each animal one eye received 100 trials per day. After the 90% correct level was reached a clear Plexiglass cap let into a textile mask was positioned over the eye. Different sections of the visual field were occluded by painting out different sectors of the cap. As figure 17.3 shows, the occlusion of the posterior 120° of the visual field did not interfere with the pattern discrimination scores, whereas of the three animals tested two required substantial retraining after occlusion of the anterior 60% of the visual field. This means that it is almost certain that a rabbit learning a monocular pattern discrimination will position the visual input on the retinal area from which the ipsilateral fibres originate.

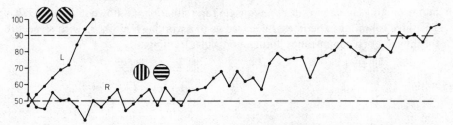

Figure 17.4. Example of monocular learning in a rabbit in which the left visual cortex was removed. On the ordinate is the percentage of correct choices, and on the abcissa the sequence of the days. Each dot represents the number of correct choices in a series of 100 trials. Per day, each eye received 100 presentations: 45° versus 135° striations to the left eye (L), vertical versus horizontal ones to the right eye (R)

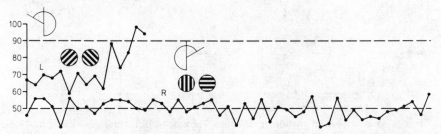

Figure 17.5. Same animal as in figure 17.4. Here the training procedure is repeated but now the anterior 60° of the visual field of the 'open' eye is occluded

However, evidence that the ipsilateral projection contributes little to memory trace formation during monocular learning comes from a study in rabbits in which the visual cortex was ablated on one side (van Hof and Lagers-van Haselen, 1975). Only 5 out of 16 animals reached the 90% criterion with the eye contralateral to the lesion. Extremely large numbers of trials were needed.

Regarding the interpretation of this study, one could argue that under the conditions of this experiment the rabbit changes its habit of looking forward. This was found not to be the case (van Hof et al., 1971). Figure 17.4 shows the graphs of a rabbit in which the left visual cortex was removed. The animal was trained to discriminate oblique striations with the left eye and vertical versus horizontal ones with the right eye. In figure 17.5, the results after covering the anterior 60° of the visual field are given. With the left eye the animal learned to look sideways, whereas the scores remained at chance level with the right eye. This was confirmed in all animals which reached criterion with the eye contralateral to the lesion, indicating that after unilateral ablation of the visual cortex the rabbit has a tendency to expose the remaining ipsilateral projection to the patterns. Thus the small contribution of the ipsilateral projection during monocular learning cannot be due to retinal misalignment.

A negligible contribution of the ipsilateral fibres to memory trace formation during monocular learning is a prerequisite for a situation, as shown in figure 17.2(A). The three following experiments will lead us to a working hypothesis with respect to the intercerebral commissures during monocular learning.

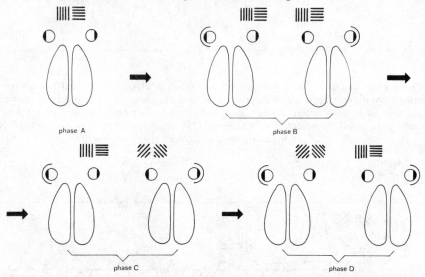

Figure 17.6.   Scheme of interocular transfer test. Phase A: binocular training with vertical versus horizontal striations. Phase B: each eye is trained separately to criterion with the same test patterns. Phase C: 45° versus 135° striations presented to the left eye, vertical versus horizontal ies to the right eye. Phase D: oblique striations to the right eye, vertical versus horizontal ones to the left eye

INTERHEMISPHERIC COMMUNICATION DURING MONOCULAR PATTERN DISCRIMINATION

Experiment 1

In the first study on interocular transfer (van Hof, 1970) the results were given in numbers of animals reaching criterion. Recently a more quantitative study was carried out (van Hof and van der Mark, 1976b). The training set-up was basically the same as the one used previously but now all manipulations were carried out by means of electropneumatic plungers controlled by a computer system (van der Mark and Meyer, (1974). The training scheme is illustrated in figure 17.6. Dutch-belted rabbits were trained binocularly to discriminate vertical versus horizontal striations (vertical stripes rewarded). One hundred exposures were given per day (phase A). After the 90% criterion was reached each eye was trained separately. Both the left and right eye received 100 exposures of vertical versus horizontal striations (phase B). The actual interocular transfer test (phases C and D) were made in 40 animals which were able to learn equally well the vertical versus horizontal discrimination with the left and right eye in phase B ('symmetrical' animals as defined by van Hof and van der Mark, 1976a). Oblique striations (45° versus 135°, 45° rewarded) were offered

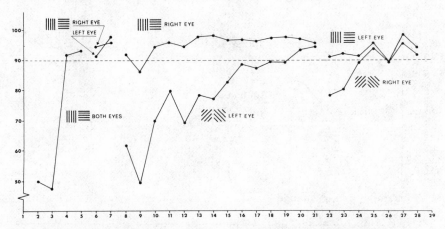

Figure 17.7. Example of learning in an animal trained as shown in figure 17.6. Percentage of correct choices on the ordinate, sequence of the days on the abcissa. Each dot represents the number of correct choices obtained during 100 trials

to the left eye in phase C and to the right eye in phase D (100 trials per day). In order to avoid position habits, the other eye received 100 presentations of vertical versus horizontal striations.

In figure 17.7 the results obtained in one animal are shown. In this particular animal, training with the oblique striations showed a considerable amount of savings in phase D compared with phase C. However, the results for all animals show savings as 22% (s.e. ± 6) for trials to criterion and 31% (s.e. ± 7) for errors to criterion. The interocular savings score was obtained using the ratio of:

$$\frac{\text{1st eye score} - \text{2nd eye score}}{\text{1st eye score} + \text{2nd eye score}} \times 100$$

In other words, this experiment confirms the conclusion that most rabbits have little interocular transfer.

Experiment 2

Does this mean that the memory trace is lateralised in the hemisphere contralateral to the trained eye (figure 17.2A)? In 12 other rabbits which were trained to discriminate vertical versus horizontal striation with the right eye and 45° versus 135° striations with the left eye, the visual cortex of the left hemisphere was ablated after criterion was reached. The operations were carried out under halothane anaesthesia and the lesions extended into the parietal and temporal areas of the hemisphere. Ten days after the operation training was started again and each eye was tested on four consecutive days. As an example the results obtained in one animal are shown in figure 17.8.

In figure 17.9 the average scores obtained after the operation are plotted for all

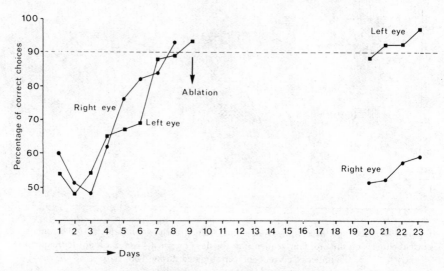

Figure 17.8. A normal rabbit was trained to discriminate 45° versus 135° striations with the left eye and vertical versus horizontal striations with the right eye. Percentage of correct choices on the y-axis, the sequence of days on the x-axis. Each dot indicates the number of correct choices per 100 trials. After criterion was reached the left visual cortex was removed. Ten days later the left eye was exposed again to the oblique striations and the right eye to the vertical versus horizontal ones

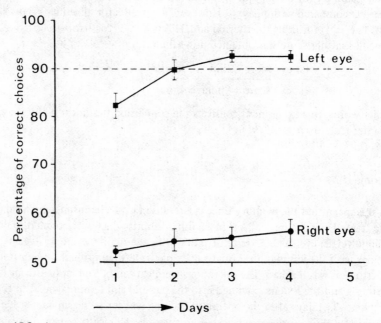

Figure 17.9. Average scores and standard errors from 12 animals which were trained in the way described in figure 17.8. Only the results obtained 10 days after the operation are shown

12 animals. As the graph shows, no appreciable retraining was required with the eye contralateral to the intact hemisphere, whereas the performance with the other eye was almost at chance level. Russell and Morgan (1976) have shown that complete removal of cortex in one hemisphere abolishes pattern discrimination in rats which were trained binocularly, from which it was concluded that the memory trace was distributed over both hemispheres. Therefore, the most likely conclusion seems that in the monocularly trained rabbit the memory trace is located in the contralateral hemisphere (figure 17.2A).

Lateralisation of the memory trace, in spite of the presence of a well-developed corpus callosum (cf. Swadlow, 1974; see also chapter 16), could be explained on the basis of the findings of Palmers and Zeier (1974) in the pigeon. These authors found that, under circumstances in which the two eyes received conflicting stimuli, one hemisphere became dominant and suppressed the other (see also Robert and Cuénod, 1969a, 1969b; Goodale, 1973). In this way a unilateral engram could be formed. This hypothesis does not explain the fact that the other hemisphere is unable to 'dial' to the memory trace via the commissures.

Experiment 3

If one considers the functional disconnection of the two hemispheres as a dynamic process based on some inhibitory mechanism, the question arises as to whether the sequences in which the patterns are presented influence the results.

In all studies found in the literature one eye is patched, occluded with a black contact lens or the eyelids are sutured. This means that for a relatively long time one eye is blinded while the other eye receives an uninterrupted series of stimulus presentations. The experiment to be described here (De Vos-Korthals and van Hof, in preparation) was a modification of that shown in figure 17.6. Here again the rabbits were first trained to discriminate vertical versus horizontal striations binocularly (phase A). Thereafter each eye was tested separately with the same patterns (phase B). In phase C the right eye was exposed to vertical versus horizontal striations and the left eye to 45° versus 135° ones. The difference with the experiment illustrated in figure 17.10 was that the rabbit wore goggles in which red or blue filters could be mounted, and at the same time the patterns consisted of either matching red or blue striations (the details of this technique have been described by van Hof and Russell, 1977).

At first, 100 presentations were offered while the animals wore goggles with a blue filter over the left eye and a red one over the right eye: 50 presentations of blue oblique striations, randomly alternated with 50 presentations of red vertical versus horizontal striations. The rewarded pattern was randomly presented to the left or right. The next day the same procedure was followed but now the left eye was covered by the red filter and the right eye with the blue filter. Vertical versus horizontal striations were now given in blue and oblique ones in red. Every day the colours were changed, but the oblique striations were presented to the left side till criterion was reached. This means that randomly the left eye was stimulated with

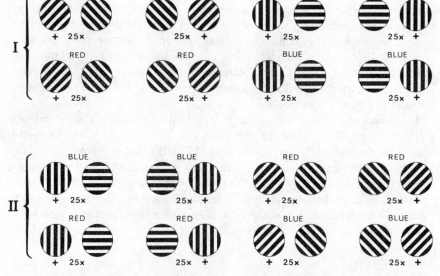

Figure 17.10. (I) the left eye was exposed to oblique striations and the right eye to vertical versus horizontal ones. On even days the left eye was covered with a blue filter and the right eye with a red one. Oblique striations (blue) and vertical versus horizontal ones (red) were presented in random sequence. On odd days the same procedure was repeated with a red filter over the left eye and a blue filter over the right eye. Oblique striations red, vertical versus horizontal ones blue. Per day, 100 presentations were offered. The various combinations which were offered randomly and the position of the rewarded pattern are indicated. (II) After criterion was reached in I the same procedure was carried out but now the right eye was exposed to the oblique striations and the left eye to the vertical versus horizontal ones

oblique striations and the right eye with vertical versus horizontal. However, neither eye received an uninterrupted series of patterns. After criterion was reached, the equivalent of phase D (figure 17.6) was given. In random sequence, either the left eye was stimulated with the vertical versus horizontal striations or the right eye with the oblique ones. The percentage of savings for the oblique striation discrimination was calculated in the same way as in experiment 1. The average percentage of savings calculated in 27 animals was 15 (s.e. ± 10) for trials to criterion and 19 (s.e ± 11) for errors to criterion. A comparison with the results obtained in experiment 1 shows that no significant difference exists. This indicates that the lateralisation process is not due to the fact that relatively long uninterrupted series are presented to one eye.

DISCUSSION

Do these results imply that during normal binocular learning dual memory traces

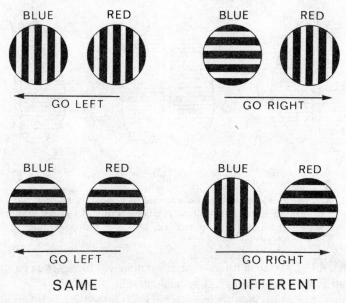

Figure 17.11.   Same–different discrimination the left pattern blue and the right one red. The left eye was covered with a blue filter and the right eye with a red one. When identical patterns are presented the left one is rewarded. The right one is rewarded when the animal is exposed to unidentical patterns. In random sequence each combination was offered 25 times per day

are formed? As a first approach to this problem a study was carried out in which the rabbit wore goggles with a blue filter over the left eye and a red filter over the right eye. The left pattern was blue and the right one red (van Hof and Russell, 1977). By these means it was possible to determine whether or not the information presented to the two eyes separately is integrated in the brain. This was found to be the case.

The most striking experiment is illustrated in figure 17.11. Before the actual experiment rabbits were trained to discriminate a 'same–different' problem. If two identical striations were offered (two vertical striations or two horizontal ones) the left pattern was rewarded, if non-identical striations were presented (horizontal versus vertical or vertical versus horizontal) the right pattern was rewarded. At first the animals were trained to solve this problem without goggles and with black–white striations. Those animals which learned this task satisfactory were also able to solve the problem when, due to the filters, each eye saw only one pattern. This means that the information offered to both eyes is integrated centrally. The experiment shows that the two eyes have access to the same memory trace.

However, this experiment does not prove that this integration takes place by way of the interhemispheric commissures. Since mutual facilitation of contralateral and ipsilateral input takes place at the cortical level (van Sluyters and Stewart, 1974), the possibility is not excluded that a memory trace is formed on each side (figure

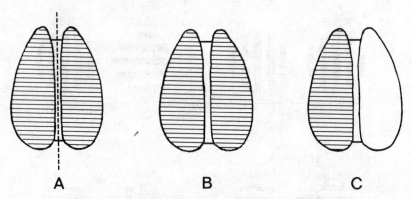

Figure 17.12. (A) Two identical engrams separated by non-conducting commissures; (B) one memory trace diffusely spread out over both hemispheres; (C) a lateralised memory trace to which the other hemisphere 'dials' by way of the commissures

17.12A). A logical step in future experimentation will therefore be to repeat the experiment shown in figure 17.11 in callosum split rabbits.

Suppose the results indicate that the binocular integration is largely abolished by this operation, the interpretation is not necessarily the one shown in figure 17.12(B): one memory trace diffusely spread out over both hemispheres. One-third of rabbits trained to discriminate vertical versus horizontal striations binocularly and thereafter tested monocularly perform well with only one of the two eyes (van Hof and van der Mark, 1976a). Therefore the possibility should be considered (figure 17.12C) that the memory trace formed during binocular training is lateralised and that the other eye 'dials' this lateralised memory tract in the ipsilateral hemisphere by way of the commissures.

The analysis of interhemispheric communication by means of pattern discrimination techniques is still incomplete but the results obtained so far indicate that it would be premature to regard the rabbit as a 'natural split-brain preparation'.

REFERENCES

De Graauw, J. G. and Van Hof, M. W. (1978). The relation between behaviour and eye refraction in the rabbit (abstr.). *Physiol. Behav.*, **21**, 257–59

Goodale, M. A. (1973). Cortico-tectal and intertectal modulation of visual responses in the rat's superior colliculus. *Expl Brain Res.*, **17**, 75–86

Hughes, A. (1971). Topographical relationships between the anatomy and physiology of the rabbit visual system. *Doc. Ophthalmol.*, **30**, 33–159

Palmers, C. and Zeier, H. (1974). Hemisphere dominance and transfer in the pigeon. *Brain Res.*, **76**, 537–41

Robert, F. and Cuénod, M. (1969a). Electrophysiology of intertectal commissures in the pigeon. I, Analysis of the pathways. *Expl Brain Res.*, **9**, 116–22

Robert, F. and Cuénod, M. (1969b). Electrophysiology of intertectal commissures in the pigeon. II, Inhibitory interaction. *Expl Brain Res.*, **9**, 123-36

Russell, I. S. and Morgan, S. C. (1969). Do single or dual memory traces subserve normal visual learning? *Brain Res.*, **107**, 212

Swadlow, H. A. (1974). Properties of antidromically activated callosal neurons responsive to callosal neurons responsive to callosal input in rabbit binocular cortex. *Expl Neurol.*, **43**, 424-44

Van Hof, M. W. (1966). Discrimination of striated patterns of different orientation in the rabbit. *Vision Res.*, **6**, 89-94

Van Hof, M. W. (1970). Interocular transfer in the rabbit. *Expl Neurol.*, **26**, 103-108

Van Hof, M.W., Treurniet-Donker, A.D. and Lagers-van Haselen, G. C. (1971). The role of the rabbit's visual cortex in the discrimination of striations of different orientation (abstr). *Pflügers Arch.*, **328**, 252

Van Hof, M. W. and Lagers-van Haselen, G. C. (1973). The retinal fixation area in the rabbit. *Expl Neurol.*, **41**, 218-21

Van Hof, M. W. and Lagers-van Haselen, G. C. (1975). Monocular pattern discrimination in rabbits after unilateral ablation of the visual cortex. *Expl Neurol.*, **46**, 257-59

Van Hof, M. W. and van der Mark, F. (1976a). Monocular pattern discrimination in normal and monocularly light-deprived rabbits. *Physiol Behav.*, **16**, 775-81

Van Hof, M. W. and van der Mark, F. (1976b). A quantitative study on interocular transfer in the rabbit. *Physiol. Behav.*, **17**, 715-17

Van Hof, M. W. and Russell, I. S. (1977). Binocular vision in the rabbit. *Physiol. Behav.*, **18**, 121-28

Van der Mark, F. and Meyer, J. H. C. (1974). Automatic control of installations for experiments relating to physiological research of the visual system. *Comput. Prog. Biomed.*, **4**, 35-41

Van Sluyters, R. C. and Stewart, D. L. (1974). Binocular neurons of the rabbit's visual cortex: receptive field characteristics. *Expl Brain Res.*, **19**, 166-95

18
COMMISSURAL CONNECTIONS OF THE VISUAL CORTEX OF THE CAT

DETLEV SANIDES

Two generalisations have commonly been made about the structure of the callosal system of the visual cortex in mammals: (a) only the line of decussation of the visual projection—in higher mammals this is the vertical meridian of the visual field—is callosally connected; (b) the callosal connections are homotopical and reciprocal (Choudhury *et al.*, 1965; Ebner and Myers, 1965; Fisken *et al.*, 1975; Garey *et al.*, 1968; Hubel and Wiesel, 1967; Innocenti and Fiore, 1976; Myers, 1962; Shatz, 1977).

These findings have been made with the use of physiological techniques and with anterograde tracing of degenerating axons. Neither technique shows the cells of origin of the projections. However, for some years this has been done by retrograde tracing with horseradish peroxidase. This technique has already been applied for the callosal system of the visual areas 17 and 18 of the cat (Innocenti and Fiore 1976; Shatz, 1977; Sanides and Donate-Oliver, 1978). It showed that the projection arises mainly in layer III and that pyramidal cells as well as stellate cells are involved. So far this is the only efferent cortical projection in which stellate cells have been found to participate.

In the present chapter I discuss some results of my own investigation of the distribution of the callosal projection. Multiple HRP injections were made in the caudal part of the lateral gyrus and the rostral end of the postlateral gyrus (figure 18.1). In this region HRP reached cortex of area 17 close to its lateral areal boundary and a large part of neighbouring area 18 except for its most lateral portion. In terms of visual field representation in area 17, the region near the projection of the vertical meridian was injected, whereas in area 18 the injected visual field representation reached from the vertical meridian up to a few degrees from the projection at the lateral border of area 18. The visual eccentricity at the lateral border of area 18 is known to be maximally 50° (Albus and Beckmann, in preparation).

In the opposite hemisphere HRP labelled cell bodies occurred in two places (figure 18.1): (a) in an area roughly homotopical to the site of injection on the lateral and on the postlateral gyrus, and (b) on the banks of the middle suprasylvian gyrus. In each of the two regions, sites with increased density of labelled cells occurred which were not caused by increased density of injected HRP in the opposite hemisphere. In the middle of the junction of the lateral and postlateral gyri there was a maximum of HRP labelled cells, and their number decreased gradually

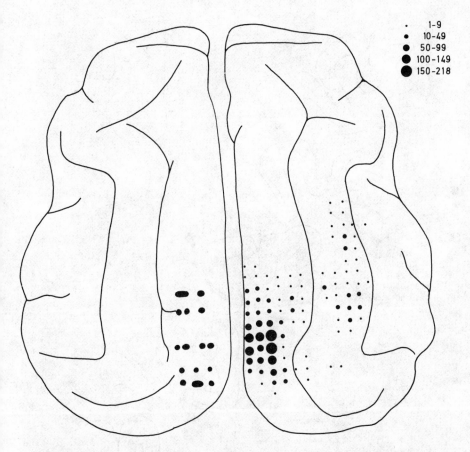

Figure 18.1. Dorsal view of a cat brain in which the HRP injection sites on the lateral gyrus of the left hemisphere are indicated by black spots. The depth of the injection was 1–3 mm. The distribution of HRP labelled cells in the right hemisphere is indicated by the black circular spots. Their size indicates the number of cells found below an area of the brain surface of about 1 mm². The cell number corresponding to the spot size is indicated to the right of the brain. All cells which are indicated in the region of the suprasylvian gyrus are located on the walls of the suprasylvian sulcus below it

from there. In the suprasylvian sulcus the density of labelled cells was somewhat increased in two spots, one rostrally the other caudally.

The following topographic distribution of HRP labelled cells has been found by comparison with Nissl stained sections of the same brain. In area 17, cells with callosal projection were most numerous along the border to area 18 and their density decreased progressively towards the suprasplenial sulcus (figure 18.2). No callosal cells were found below the suprasplenial sulcus. In area 18 the distribution of cells with callosal projection looked like a mirror image of area 17. Most cells lay

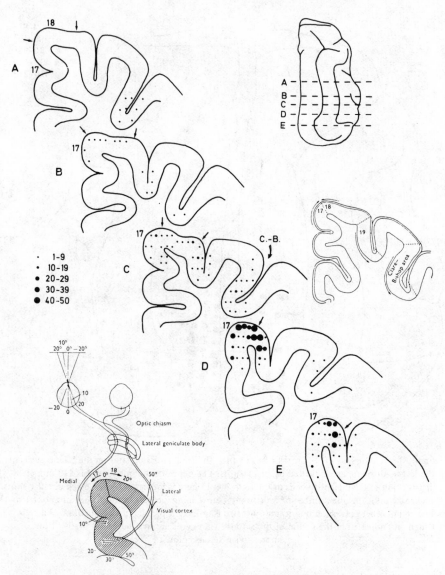

Figure 18.2. The right hemisphere of the same brain as in figure 18.1. is shown in a rostro-caudal sequence of frontal slices. The level of each slice (letters A to E) is indicated on the drawing of the entire hemisphere on the upper right of the figure. The black spots indicate the cell number found below a cortical area of about 1 mm². The thickness of the cortical slices is about 0.5 mm. The cell number corresponding to the spot size is indicated on the middle left side. Arrows show the lateral borders of areas 17 and 18. C.-B. in section C shows the location of the Clare–Bishop area. The physiological defined limits of the Clare–Bishop area are shown in the drawing to the right of section C (from Hubel and Wiesel, 1969). It corresponds very well to the location of labelled cells. The representation of the visual field in areas 17 and 18 is indi-cated in the drawing on the lower left side (from Hubel and Wiesel, 1971)

near the medial border to area 17 and laterally the density decreased gradually. However, in contrast to area 17, at least in some places, HRP labelled cells spread as far as the lateral border of area 18 and even beyond it into area 19 (figure 18.2C).

In terms of visual field representations the distribution is such that in both areas 17 and 18 the densest callosal projection arises along the representation of the vertical meridian. The maximum lay in the vicinity of the representation of the vertical meridian in the centre of the visual field. With increasing distance from the vertical meridian the projection decreases.

At least part of the cell groups in the middle suprasylvian gyrus corresponds very well with the physiologically defined location of the Clare-Bishop area (figure 18.2C; Clare and Bishop, 1954). The appearance of two cell concentrations in this region

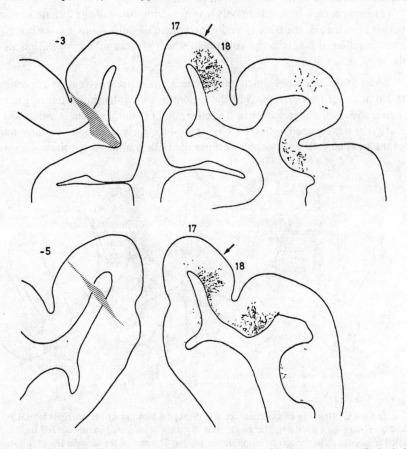

Figure 18.3.   Camera lucida drawings of two coronal sections of both hemispheres of a brain in which the left lateral and postlateral gyri had been undercut. The cut is indicated by shading. The sections are taken from the rostral part of the postlateral gyrus. The numbers on the upper left indicate the Horsley-Clarke co-ordinate levels of the sections. Degenerating terminals in the right hemisphere are dotted. The arrows indicate the lateral border of area 17 as seen in neighbouring Nissl stained sections

may be an indication that several separate areas are involved. Palmer *et al.* (1978) have found four complete visual field representations in the suprasylvian sulcus.

The wide spread of the origin of the callosal projection in area 17 and to a greater extent in area 18 is puzzling from two points of view:

(1) The region with callosal terminations appears to be much more restricted. Most investigators have described callosal terminals that are restricted to a strip on top of the lateral and postlateral gyri which barely reaches area 17 and only to the medial part of area 18 (Ebner and Myers 1965; Fisken *et al.*, 1975; Garey *et al.*, 1968; Hubel and Wiesel, 1967). This distribution has been confirmed by a degeneration study of our own (figure 18.3). This means that there must be some heterotopic convergence of the callosal projections.

(2) Since in each hemisphere only a very narrow stripe of the ipsilateral visual field is represented, the wide spread of the origin of callosal input must bring about a combination of points in the visual field which are located on opposite sides of the vertical meridian.

Some of the cell types which participate in the callosal projection are concentrated in rather restricted parts of the regions in which the projection originates. This is shown in a representative frontal section of another brain in which the lateral gyrus was injected with HRP (figure 18.4A). A classification of a large number of the labelled cells was possible because the HRP granules often show the outlines

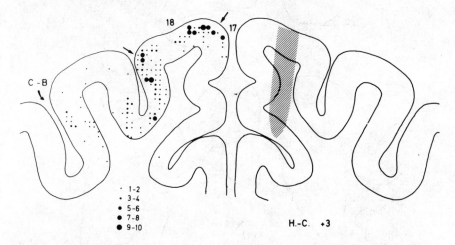

Figure 18.4A. Drawing of a coronal section through a brain in which the right lateral gyrus had been injected with HRP. The position of the track is indicated by the shaded region. All HRP labelled cells in the left hemisphere are shown. The size of the circular dots indicates the number of cells found in an area of about 1 mm² in the 60 μm section. The cell number corresponding to the spot size is indicated on the lower left. The lateral borders of areas 17 and 18 were identified in neighbouring Nissl stained sections and are indicated by arrows. C.-B. refers to the Clare-Bishop area.

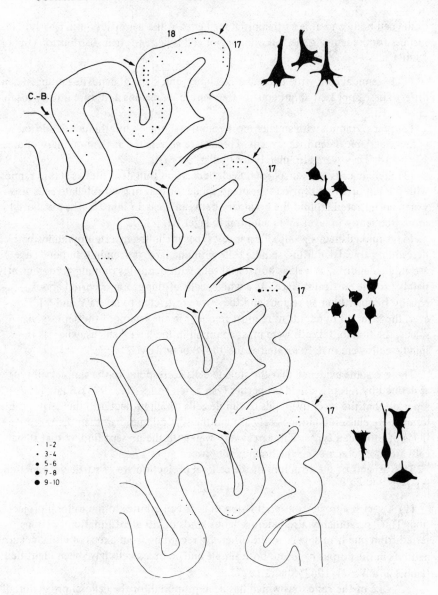

Figure 18.4B. The right half of the section as in figure 18.4A, with the distribution of those cells which could be identified as one of several cell types. Camera lucida drawings of the corresponding cell types are shown to the right of each drawing of the section. They are, from top to bottom, (1) pyramidal cells, (2) star-pyramids, (3) stellate cells and (4) miscellaneous rarer cell types: inverted pyramids, spindle cells and horizontal cells

of the cell body and at least the initial segments of the dendrites quite clearly. This suffices for recognising the following major cell types and their distribution (figure 18.4B):

(1) Pyramidal cells with triangular cell body, thick apical dendrite and basal dendrites. These appeared about equally frequent in all regions and were mostly located in layer III.

(2) Star-pyramids with smaller more round cell bodies and thinner dendrites, with a clear apical dendrite present. These were aggregated at the boundary of areas 17 and 18. They were also mainly located in layer III.

(3) Stellate cells with small round cell bodies and thin dendrites as star-pyramids with the important exception that no apical dendrite is present. Stellate cells also were concentrated around the boundary between areas 17 and 18. They occurred more frequently in layer IV in addition to layer III.

(4) A miscellaneous group of rarer cell types including inverted pyramids with descending apical dendrites, spindle cells with one large descending and one large ascending dendrite, as well as horizontal cells with dendrites running predominantly parallel to the cortical surface. As a whole, cells of this group occurred about equally frequently in all regions and they were restricted to layers V and VI. However, the inverted pyramids were most frequent in the region of the suprasylvian sulcus, the horizontal cells were most common in the lateral sulcus, whereas the spindle cells were mainly located at the 17–18 boundary.

There is some evidence that the stellate cells correspond to the simple cell type as defined by receptive field properties (van Essen and Kelly, 1973). Shatz (1977) reported that the receptive fields of simple cells which project into the corpus callosum were clustered more closely around the vertical meridian than the receptive fields of other cell types. This agrees very well with the present finding that stellate cells are most common at the boundary between areas 17 and 18.

Two aspects of the structure of the callosal projection are of particular functional interest:

(1) A very heterogeneous population of cells contributes to the callosal projection. Thus, presumably also heterogeneous kinds of visual information are transferred from one hemisphere to the other. By recording from axons of visual cortical neurons in the corpus callosum both simple and complex cells have been identified (Hubel and Wiesel, 1967; Shatz, 1977).

(2) One of the functions which has been proposed for the callosal projection of the visual cortical areas is to unite the representations of the two hemiretinae along the vertical meridian (Choudhury et al., 1965; Whitteridge, 1965). However, since the origin of the callosal projection covers such a wide region of the visual field representations, especially in areas 18 and 19, its function probably goes beyond this.

REFERENCES

Albus, K. and Beckmann, R. (in preparation). The second and the third visual area of the cat: interindividual variability in retinotopic arrangement and cortical location.

Choudhury, B. P., Whitteridge, D. and Wilson, M. E. (1965). The function of the callosal connections of the visual cortex. *Q. Jl exp. Physiol.*, **50**, 214–19

Clare, M. H. and Bishop, G. H. (1954). Responses from an association area secondarily activated from optic cortex. *J. Neurophysiol.*, **17**, 271–77

Ebner, F. F. and Myers, R. E. (1965). Distribution of corpus callosum and anterior commissure in cat and raccoon. *J. comp. Neurol.*, **124**, 353–66

Fisken, R. A., Garey, L. J. and Powell, T. P. S. (1975). The intrinsic, association and commissural connections of area 17 of the visual cortex. *Phil. Trans. R. Soc. Lond. B*, **272**, 487–536

Garey, L. J., Jones, E. G. and Powell, T. P. S. (1968). Interrelationship of striate and extrastriate cortex with the primary relay sites of the visual pathway. *J. Neurol. Neurosurg. Psychiat.*, **31**, 135–57

Hubel, D. H. and Wiesel, T. N. (1967). Cortical and callosal connections concerned with the vertical meridian of visual fields in the cat. *J. Neurophysiol.*, **30**, 1561–73

Hubel, D. H. and Wiesel, T. N. (1969). Visual area of the lateral suprasylvian gyrus (Clare–Bishop Area) of the cat. *J. Physiol., Lond.*, **202**, 251–60

Hubel, D. H. and Wiesel, T. N. (1971). Aberrant visual projections in the Siamese cat. *J. Physiol., Lond.*, **218**, 33–62

Innocenti, G. M. and Fiore, L. (1976). Morphological correlates of visual field transformation in the corpus callosum. *Neurosci. Lett.*, **2**, 245–52

Myers, R. E. (1962). Commissural connections between occipital lobes of the monkey. *J. comp. Neurol.*, **118**, 1–16

Palmer, L. A., Rosenquist, A. C. and Tusa, R. J. (1978). The retinotopic organization of lateral suprasylvian visual areas in the cat. *J. comp. Neurol.*, **177**, 237-56.

Sanides, D. and Donate-Oliver, F. (1978). Identification and localization of some relay cells in cat visual cortex. In *Architectonics of the Cerebral Cortex*, IBRO Monographs Series, vol. 3 (M. A. B. Brazier and H. Petsche, eds.), Raven Press, New York

Shatz, C. (1977). Abnormal interhemispheric connections in the visual system of Boston Siamese cats. *J. comp. Neurol.*, **171**, 229–46

Van Essen, D. and Kelly, J. (1973). Morphological identification of simple, complex and hypercomplex cells in the visual cortex of the cat. In *Intracellular Staining in Neurobiology* (S.B. Kater and C. Nicholson, eds.), Springer Verlag, Heidelberg, pp. 189–98

Whitteridge, D. (1965). In *Functions of the Corpus Callosum* (E. G. Ettlinger, ed.), Churchill, London

19

ADULT AND NEONATAL CHARACTERISTICS OF THE CALLOSAL ZONE AT THE BOUNDARY BETWEEN AREAS 17 AND 18 IN THE CAT

G. M. INNOCENTI

To an anatomist and physiologist the system of connections established through the corpus callosum is interesting for two main reasons. The first is the possibility of discovering the morphological and electrophysiological basis for the behavioural performance mediated by the cerebral commissure; the second comes from the fact that it offers an excellent paradigm for the analysis of a cortical network *in statu nascendi* and in its fully developed form. One hopes that this analysis will yield answers suitable for generalisation to other aspects of cortical organisation.

In several mammalian species, callosal axons have been seen to terminate at the boundary between cyto-architectonic areas 17 and 18 (cf. chapter 10). Injections of horseradish peroxidase (HRP) at or near the boundary allow the visualisation of the neurons of origin of the corpus callosum (they will be called 'callosal neurons') in the contralateral visual cortex (Innocenti and Fiore, 1976; Jacobson and Trojanowski, 1974; Shatz, 1977b; Winfield *et al.*, 1975; Wong-Riley, 1974; Yorke and Caviness, 1975). HRP stained axons can be followed through the splenium of the corpus callosum from the injection site to the contralateral hemisphere (figure 19.1a). There, in fortuitous sections, some of the axons can be traced from the white matter to their neurons of origin.

In the cat, most of the HRP filled callosal neurons appear to be located at sites roughly homotopic to those which have been injected. The injection at the 17/18 boundary of retrograde–anterograde cocktails (HRP and radioactive leucine) and the combined use of autoradiographic and diaminobenzidine processing (Colwell, 1975), can show at the homotopic site in contralateral cortex both callosal neurons and callosal terminals (figure 19.1b., c).

Although it has been known for years that the corpus callosum connects homotopic cortical points on the two hemispheres (Curtis, 1940), we do not yet know how precisely and completely the regions of origin and termination of callosal fibres overlap each other in any given cortical area (cf. chapter 18).

However, from anatomical, functional and embryological points of view, the origin and termination of the corpus callosum are distinct entities.

(1) It is well established that, at least in the higher mammalian species (including the cat), heterotopic, non-reciprocal callosal connections exist (Boyd *et al.*, 1971;

244

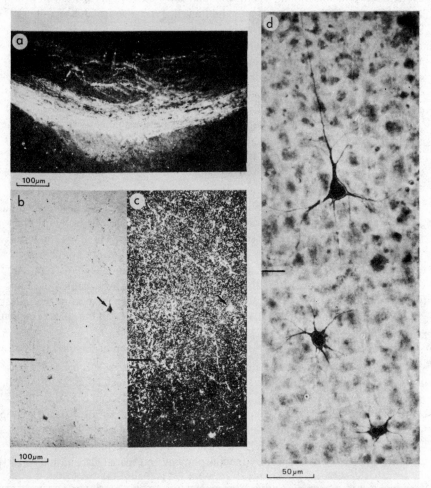

Figure 19.1.(a) Dark-field photomicrograph of HRP stained axons in the splenium of the corpus callosum of an adult albino mouse after HRP injection into the 17/18a boundary region.
(b, c) A combined HRP–autoradiography experiment in an adult cat. HRP filled neurons
(bright-field photomicrograph on the left) and leucine filled terminals and preterminal fibres
(dark-field photomicrograph on the right) in the same location in the cortex homotopic to the
injection site (17/18 boundary). The arrow points to the same neuron in both pictures. The
small horizontal bars mark the boundary between layers III and IV (pial surface up), as determined on an adjacent section that was counterstained with toluidine blue. (d) Phase-contrast
photomicrograph of three callosal neurons (one pyramid and two stellate cells) in area 18 stained
in a Golgi-like way by HRP. The horizontal bar marks the boundary between layers III and IV
(pial surface up). Camera lucida drawings of the same neurons are shown in figure 19.4. The
sections (a, d) and (b, c) are 80 and 40 μm thick, respectively, treated for HRP as described elsewhere (Innocenti and Fiore, 1976); (a) and (d) were counterstained with toluidine blue

Curtis, 1940; Diamond *et al.*, 1968; Goldman and Nauta, 1977; Heath and Jones, 1970; Hubel and Wiesel, 1965; Jones and Powell, 1968; Pandya and Vignolo, 1971; Shanks *et al.*, 1975).

(2) Electrophysiological experiments have shown that callosal neurons and neurons which are activated through the callosal pathway form, in the primary sensory areas, two separate populations (Innocenti *et al.*, 1972, 1973, 1974; Robinson, 1973; Swadlow, 1974; Toyama *et al.*, 1974), with different receptive field properties (Innocenti *et al.*, 1972, 1973, 1974; Robinson, 1973; Swadlow, 1974).

(3) During ontogenesis, the neurons of origin and the connections made by the corpus callosum must obviously appear at different times (Wise and Jones, 1976). They probably follow different developmental courses since it seems likely that different laws control the growth of the somadendritic and axonal parts of the neuron (van der Loos, 1976).

I propose, therefore to call 'callosal zone' the district of cortex limited both tangentially and radially within a given cortical area (cyto-architectonically or otherwise defined) which includes the somata of callosal neurons. I shall use the term 'callosal terminal territory' to indicate the district of cortex which contains the termination of the callosal axons. I would like to stress that one major feature in the organisation of neocortex is the existence in it of spatially separated outputs (Gilbert and Kelly, 1975). The questions approached here in relation to the callosal zone could be also applied to other, similarly defined, zones in the cortex: collicular, geniculate, etc.

In the callosal zone the final elaboration and transmission of the message that one visual cortex sends to its contralateral homologue takes place. This message has two main aspects. One concerns the transformation of the cortical representation of the visual field which takes place in the callosal zone, and the second concerns the receptive field properties of the callosal neurons. Both aspects of the message are represented in the morphological features of the callosal zone—the first aspect by the number of neurons which encode, in the callosal message, different parts of the visual field, and the second aspect by the morphology and spatial distribution of these

Figure 19.2. Extent and location of the callosal zone at the 17/18 boundary in the adult cat. (Left) Computer-microscope (Glaser and Van der Loos, 1965) reconstruction (from 80 μm thick sections) indicating positions of HRP positive neurons at different coronal levels of lateral gyrus. Only cells found in areas 17 and 18 are shown. In each section, broken lines indicate the lower borders of layers I, III, IV, V and VI, respectively. Arrows point at the 17/18 boundary (17 on the right, 18 on the left). Letters relate each section to the lateral gyrus (see inset figure). (Right) Number of HRP positive cell bodies per section at different anteroposterior levels. Degrees of visual field representation are indicated according to the results obtained in animals in which electrophysiological controls at the injection site were performed (cf. Innocenti and Fiore, in preparation) and to the map of Bilge *et al.*, 1967. The letters refer to the sections shown on the left. The 'bumps' in the curve, at A, B, C, and D, correspond to the points of highest HRP density at the injection site. In brain figure (inset), dots mark the position of injections; arrows point to lateral (lat), suprasylvian (sups), entolateral (entolet); and postlateral (postl) sulci. Reproduced from Innocenti and Fiore, 1976, with kind permission of Elsevier

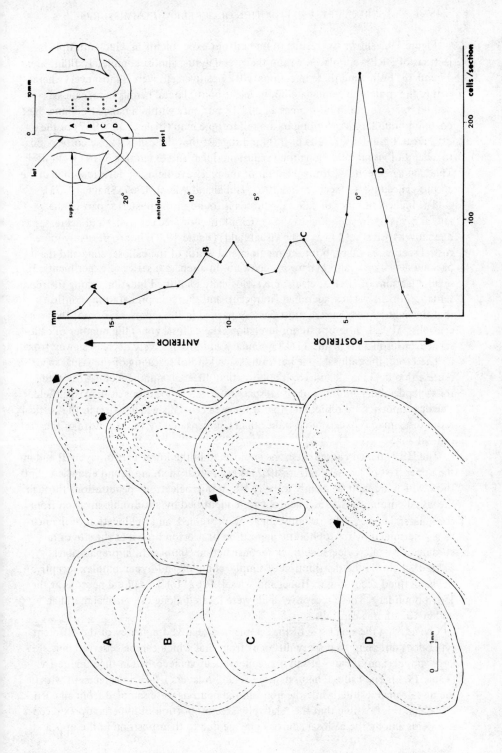

Figure 19.2 shows the results of one of four experiments in which multiple injections of HRP were placed within the lateral gyrus, almost completely filling areas 17 and 18. Following these injections, HRP positive cells were almost everywhere within the ipsilateral geniculate body. In the contralateral hemisphere, callosal neurons were found in both areas 17 and 18 but only within a band straddling their common boundary. According to the retinotopic map (Bigle *et al.,* 1967) of the cat's areas 17 and 18, results of this kind suggest that the callosal zone corresponds to a band of visual field along the vertical meridian and extending 5–10° from it. This is in agreement with the position of the receptive fields of units recorded in the corpus callosum (Berlucchi *et al.,* 1967; Hubel and Wiesel, 1967; Shatz, 1977a).

The highest number of callosal neurons is found in the posterior part of the lateral gyrus (corresponding to the representation of area centralis) and decreases as one moves rostrally (down in the visual field) (figure 19.2). In progressively more rostral sections, in fact, both the mediolateral width of the callosal zone and the packing density of callosal neurons decrease. In a separate series of experiments, small injections of HRP at electrophysiologically identified locations along the representation of the vertical meridian (Innocenti and Fiore, in preparation) confirm that the callosal neurons are most densely packed in the representation of the area centralis. At each anteroposterior level along the callosal zone, the number of callosal neurons is highest at the 17/18 boundary and progressively decreases away from it. Therefore, the callosal zone performs some kind of rescaling of the visual space represented in areas 17 and 18. It appears that different numbers of callosal neurons encode equal amounts of visual space at different locations in the visual field. The disproportionate representation of the area centralis which exists in the cortical retinotopic map is exaggerated rather than compensated by the structure of the callosal zone.

The HRP stained callosal neurons are located in the lower part of layer III and in the upper part of layer IV (figure 19.2). Very few of them are found elsewhere, but those which are, appear mainly in layer VI. In microelectrode penetrations through the visual cortex, the callosal neurons were identified by antidromic invasion from contralateral cortex. The receptive fields were studied, and the location of the neurons determined by iontophoretic deposition of procion brown at the site of recording or by microelectrode track reconstruction (Innocenti, in preparation). Table 19.1 shows the distribution of simple, complex and hypercomplex receptive fields (defined according to Hubel and Wiesel, 1962) for 15 callosal neurons at the 17/18 boundary. These receptive fields were located along the vertical meridian within 10° of area centralis.

Considering the small size of the sample, the relative frequency of the different types does not seem to be very different from that which can be observed in a larger population of callosal and non-callosal neurons recorded in the same region (Table 19.1). The callosal neurons were found in layers III–IV in agreement with the histological results, while the non-callosal neurons were sampled from all cortical layers. It is possible that the relatively large proportion of hypercomplex receptive fields among the callosal neurons may be due to their position in the upper

Table 19.1.
Receptive field of properties of callosal neurons at the
17/18 boundary

Receptive field type	Callosal neurons (n = 15)	Total population (n = 62)
Simple	2 (13.3%)	10 (16.3%)
Complex	9 (60%)	45 (72.4%)
Hypercomplex	4 (26.7%)	7 (11.3%)

half of the cortex where a prevalence of these receptive fields exists (Camarda and Rizzolatti, 1976; Hubel and Wiesel, 1962; Kelly and van Essen, 1974). An example of the responses to moving slits of different lengths of a callosal neuron with hypercomplex receptive field properties is shown in figure 19.3.

A broad range of receptive field orientations was observed among the callosal neurons, as well as various degrees of directional selectivity and ocular dominance. The receptive field ('minimum response field': Barlow et al., 1967) of the callosal neurons is, on the average, relatively small (1.35 (degrees of arc)^2 ± 1.04 s.d.).

These results indicate that the variety of receptive field types that others (Berlucchi et al., 1967; Hubel and Wiesel, 1967; Shatz, 1977a) have observed among callosal fibres reflect the properties of the callosal neurons at the 17/18 boundary, although callosal neurons in area 19 and in the area of Clare–Bishop may contribute to it.

The variety of receptive field types has a possible correlate in the variety of histological types among the callosal neurons. In some cases, the HRP technique allows a very complete, Golgi-like visualisation of the dendritic tree; when this happens dendritic spines and the axon can often be seen (Innocenti and Fiore, 1976). The histological type of neurons stained in this way can be recognised (when the orientation of the cut is parallel to the local radial axis; Molliver and van der Loos, 1970) with no greater difficulty than in Golgi preparations. One can commonly find the following among the callosal neurons: typical pyramidal cells (figure 19.1d and figure 19.4) with triangular cell bodies and long apical dendrites ascending to ramify in layer I (layer III); typical stellate cells with round cell bodies and dendrites ramifying within a few cell body diameters (layers III, IV) (figure 19.1d and figure 19.4), as well as several intermediate types. The existence among the callosal neurons of typical layer IV stellate cells and of typical pyramidal cells is particularly meaningful since these neuronal types may account, respectively, for the simple and complex receptive fields (cf. Kelly and van Essen, 1974) found among the callosal neurons studied in our electrophysiological experiments and described by others (Berlucchi et al., 1967; Hubel and Wiesel, 1967; Shatz, 1977a) among callosal fibres.

One may speculate that the two main morphological features of the callosal zone have probably opposite consequences on the receptive field properties of callosal neurons. The callosal zone occupies a limited region along the radial axis of the cor-

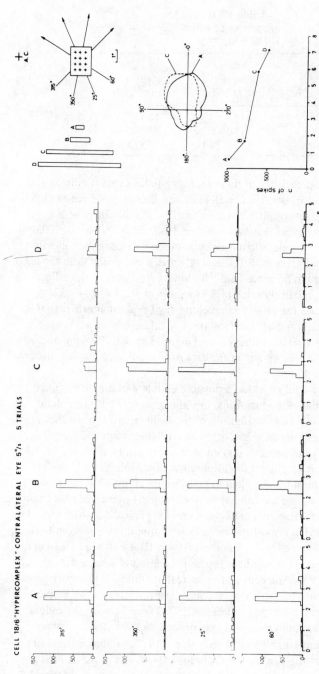

Figure 19.3 Response pattern of a callosal neuron with 'hypercomplex' receptive field. Graphs A, B, C, D, on the left-hand side, are peristimulus-time histograms (bin wide 200 ms) of the responses, elicited by moving slits of different length each tested at four different orientations. The scheme on the top right shows: the size of the slits; the direction of movement (in degrees from the horizontal); the size of the receptive field and its location with respect to the right area centralis (A.C.). 'On' responses (+) to stationary stimuli could be evoked throughout this receptive field. The slits were moved perpendicular to their long axis. The middle graph on the right shows two computer-derived polar plots (cf. Daniels and Pettigrew, 1975) of the response to two different slit lengths (A and C) of varying orientation. The vector that connects each point of the contour with the centre of the co-ordinates represents the direction of the stimulus; its length represents the magnitude of the response as a percent (for each contour) of the optimal one. Note that, after an increase in slit length, the neuron remains optimally responsive to roughly the same orienta-tion although it becomes more sharply tuned. The bottom graph on the right shows the magnitude of the response as a function of slit length. Spikes fired during presentation of slits of the same length at different orientations (histograms of columns A, B, C and D were separately added). The neuron was recorded in the left visual cortex, stimulated through the contralateral eye, with stimulus speed at 5° /s

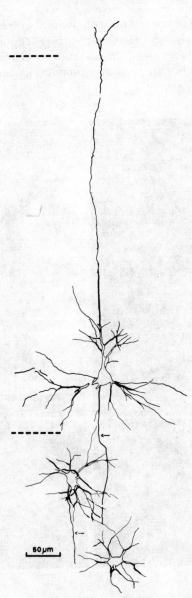

Figure 19.4. Camera lucida drawings of the pyramidal and stellate cells shown in figure 19.1(d). The horizontal bars show the lower boundaries of layers I and III. The arrows point to the axons

tex. The callosal neurons, therefore, are likely to share with each other a certain amount of thalamocortical and 'local' connections. A certain uniformity in the receptive field properties would, therefore, result if the consequence of similar cell position were not counteracted by the existence of very different dendritic domains among the callosal neurons. If the receptive field properties of a cortical neuron are related to the morphology of its dendritic tree (Kelly and van Essen, 1974), then the variety of cell types among the callosal neurons would be the means by which the visual cortex solves the problem of providing its callosal message with a variety of receptive field types.

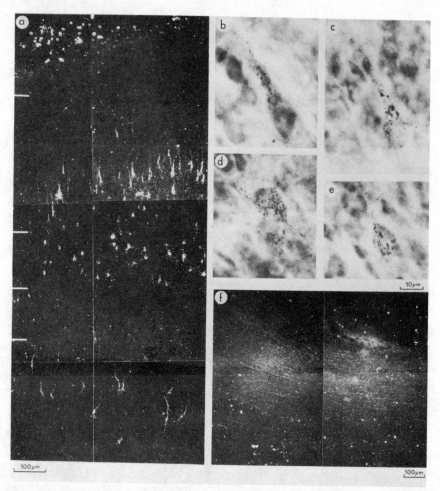

Figure 19.5.(a) Collage of dark-field photomicrographs showing callosal neurons of a kitten injected at three days of age. The photos are from area 18 close to the boundary with area 17. The small horizontal lines mark the lower boundaries of layers I, III, IV and V. (b–e) Phase-contrast photomicrographs of HRP filled callosal neurons at the 17/18 boundary. Two pyrami-dal cells (b and c; layer III) and two non-pyramidal cells (d and e; layer IV) are shown. The neu-rons are oriented in the same manner with respect to the pia mater, which is at the top/left. (f) Dark-field photomicrograph showing HRP stained axons in the splenium of the corpus callosum. All the preparations (80 μm thick sections counterstained with toluidine blue) were taken from the animal (D7) which is shown in figure 19.6

During ontogenetic development, exigencies other than those imposed by function may be operant on the morphology of the callosal zone which, therefore, could also be expected to be different.

HRP was injected into the visual cortex of four kittens (from three different litters) at two, three (two animals) and four days postnatally. The two- and four-day-old kittens survived 24 h after the injection, the three-day-old ones survived, respectively, 18 and 48 h. The results of these experiments are very similar and will be described together.

In the first postnatal week, the occipital cortex of the cat shows both macroscopical and microscopical signs of immaturity (Innocenti *et al.,* 1977). The layering, the existence of different cyto-architectonic fields and of different cell types, can however already be recognised in Nissl stained material.

At the injection site, where two 0.5 μl injections had been placed, the HRP filled most of areas 17 and 18 and diffused into the lateral suprasylvian cortex (figure 19.6). Retrograde transport of HRP was observed to most of the ipsilateral geniculate nucleus and to the pulvinar. The relative size of the region of HRP uptake was therefore comparable to that which had been achieved with multiple injections in the adult. HRP filled callosal neurons can be seen contralateral to the injection as early as the second postnatal day, although they are rather faintly stained (figure 19.5a–e). The dark homogeneous precipitate, which in the adult yields a Golgi-like image of the dendritic tree, was never observed.

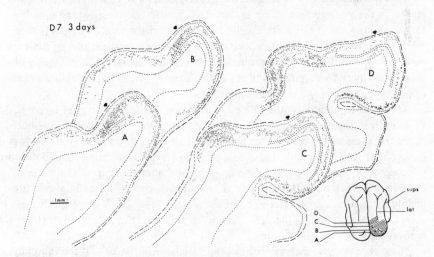

Figure 19.6.   The extent and location of the callosal zone in a kitten injected at three days of age. (A–D) Computer microscope reconstructions showing the location of HRP stained cell bodies at four different coronal planes (cf. inset). The arrows point to the 17/18 boundary (17 on the right, 18 on the left). Unlike in the adult, the callosal zone at the 17/18 boundary continues without interruption up to the suprasylvian sulcus. Dashed lines mark the lower limits of layers I, IV, V and VI in area 18. In the brain figurine (inset) the planes of section are indicated. Two dots mark the position of the injection and the hatched area, the region of HRP diffusion; sups and lat indicate the suprasylvian and lateral sulci, respectively

Both pyramidal and non-pyramidal cell bodies can be recognised among the callosal neurons in neonatal areas 17 and 18, although the faint staining makes the exact differentiation of cell type more difficult than in the adult (figure 19.5a–e). The pyramidal cells show signs of immaturity. In particular, the apical dendrite is very thick, especially at its base, and sits on the nucleus as a Phrygian cap. There is little cytoplasm around the nucleus and few or no basal dendrites can be seen. Some of the non-pyramidal neurons have round cell bodies and a few dendrites radiate from them more or less symmetrically. These neurons are preferentially located in layer IV, although a few of them can also be seen in layer III. Their morphology (reminiscent of the stellate cells seen in the adult) and their depth of location suggest that they may be immature stellate cells. It seems, therefore, that at two days of age both pyramidal and stellate cells have already sent axons to the contralateral hemisphere. In layer VI, a third neuronal type can be identified (figure 19.5a), which has a fusiform, often radially oriented, cell body. In the adult visual cortex, few cells are stained with HRP in layer VI. Often they are fusiform in shape and sometimes show a long apical dendrite which can be followed to layer I.

The callosal zone in area 17/18 differs in other ways in the first postnatal week and at maturity (figure 19.6). In the first postnatal week, it appears to have no clear-cut mediolateral boundaries. Laterally, it continues without interruption throughout areas 18 and 19 up to the lateral suprasylvian cortex. Medially, it extends throughout most of area 17, down the medial bank of the hemisphere and into the splenial sulcus. In addition, the packing density of callosal neurons appears greater in the young animals than in the adult. This seems to reflect the overall higher packing density of cortical cells, typical of immature visual cortex (Cragg, 1975). The packing density of callosal neurons is highest in the region of the 17/18 boundary and in the lateral suprasylvian cortex, and decreases with increasing distance from these two regions. A high packing density of callosal neurons also exists in the upper bank of the suprasplenial sulcus.

At the 17/18 boundary, the callosal neurons are found over most of layers III, IV and VI. In the neonate the callosal zone is, therefore, more broadly distributed in the thickness of the cortex than in the adult where only a few neurons are found in the lower part of layer IV and inconstantly in layer VI. A strong contribution to the corpus callosum comes also from layer VI of the lateral suprasylvian cortex. Outside the 17/18 boundary and lateral suprasylvian cortex, the callosal cells are mainly located in layer III and a few of them are in layer IV. A thin superficial sheet of cortex, including the darkly stained remnant of the cortical plate (layer II), is always free of callosal neurons.

These results show that, at birth, all the visual cortical areas that are callosally connected in the adult have already sent their axons to the contralateral hemisphere. It is not known, though, whether the axons have reached their final position, have elaborated their telodendria or participated in the formation of functioning synapses. There are, however, callosal neurons outside the boundary of the adult callosal zones.

This latter, rather surprising, finding is *not* due to diffusion of HRP from the injection site. The non-injected hemisphere appears completely free of extracellular HRP and of HRP included within endothelial or glial cells. The presence of HRP filled glial cells (recognisable by their small size and their typical processes) seems to be a particularly sensitive sign of HRP diffusion. HRP filled glia can be identified at the periphery of an injection site where no extracellular HRP can be seen. In a kitten of this series (eight days old at time of injection, not included in this chapter), diffusion of HRP from the injection site provoked staining of glial elements in a limited portion of contralateral cortex in the bank of the interhemispheric fissure. However, no neurons were stained in this region. Neither in this animal nor in the others of this series were HRP-stained neurons found in the thalamic nuclei contralateral to the injection site. The specific laminar location of HRP positive neurons in the cortex also seems incompatible with the possibility that they have been stained by diffusion from the injection hemisphere.

The last two arguments (absence of HRP positive neurons in the thalamus contralateral to the injection, and the laminar specificity of HRP stained neurons in the cortex) also speak against the possibility that retrograde transsynaptic transport of HRP may have occurred in these animals, resulting in the presence of callosal neurons outside the adult boundaries of the callosal zone. The existence of fibres faintly stained with HRP, in the splenium of the corpus callosum (figure 19.5f) indicates that a normal transport of HRP took place through the commissure.

It seems, therefore, that in the newborn kitten, a wider portion of the visual cortex projects to the corpus callosum than in the adult. If one assumes that similar retinotopic maps exist in newborn and adult cats then the conclusion is that, in the former, fibres from parts of the visual field other than the vertical meridian pass through the callosum. The callosal zone at the 17/18 boundary undergoes a postnatal remodelling, during which either neurons must die or axons must be retracted. The reason for this apparently wasteful course of neuronal development, which has also been observed in other parts of other nervous systems (Clarke and Cowan, 1976; Cowan, 1973), is unknown. Are the neurons or the axons which shall die during development only used as ephemeral instruments in the formation of permanent connections or do they have some other role? Certainly, the morphology of a growing nervous system is dictated by exigencies which are different from those which determine a stabilised adult morphology. Although the ultimate requirement of an adult nervous system is that its morphology serves the necessary functions (in this we were led to consider the callosal zone as a good example of consonance of structure and function), the developmental process may, at least temporarily, impose its own morphogenetic rules. Further studies on the callosal system of connections may determine the degrees of freedom that the genetic developmental rules allow to a cortical structure in order for it to match changes occurring during development in the sensory organs or in the sensory environment of the animal.

ACKNOWLEDGEMENTS

I am not the only one responsible for this paper. Drs L. Fiore, R. Caminiti and J. Orsoni collaborated on different parts of the experiments. The Swiss National Science Foundation gave most of the money. My colleagues at the Institut d'Anatomie helped me with their discussions. Dr D. Frost was my *arbiter elegantiarum* for the English form of the text. Throughout this research, Hendrik Van der Loos, to whom I am most indebted, pestered me with all sorts of pedantic criticisms!

REFERENCES

Barlow, H. B., Blakemore, C. and Pettigrew, J. D. (1967). The neural mechanism of binocular depth discrimination. *J. Physiol., Lond.,* **193**, 327-42

Berlucchi, G., Gazzaniga, M. S. and Rizzolatti, G. (1967). Microelectrode analysis of transfer of visual information by the corpus callosum. *Arch. Ital. Biol.,* **105**, 583-96

Bilge, M., Bingle, A., Seneviratne, K. N. and Whitteridge, D. (1967). A map of the visual cortex in the cat. *J. Physiol., Lond.,* **191**, 116P-118P

Boyd, E. H., Pandya, D. N. and Bignall, K. E. (1971). Homotopic and nonhomotopic interhemispheric cortical projections in the squirrel monkey. *Expl Neurol.,* **32**, 256-74

Camarda, R. and Rizzolatti, G. (1976). Receptive fields of cells in the superficial layers of the cat's area 17. *Expl Brain Res.,* **24**, 423-27

Clarke, P. G. H. and Cowan, W. M. (1976). The development of the isthmo-optic tract in the chick, with special reference to the occurrence and correction of developmental errors in the location and connections of isthmo-optic neurons. *J. comp. Neurol.,* **167**, 143-64

Colwell, S. A. (1975). Thalamocortical-corticothalamic reciprocity: a combined anterograde-retrograde tracer technique. *Brain Res.,* **92**, 443-49

Cowan, W. M. (1973). Neuronal death as a regulative mechanism in the control of cell number in the nervous system. In *Development and Aging in the Nervous System* (M. Rockstein, ed.), Academic Press, New York

Cragg, B. G. (1975). The development of synapses in the visual system of the cat. *J. comp. Neurol.,* **160**, 147-66

Curtis, H. J. (1940). Intercortical connections of corpus callosum as indicated by evoked potentials. *J. Neurophysiol.,* **3**, 407-13

Daniels, J. D. and Pettigrew, J. D. (1975). A study of inhibitory antagonism in cat visual cortex. *Brain Res.,* **93**, 41-62

Diamond, I. T., Jones, E. G. and Powell, T. P. S. (1968). Interhemispheric fiber connections of the auditory cortex of the cat. *Brain Res.,* **11**, 177-93

Gilbert, C. D. and Kelly, J. P. (1975). The projections of cells in different layers of the cat's visual cortex. *J. comp. Neurol.,* **163**, 81-106

Glaser, E. M. and Van der Loos, H. (1965). A semi-automatic computer-microscope for the analysis of neuronal morphology. *I.E.E.E. Trans. Biomed. Eng.,* **BME-12**, 22-31

Goldman, P. S. and Nauta, W. J. H. (1977). Columnar distribution of cortico-cortical fibers in the frontal association, limbic, and motor cortex of the developing rhesus monkey. *Brain Res.,* **122,** 393-413

Heath, C. J. and Jones, E. G. (1970). Connexions of area 19 and the lateral suprasylvian area of the visual cortex of the cat. *Brain Res.,* **19,** 302-305

Hubel, D. H. and Wiesel, T. N. (1962). Receptive fields, binocular interaction and functional architecture in the cat's visual cortex. *J. Physiol., Lond.,* **160,** 106-54

Hubel, D. H. and Wiesel, T. N. (1965). Receptive fields and functional architecture in two nonstriate visual areas (18 and 19) of the cat. *J. Neurophysiol.,* **28,** 229-89

Hubel, D. H. and Wiesel, T. N. (1967). Cortical and callosal connections concerned with the vertical meridian of visual fields in the cat. *J. Neurophysiol.,* **30,** 1561-73

Innocenti, G. M. and Fiore, L. (1976). Morphological correlates of visual field transformation in the corpus callosum. *Neurosci. Lett.,* **2,** 245-52

Innocenti, G. M., Manzoni, T. and Spidalieri, G. (1972). Peripheral and transcallosal reactivity of neurones within SI and SII cortical areas. Segmental division. *Arch. Ital. Biol.,* **110,** 415-43

Innocenti, G. M., Manzoni, T. and Spidalieri, G. (1973). Relevance of the callosal transfer in defining the peripheral reactivity of somesthetic cortical neurones. *Arch. Ital. Biol.,* **111,** 187-221

Innocenti, G. M., Manzoni, T. and Spidalieri, G. (1974). Patterns of the somesthetic messages transferred through the corpus callosum. *Expl Brain Res.,* **19,** 447-66

Innocenti, G. M., Fiore, L. and Caminiti, R. (1977). Exuberant projection into the corpus callosum from the visual cortex of newborn cats. *Neurosci. Lett.,* **4,** 237-42

Jacobson, S. and Trojanowski, J. Q. (1974). The cells of origin of the corpus callosum in rat, cat and rhesus monkey. *Brain Res.,* **74,** 149-55

Jones, E. G. and Powell, T. P. S. (1968). The commissural connexions of the somatic sensory cortex in the cat. *J. Anat.,* **103,** 433-55

Kelly, J. P. and van Essen, D. C. (1974). Cell structure and function in the visual cortex of the cat. *J. Physiol., Lond.,* **238,** 515-47

Molliver, M. E. and van der Loos, H. (1970). The ontogenesis of cortical circuitry: the spatial distribution of synapses in somesthetic cortex of newborn dog. *Ergebn. Anat.,* **42,** 1-54

Pandya, D. N. and Vignolo, L. A. (1971). Intra- and interhemispheric projections of the precentral, premotor and arcuate areas in the rhesus monkey. *Brain Res.,* **26,** 217-33

Robinson, D. L. (1973). Electrophysiological analysis of interhemispheric relations in the second somatosensory cortex of the cat. *Expl Brain Res.,* **18,** 131-44

Shanks, M. F., Rockel, A. J. and Powell, T. P. S. (1975). The commissural fibre connections of the primary somatic sensory cortex. *Brain Res.,* **98,** 166-71

Shatz, C. (1977a). Abnormal interhemispheric connections in the visual system of Boston Siamese cats: a physiological study. *J. comp. Neurol.,* **171,** 229-46

Shatz, C. J. (1977b). Anatomy of interhemispheric connections in the visual system of Boston Siamese and ordinary cats. *J. comp. Neurol.,* **173,** 497-518

Swadlow, H. A. (1974). Properties of antidromically activated callosal neurons and neurons responsive to callosal input in rabbit binocular cortex. *Expl Neurol.,* **43,** 424-44

Toyama, K., Matsunami, K., Ohno, T. and Tokashiki, S. (1974). An intracellular study of neuronal organization in the visual cortex. *Expl Brain Res.*, **21**, 45–66

Van der Loos, H. (1976). Neuronal circuitry and its development. In *Perspectives in Brain Research* (M. A. Corner and D. F. Swaab, eds.), Progress in Brain Research, vol. 45, Elsevier, Amsterdam

Winfield, D.A., Gatter, K.C. and Powell, T.P.S. (1975). Certain connections of the visual cortex of the monkey shown by the use of horseradish peroxidase. *Brain Res.*, **92**, 456–61

Wise, S. P. and Jones, E. G. (1976). The organization and postnatal development of the commissural projection of the rat somatic sensory cortex. *J. comp. Neurol.*, **168**, 313–44

Wong-Riley, M. T. T. (1974). Demonstration of geniculocortical and callosal projection neurons in the squirrel monkey by means of retrograde axonal transport of horseradish peroxidase. *Brain Res.*, **79**, 267–72

Yorke Jr., C. H. and Caviness Jr., V. S. (1975). Interhemispheric neocortical connections of the corpus callosum in the normal mouse: a study based on anterograde and retrograde methods. *J. comp. Neurol.*, **164**, 233–46

20
TRANSFER OF VISUAL INFORMATION ACROSS THE MIDLINE TO THE SUPERIOR COLLICULUS IN THE SPLIT-CHIASM CAT

A. ANTONINI, G. BERLUCCHI, C. A. MARZI and J. M. SPRAGUE

INTRODUCTION

The importance of subcortical centres, such as the superior colliculus, for learning visual pattern discriminations in the cat has been clearly demonstrated (Berlucchi *et al.*, 1972; Sprague, 1972; Sprague *et al.*, 1973). Less is known about the importance of these centres for the interhemispheric transfer of learned, visually guided behavioural responses.

We have begun to investigate this problem by an electrophysiological analysis of the transfer of visual information from one eye to the contralateral superior colliculus, after interrupting the crossed retinotectal connections, along with all other crossed projections of the retinae, by a mid-sagittal section of the optic chiasm. It will be recalled that split-chiasm cats are capable of transferring monocularly learned pattern discriminations between their eyes, whereas this interocular transfer is absent following an additional section of the corpus callosum (Myers, 1956; Sperry, 1961).

Figure 20.1 shows the relations between the visual field, the retinae and the superior colliculi in cats with intact optic pathways. Figure 20.2 illustrates how a mid-sagittal section of the optic chiasm disrupts the normal pattern of retinotectal connections. The splitting of the chiasm destroys all the optic fibres crossing in the midline, thereby totally de-efferenting the nasal hemiretinae and sparing only the connections between each temporal hemiretina and the ipsilateral half of the brain. As a consequence, if neurons in one superior colliculus of a split-chiasm cat respond to visual stimuli presented to the contralateral eye, such a response must be mediated by an indirect connection relaying visual information from one side of the brain to the contralateral superior colliculus.

Anatomical data indicate that the following pathways may transfer visual information from one side of the brain to the contralateral superior colliculus in the cat:

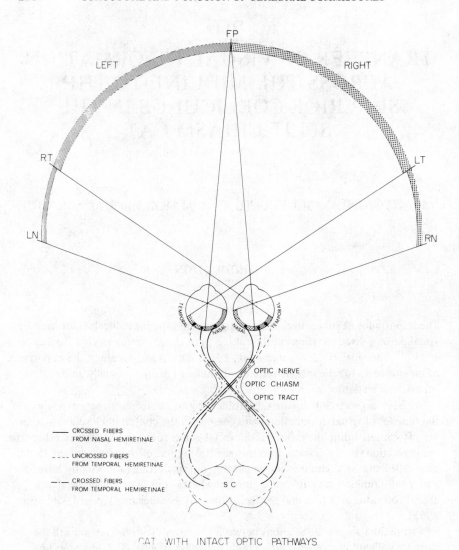

Figure 20.1. Relationships between the visual fields, the nasal and temporal hemiretinae and the SC in cats with intact visual pathways. Each SC receives a direct input from the temporal hemiretina of the ipsilateral eye and the whole retina of the contralateral eye. Each nasal hemi- retina projects only contralaterally, whereas each temporal hemiretina projects both ispilater- ally and contralaterally. The extent of the visual field of each hemiretina is shown in accord with Hughes (1976). Abbreviations: LN, lateral border of visual field of left nasal hemiretina; RT, lateral border of visual field of right temporal hemiretina; FP, fixation point; LT, lateral border of visual field of left temporal hemiretina; RN, lateral border of visual field of right nasal hemiretina

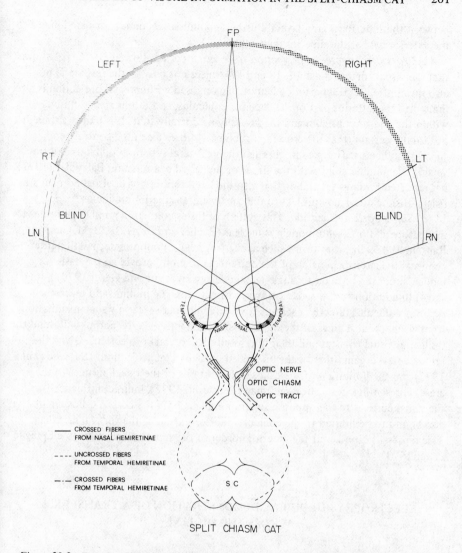

Figure 20.2. Relationships between the visual fields, the temporal hemiretinae and the SC in split-chiasm cats. After splitting of the chiasm, direct projections from retina to SC are constituted only by uncrossed fibres from temporal hemiretina. The nasal hemiretinae are de-efferented, and the crossed projections from temporal hemiretinae are also interrupted. Same abbreviations as figure 20.1

(1) *Commissure of the superior colliculi*. Edwards (1977) has recently shown that this commissure originates from and terminates in collicular layers which lie deeper than the stratum opticum. This latter layer may also give rise to or receive a minimal number of commissural fibres, but there are no commissural connections

between the superficial grey layers. Further, commissural connections are limited to the anterior half of the superior colliculus.

(2) *Crossed corticotectal projection from visual cortex*. Powell (1976) has shown that the visual cortical areas 17, 18 and 19 project not only to the ipsilateral but also the contralateral superior colliculus. This crossed corticotectal projection is also limited to the anterior part of the superior colliculus, and terminates exclusively within the stratum opticum and the layers lying dorsally to it. It is likely, although not totally certain, that the crossed corticotectal fibres reach the contralateral superior colliculus after passing through the ipsilateral superior colliculus and traversing the midline along with the fibres of the tectal commissure. Baleydier (1977) has reported findings suggesting that also the lateral suprasylvian visual cortical area (Clare–Bishop area) may project to the contralateral superior colliculus.

(3) *Supra-optic decussation*. This system of fibres contains a number of decussating tectopetal fibres whose origin is unclear (Bucher and Bürgi, 1953; Magoun and Ranson, 1942). In lower forms such as the frog, the supra-optic decussation interconnects the anterior portion of the optic tecta, thereby providing the basis for binocular convergence on to single tectal neurons (Keating and Gaze, 1970).

(4) In addition to the above pathways which cross the midline and reach the superior colliculus directly, each superior colliculus may receive visual information from visual cortical areas of the opposite side indirectly, via the corpus callosum, the ipsilateral visual cortices and their uncrossed corticotectal projections. Given the retinotopical organisation of the uncrossed corticotectal projections (Sprague *et al.*, 1973) and the limitation of the callosal connections of the visual cortices to the areas representing the vertical meridian (Berlucchi, 1972), indirect influence from the visual cortices to the opposite superior colliculus via the corpus callosum are also bound to be limited to the collicular representation of the vertical meridian. This representation lies at the anterior border of the superior colliculus (see Sprague *et al.*, 1973).

ELECTROPHYSIOLOGICAL DEMONSTRATION OF A TRANSFER ACROSS THE MIDLINE

We have recorded from single superior collicular neurons in unanaesthetised, curarised split-chiasm cats after a midpontine transection (Batini *et al.*, 1959). The experiments involved the mapping of the visual receptive fields of these neurons by presenting appropriate visual stimuli to either eye. We found that visual stimuli presented to the ipsilateral eye were effective in exciting neurons throughout the superior colliculus except at its caudal pole, a region which normally receives fibres exclusively from the extreme periphery of the contralateral nasal retina and therefore is bound to be de-afferented by splitting of the chiasm. Of 192 units which could be driven by the ipsilateral eye, 111 (57.8%) could also be driven by the contralateral eye.

This finding demonstrates that the ipsilateral visual input converges with the across-the-midline visual input on to a substantial proportion of the collicular neurons. These binocularly activated neurons were not spread throughout the superior colliculus, but were restricted to its anterior half. Within this portion of the superior colliculus, virtually all neurons had a receptive field in either eye; and, for each of these binocular units, both receptive fields abutted the vertical meridian of the visual field.

As should be expected from the laws of optics, the receptive field in the ipsilateral eye lay in the contralateral visual field, whereas the receptive field in the contralateral eye lay in the ipsilateral visual field. Since, in addition, the receptive field in one eye had about the same elevation relative to the horizontal meridian and the same vertical extension as the receptive field in the other eye, the two receptive fields of each binocular unit matched each other at the vertical meridian and formed

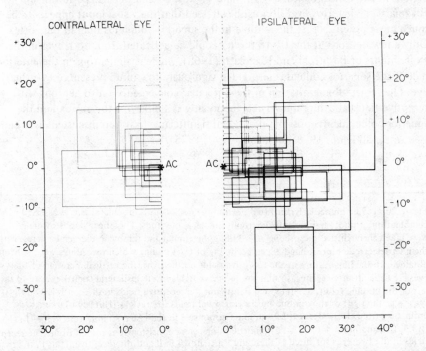

Figure 20.3. Maps of receptive fields in the ipsilateral and contralateral eye for 12 binocular and 8 monocular units in the SC of split-chiasm cats. All receptive fields are shown as if they belonged to units in the left SC. Receptive fields are shown schematically as squares or rectangles; for each of them the length of the border near the vertical meridian and of the maximal horizontal axis was carefully assessed on the tangent screen and converted to spherical co-ordinates. Thin lines mark borders of receptive fields of binocular units and thick lines mark borders of receptive fields of monocular units. Note that most receptive fields of monocular units are located away from the vertical meridian, whereas all the receptive fields of binocular units abut the vertical meridian in both eyes. Negative ordinate points indicate lower visual field; positive ordinate points correspond to upper visual field. AC, projection of the area centralis

a combined receptive field straddling the midline of the horopter. Units in the posterior half of the superior colliculus responded only to stimulation of the ipsilateral eye and had receptive fields detached from the vertical meridian. These findings are illustrated in a number of figures taken from the original report (see Antonini *et al.,* 1978).

Figure 20.3 shows a number of receptive fields of monocular and binocular units and their relations with the vertical meridian. Figure 20.4 shows the location in the superior colliculus of units with binocular and monocular receptive fields. Figure 20.5 shows the response of a direction-sensitive binocular unit to a stimulus moved along the preferred and the null direction across the receptive fields in both eyes. It can be seen that the preferred direction is the same for both receptive fields.

This finding of a binocular convergence in the superior colliculus, in spite of the splitting of the chiasm, is comparable with that on the survival of binocular interactions in the visual cortical areas 17 and 18 of split-chiasm cats (Berlucchi and Rizzolatti, 1968). However, it must be stressed that the visual input appears to be much more potent across the midline in the superior colliculus than in the cortex. Only a few neurons at the 17–18 border could be activated from both eyes in the experiments of Berlucchi and Rizzolatti (1968), whereas all neurons in the anterior half of the superior colliculus responded vigorously to stimuli presented to either eye. The remarkable limitation of the binocular convergence on to neurons with receptive fields abutting the vertical meridian was similar for the cortex and the superior colliculus. Its possible functional significance has been discussed elsewhere (see Antonini *et al.,* 1978; Berlucchi, 1972; 1975).

Figure 20.4. The binocularly activated portion of the SC of a split-chiasm cat, as assessed by a combination of photographic and electrophysiological methods. The photographs of the SC were taken through the microscope after killing the animal and removing the hemispheres, with the microelectrode repositioned at the beginning of tracks along which recordings were previously obtained. In the illustrations of the receptive fields on the right, the vertical meridian of the two eyes are brought into register, so that the receptive fields in the ipsilateral (right) eye are to the left of the midline (contralateral visual field), and the receptive fields in the contralateral (left) eye are to the right of the midline (ipsilateral visual field). In track A (Horsley-Clarke coordinates of the electrode: A4, L2) no units responsive to the visual stimuli were found. In track B (A3.5, L2) and in track C (A3, L2) binocular units were consistently recorded from. The receptive fields in the two eyes for three of these units are shown in B and the receptive fields in the two eyes for another unit are shown in C. Unit 1 in B was somewhat exceptional because of the large difference in size between the receptive fields in the two eyes. In track D (A2, L2) two superficial units had receptive fields only in the ipsilateral eye, and these fields were somewhat detached from the vertical meridian (units 5 and 6). Unit 7 was encountered deeper in the tract, was binocular and had receptive fields bordering on the vertical meridian in both eyes. In track E (A1.5, L2) all units from which recordings could be obtained had receptive fields only in the ipsilateral eye. These receptive fields were considerably distant from the vertical meridian (see units 8, 9, 10). The interrupted line traced on the SC surface is based on similar explorations with more medial or lateral sequences of tracks. It indicates the posterior border of the binocular SC portion. IC, inferior colliculus

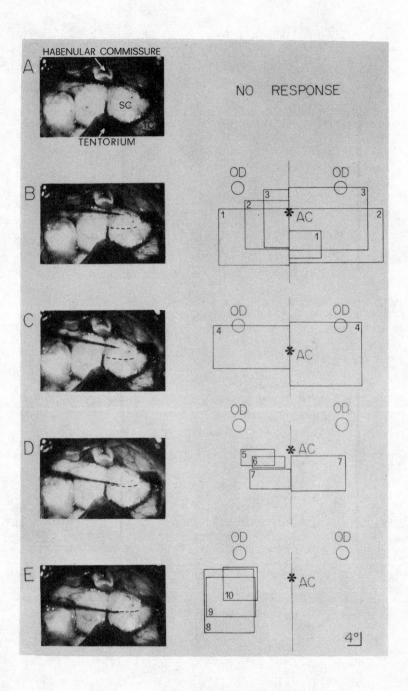

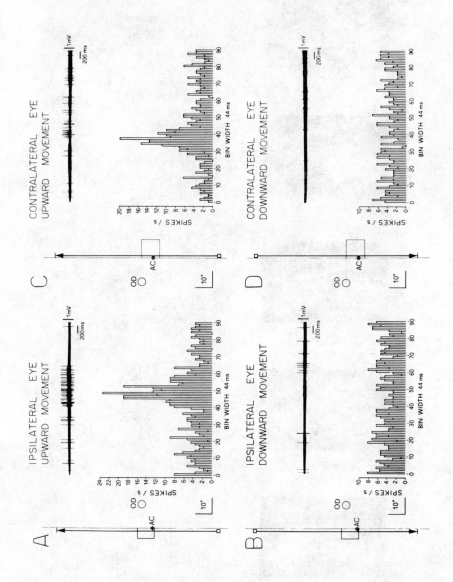

EXPERIMENTS ON CATS WITH A UNILATERAL OPTIC TRACT SECTION

Additional evidence on the transmission of visual information across the midline to the superior colliculus has been obtained in cats with a unilateral section of the optic tract (Antonini *et al.*, in preparation). This operation obviously causes a complete de-afferentation of the visual centres on one side of the brain, including the superior colliculus. Responses to visual stimuli recorded in the de-afferented superior colliculus (SC) must therefore depend on information transmitted from the other side of the brain (see figure 20.6).

In agreement with the experiments on split-chiasm cats, we found such responses only for neurons in the anterior half of the superior colliculus. Binocular activation was the rule for these neurons, but in this case the receptive fields were in homonymous halves of the visual field, i.e. ipsilateral to the side of recording. This reflects the fact that the remaining visual input originated from the nasal retina ipsilateral to the section and the temporal retina contralateral to the section. This finding establishes that both nasal and temporal hemiretinae can be represented in the SC via an indirect projection across the midline.

Previously, the representation of the ipsilateral visual field in the superior colliculus had been attributed solely to the direct projection from the temporal retina to the contralateral superior colliculus, a projection whose existence is well documented both anatomically (Harting and Guillery, 1976; Laties and Sprague, 1966; Stone, 1966) and electrophysiologically (Feldon *et al.*, 1970; Kirk *et al.*, 1976a, 1976b; Stone and Fukuda, 1974).

We have studied the importance of this projection for visually guided behaviour by perimetry tests in cats with a unilateral section of the optic tract. Briefly, these cats were trained both pre- and postoperatively to fixate on a central stimulus and to make a food-motivated orientation response on another stimulus introduced in different points of their visual field. As shown in figure 20.1, each optic tract contains fibres coming from the ipsilateral temporal retina and both halves of the contralateral retina. On the reasonable assumption that the ability to perform in a

Figure 20.5. Binocular unit in the right SC of a split-chiasm cat showing congruent directional selectivity in the two eyes. The stimulus was a square patch of light, one square degree in area and about 10 times brighter than the screen background luminance which crossed the receptive field in either direction along the vertical axis with a constant speed of 24.6 deg/s. The cell response to this stimulus is shown both as an oscilloscopic recording of the action potentials appearing during a single crossing of the receptive field by the stimulus, and as an average response histogram constructed with 25 crossings of the receptive field. The receptive field and the responses for the ipsilateral eye are shown in A and B, and the receptive field and the responses for the contralateral eye are shown in C and D, along with the trajectories of the stimulus across the receptive field. Note that there is a response to the stimulus moving upwards and no response to the stimulus moving downwards in either eye (congruent directional selectivity in the two eyes). This unit was in the stratum opticum. AC, projection of the area centralis; OD, projection of the optic disc

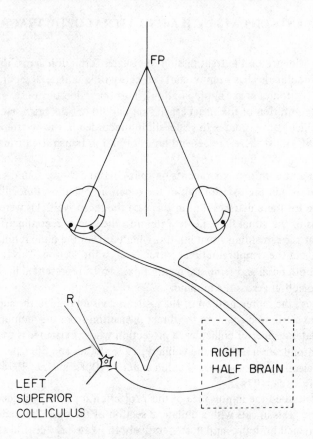

Figure 20.6. Recording from a superior colliculus de-afferented by a section of the ipsilateral optic tract. All visual responses in the de-afferented superior colliculus must originate in the ipsilateral nasal retina and contralateral temporal retina and be mediated by indirect connections across the midline

perimetry test depends to a large extent on the retinal input to the superior colliculus and pretectum (Sprague, 1966; Sprague and Meikle, 1965), one would expect that the animal should remain responsive not only to stimuli presented to the temporal retina contralateral to the section and the nasal retina ipsilateral to the section, but also to stimuli presented to the temporal retina ipsilateral to the section. This expectation was contradicted by the result of the experiment, which showed a complete unresponsiveness for stimuli presented to the temporal retina ipsilateral to the section and the nasal retina contralateral to the section.

It is interesting to compare these results in ordinary cats and the findings obtained in similar perimetry tests after unilateral optic tract section in Siamese cats. As indicated in chapter 24, the retinotectal projections are almost entirely crossed in the Siamese cat. In accord with this, we found in three Siamese cats of the Boston

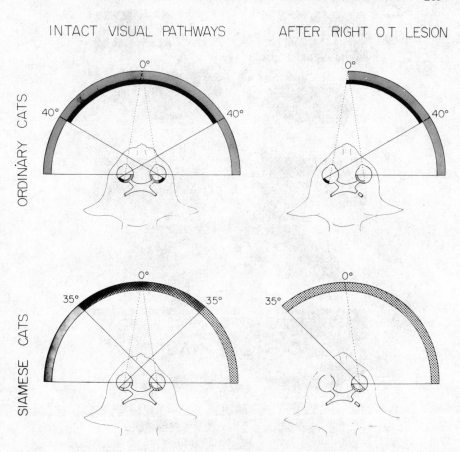

Figure 20.7. Visual fields in ordinary and Siamese cats before and after a unilateral optic tract section

type that a unilateral optic tract section causes blindness in the eye contralateral to the section, while the eye ipsilateral to the section had a virtually normal visual field (see figure 20.7).

There is therefore a substantial difference between the crossed projections from the temporal retina in the ordinary cat and those in the Siamese cat, in that such projections can mediate visually guided orientation in the Siamese but not in the ordinary cat. Whether this difference is due to the fact that there are more crossing fibres from temporal retina in the Siamese cat, or to a more fundamental dissimilarity between the two breeds in the organisation of their visual pathways, remains to be determined. It is possible that the crossed fibres from temporal retina in the ordinary cat and the uncrossed fibres from temporal retina in the Siamese cat are too few to sustain performance in a perimetry test.

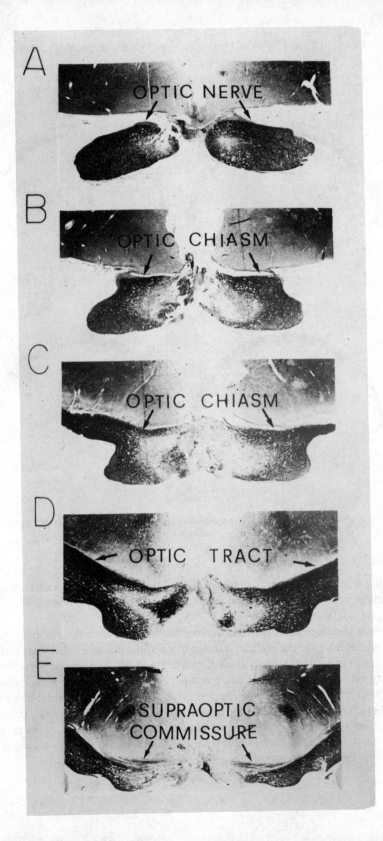

CALLOSAL SECTION AND TRANSFER ACROSS THE MIDLINE OF VISUAL INFORMATION TO THE SUPERIOR COLLICULUS

The anatomical pathways which may be responsible for the transmission of visual information from one side of the brain to the contralateral superior colliculus, have been listed in the introduction to this chapter. We can immediately exclude the supra-optic commissure as the only pathway underlying such a transmission, since our chiasmatic sections were usually deep enough to interrupt this decussation, which lies just above the chiasm (see figure 20.8). Indirect considerations are also against the commissure of superior colliculi as being the principal route for transfer of visual information across the midline. Whereas there is a striking correspondence between the binocular portion of the superior colliculus in split-chiasm cats, as shown in this experiment, and the collicular portion provided with commissural interconnections, as shown by Edwards (1977), it must however be pointed out that the binocular units found in our experiments on split-chiasm cats were all located in or above the stratum opticum, i.e. above the layers of origin and termination of the commissural fibres (Edwards, 1977).

The crossed corticotectal pathway described by Powell (1976) is more likely to be involved in the binocular convergence which we have described for neurons in the anterior half of the superior colliculus of split-chiasm cats, since its termination is restricted to the superficial layers of the vertical meridian representation in the superior colliculus. However, if one grants that the crossed corticotectal pathway does not course in the corpus callosum (Powell, 1976), the following results suggest a different possibility.

We have recorded from the superior colliculus of split-chiasm cats with an additional section of the corpus callosum. The results were striking: the response to stimulation of the contralateral eye was virtually abolished (see figure 20.9). In agreement with this, we also found in cats with a unilateral optic tract section that callosotomy suppressed all visual responses in the de-afferented superior colliculus. The most parsimonious interpretation of these findings is that, as suggested in the introduction, the main route for the conveyance of visual information from the visual cortex on one side to the contralateral superior colliculus is by way of the corpus callosum, the opposite visual cortex and its uncrossed corticotectal projection. However, the possibility that the corpus callosum contains non-commissural, crossed corticotectal projections cannot be excluded. Another alternative is that the cells of origin of the non-callosal, crossed corticotectal pathway of Powell (1976) can be disturbed by a callosal section.

Figure 20.8. Serial frontal sections showing the optic chiasm split along the midline (Weil preparation). The optic chiasm was sectioned one week before the experiment, so that myelin degeneration was still very incomplete at the time of fixation. Sections A–E are shown in a rostrocaudal sequence, the distance between two consecutive sections being approximately 250 μm. Note in E that the supra-optic commissure was transected along with the chiasm

MONOCULAR   BINOCULAR

	MONOCULAR	BINOCULAR	
SPLIT CHIASM CATS	81	111	192
SPLIT BRAIN CATS	154	7	161

$x^2 = 112.4$

$p < 5 \cdot 10^{-10}$

Figure 20.9. Effects of a callosal section in binocular convergence in the superior colliculus of split-chiasm cats. This figure shows the number of units driven by either eye in the superior colliculus of split-chiasm cats with intact commissures and after callosotomy. It can be seen that the response to the contralateral eye is almost suppressed following callosotomy

IMPLICATIONS OF THE FINDINGS FOR VISUALLY GUIDED BEHAVIOUR

Theoretical interpretations of the striking absence of interocular transfer of visual pattern discriminations in split-chiasm cats and monkeys with an additional section of the forebrain commissures have typically stressed the importance of the cortex for the interhemispheric transfer of complex learned response (see, for example, Sperry, 1961; Thompson, 1965). Forebrain commissures are cortical in both origin and termination, and it has generally been assumed that their section would abolish communication between the cortical areas of the two sides while leaving unaffected interactions across the midline between subcortical centres. These subcortical interactions surviving callosal sections have been held responsible for the interhemispheric transfer of lower forms of learning, such as a simple brightness discrimination (Meikle, 1964), as well as for elementary patterns of visuomotor behaviour requiring the activity of the two sides of the brain (Voneida, 1963).

The present findings force us to reconsider these conceptions, since they have made clear that section of the corpus callosum nearly abolishes the transmission of visual information from one eye to the contralateral superior colliculus in split-chiasm cats. Thus it is not only the visual cortical areas of the two sides that are functionally disconnected by a callosal section; the superior colliculi and perhaps other subcortical centres are also deprived of their visual input from the other side of the brain. This fact can no longer be overlooked when trying to understand the neural bases of the interhemispheric transfer of visual discriminations. The concept that both cortical and subcortical visual contres are crucially involved in learning visual pattern discriminations (Sprague et al., 1973) therefore becomes applicable also for the neurological interpretation of the interhemispheric transfer of these discriminations.

The present findings should also be discussed in relation to the report of Sprague (1966) on the role of the intertectal connections in visually guided behaviour. He has observed that section of these connections restores visual orienting to a hemifield previously blinded by ablation of the contralateral occipitotemporal cortex, and has attributed this effect to the removal of an inhibition exerted by the superior colliculus of the intact side on the superior colliculus ipsilateral to the cortical lesion. Sherman (1977) has confirmed this observation in a somewhat different experimental situation, and has supported Sprague's hypothesis of an intertectal inhibition. The electrophysiological experiments of Rizzolatti *et al.* (1974) have shown that the response of superior collicular neurons to visual stimuli presented within their receptive fields could be suppressed or reduced by other visual stimuli concurrently appearing outside the receptive field. This suppressive effect could be seen also when the stimulus activating the receptive field and the competing stimulus were in different halves of the visual field, thus suggesting an inhibition across the midline.

The anatomical pathways involved in the behavioural effects described by Sprague (1966) and Sherman (1977) and in the electrophysiological suppression observed by Rizzolatti *et al.* (1974) are unknown, but it is very likely that they are different from the pathway mediating the excitatory responses of superior colliculus neurons to the contralateral eye in our split-chiasm cats. A testable hypothesis is that while the visual responses across the midline observed in the present experiment depend on corticotectal crossed interactions, whether direct or mediated by the callosum, the inhibitory effects of Sprague (1966) and Rizzolatti *et al.* (1974) are effected by the commissure of the superior colliculus.

ACKNOWLEDGEMENT

This research was supported by a grant (RO1 EY00577-11) from the Department of Health, Education and Welfare, Public Health Service.

REFERENCES

Antonini, A., Berlucchi, G. and Sprague, J. M. (1978). Indirect, across-the-midline retinotectal projections and the representation of the ipsilateral visual field in the superior colliculus of the cat. *J. Neurophys.*, **41**, 285-304

Baleydier, C. (1977). A bilateral cortical projection to the superior colliculus in the cat. *Neurosci. Lett.*, **4**, 9-14

Batini, C., Moruzzi, G., Palestini, M., Rossi, G. F. and Zanchetti, A. (1959). Effects of complete, pontine transection on the sleep–wakefulness rhythm: the midpontine pretrigeminal preparation. *Arch. Ital. Biol.*, **97**, 1-32

Berlucchi, G. (1972). Anatomical and physiological aspects of visual functions of corpus callosum. *Brain Res.*, **37**, 371-92

Berlucchi, G. (1975). Some features of interhemispheric communication of visual information in brain damaged cats and normal humans. In *Les Syndromes de disconnexion calleuse chez l'homme* (F. Michel and B. Schott, eds.), Colloque international de Lyon, pp. 123-36

Berlucchi, G. and Rizzolatti, G. (1968). Binocularly driven neurons in visual cortex of split-chiasm cats. *Science,* **159**, 308-10

Berlucchi, G., Sprague, J. M., Levy, J. and Di Berardino, A. (1972). The pretectum and superior colliculus in visually guided behavior and in flux and form discrimination in the cat. *J. comp. physiol. Psychol.,* **78**, 123-72

Bucher, V. M. and Bürgi, S. M. (1953). Some observations on the fiber connections of the di-and mesencephalon in the cat. III. The supra-optic decussation. *J. comp. Neurol.,* **98**, 355-80

Edwards, S. B. (1977). The commissural projection of the superior colliculus in the cat. *J. comp. Neurol.,* **173**, 23-40

Feldon, S., Feldon, P. and Kruger, L. (1970). Topography of the retinal projection upon the superior colliculus of the cat. *Vision Res.,* **10**, 135-43

Harting, J. K. and Guillery, R. W. (1976). Organization of the retinocollicular pathway in the cat. *J. comp. Neurol.,* **166**, 133-44

Hughes, A. (1976). A supplement to the cat schematic eye. *Vision Res.,* **16**, 121-28

Keating, M. J. and Gaze, R. M. (1970). The ipsilateral retinotectal pathway in the frog. *Q. Jl exp. Physiol.,* **55**, 284-92

Kirk, D. L., Levick, W. R., Cleland, B. G. and Wässle, H. (1976a). Crossed and uncrossed representation of the visual field by brisk-sustained and brisk-transient cat retinal ganglion cells. *Vision Res.,* **16**, 225-31

Kirk, D. L., Levick, W. R. and Cleland, B. G. (1976b). The crossed or uncrossed destination of axons of sluggish-concentring and non-concentring cat retinal ganglion cells, with an overall synthesis of the visual field representation. *Vision Res.,* **16**, 233-36

Laties, A. M. and Sprague, J. M. (1966). The projection of the optic fibers to the visual centers in the cat. *J. comp. Neurol.,* **127**, 37-70

Magoun, H. W. and Ranson, M. (1942). The supraoptic decussation in the cat and monkey. *J. comp. Neurol.,* **76**, 435-59

Meikle, T. H. (1964). Failure of interocular transfer of brightness discrimination in split-brain cats. *Nature (Lond.),* **202**, 1243-44

Myers, R. (1956). Function of corpus callosum in interocular transfer *Brain,* **79**, 358-63

Powell, T. P. S. (1976). Bilateral cortico-tectal projection from the visual cortex in the cat. *Nature (Lond.),* **260**, 526-27

Rizzolatti, G., Camarda, R., Grupp, A. and Pisa, M. (1974). Inhibitory effect of remote visual stimuli on visual responses of cat superior colliculus: spatial and temporal factors. *J. Neurophys.,* **37**, 1262-75

Sherman, S. M. (1977). The effect of superior colliculus lesions upon the visual fields of cats with cortical ablation. *J. comp. Neurol.,* **172**, 231-46

Sperry, R. W. (1961). Some developments in brain lesion studies of learning. *Fedn. Proc.,* **20**, 609-16

Sprague, J. M. (1966). Interaction of cortex and superior colliculus in mediation of visually guided behavior in the cat. *Science,* **153**, 1544-47

Sprague, J. M., (1972). The superior colliculus and pretectum in visual behavior. *Invest. Ophthalmol.,* **11**, 473-82

Sprague, J. M. and Meikle, T. H., Jr. (1965). The role of the superior colliculus in visually guided behavior. *Expl Neurol.,* **11**, 115-46

Sprague, J. M., Berlucchi, G. and Rizzolatti, G. (1973). The role of the superior colliculus and pretectum in vision and visually guided behavior. In *Handbook of Sensory Physiology*, vol. VII/3. Springer Verlag, Berlin, pp. 27–101

Stone, J. (1966). The naso-temporal division of the cat's retina. *J. Comp. Neurol.*, **126**, 585–99

Stone, J. and Fukuda, Y. (1974). The naso-temporal division of cat's retina re-examined in terms of Y-, X- and W-cells. *J. comp. Neurol.*, **155**, 377–94

Thompson, R. (1965). Centrencephalic theory and interhemispheric transfer of visual habits. *Psychol., Rev.*, **72**, 385–98

Voneida, T. J. (1963). Performance of visual conditioned response in split-brain cats. *Expl Neurol.*, **8**, 493–504

21

ALTERED INCORPORATION OF LABELLED URIDINE INTO RNA IN SECONDARY EPILEPTIC FOCI CONTRALATERAL TO PRIMARY EPILEPTIC LESIONS IN THE CAT'S CORTEX

A. CUPELLO, R. AMORE, F. FERRILLO, G. LAZZARINI
and G. ROSADINI

INTRODUCTION

Morrell (1959) described the appearance of a secondary epileptic focus in the rabbit cortical area contralateral and homotopic to a primary epileptic lesion induced by freezing. Such a secondary epileptic lesion is called mirror focus.

This secondary focus is at first dependent on primary focus discharges but after a certain time it becomes independent in that it can generate autonomously epileptic discharges.

The mechanism by which the mirror focus becomes autonomously epileptogenic is not known yet with certainty; a hypothesis suggests a plasticity model where the mirror focus 'learns' to be epileptogenic (Barondes, 1969).

Taking into account that RNA seemed to be involved in learning and memorisation processes (Hydén and Egyhazi, 1962, 1964), Morrell studied the RNA content in the cortical neurons of the mirror focus. He found densely stained basophilic neurons, where the increased dye-binding of such neurons was abolished by RNAse treatment (Morrell, 1964).

A first interpretation of the data was that RNA content increased in the mirror focus nerve cells. Later, the same group (Engel and Morrell, 1970) took into account the possibility that such dense neurons were in reality inhibited or dying cells; they found indeed a very low incorporation of labelled RNA precursors in those neurons.

No modification of incorporation into RNA of labelled precursor was found by Dewar et al. (1972) in mirror foci induced by cobalt application on rat cortex. Westmoreland et al. (1972), on the other hand, found by use of micromethods an RNA decrease in all cortical layers in cobalt-induced mirror foci in rat cortex.

In view of these contradictory results we tried to re-investigate the problem of

276

RNA and, in particular, of messenger RNA synthesis in secondary epileptic foci, analysing by micromethods the incorporation of [^{3}H]uridine in cat's cortex mirror foci. The use of micromethods was necessary due to the extremely small amount of tissue corresponding to the mirror focus proper (a few mg).

MATERIALS AND METHODS

Production of epileptic lesions and EEG recording

Experiments were performed on four adult cats weighing about 3.5 kg; animals were operated under barbiturate anaesthesia (Nembutal 30 mg/kg) using aseptic surgical techniques.

Pairs of screw electrodes were threaded into the skull overlying sensorimotor, occipital and temporal cortices of both hemispheres.

Epileptogenic foci were produced by intracortical injection of alumina cream into the right sensorimotor cortex. EEG recording sessions were taken weekly.

Injection of the labelled precursor and sampling of tissue

5, 6-[^{3}H] Uridine (20 μCi), 48 Ci/m mol (Radiochemical Centre, Amersham) was injected subarachnoidally and locally on the cortex surface in 10 μl volumes at the level of the electrode recording the mirror activity and in the corresponding areas of four control animals, under light pentobarbital anaesthesia.

The animals were sacrificed 1 h after the injections by a large dose of pentobarbital and the brains removed and quickly put on ice. The cortical regions just underlying the electrodes recording the mirror focus activity (1–4 mm^2 areas) were removed from the epileptic brains. Corresponding homotopic regions were taken by the same procedure from controls.

Homogenisation of tissue and determination of precipitable and soluble radioactivity

The tissue samples (a few mg in weight), after extensive washing in buffer 1 (sucrose 0.32 M; Tris-HCl 10 mM, pH 7.5), were homogenised in 100 μl of buffer 2 (Tris-HCl 10 mM, pH 7.5; SDS 0.5%) in a small Dounce homogeniser (0.5 ml volume).

From the total homogenate 10 μl aliquots were taken for soluble and precipitable radioactivity determination. The aliquots were precipitated together with albumin as a carrier by 0.2 ml of 5% TCA. The suspensions were then centrifuged and the supernatants recovered. The pellets were washed twice with 0.1 ml of 5% TCA, the washing supernatants saved and put together with the first ones and counted for TCA soluble radioactivity determination.

The final pellets were resuspended in 1 ml of 5% TCA and filtered on Millipore filters for the determination of the TCA insoluble radioactivity. The pool-corrected incorporations (PCI) were calculated by the ratio TCA precipitable: TCA soluble radioactivity.

Extraction of RNA from homogenates and determination of oligo(dT)-cellulose binding poly(A)-associated RNA

RNA extraction from the homogenates was performed by a phenol–SDS treatment. The extracted RNA was precipitated by ethanol and after collection by centrifugation, dissolved in 0.5 ml of binding buffer (400 mM NaCl; 1 mM EDTA; 10 mM Tris-HCl, pH 7.8; 0.2% SDS). Then it was treated with 0.2 ml of 5% oligo(dT)-cellulose for 30 min at 20 °C.

After the treatment, the cellulose was collected as a pellet and washed five times with 0.5 ml of binding buffer.

The first supernatant was put together with the washing supernatants and this solution was then TCA-precipitated, filtered on Millipore filters and counted.

The cellulose pellet was then washed four times with 0.5 ml of elution buffer (1 mM EDTA; 10 mM Tris-HCl, pH 7.8; 0.2% SDS). The washing supernatants were pooled, TCA-precipitated, filtered on Millipore filters and counted for the determination of the poly(A)-associated radioactivity.

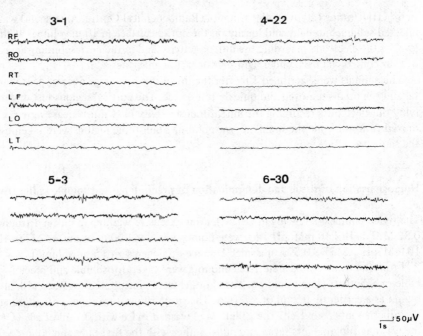

Figure 21.1. EEG pattern of the development of the mirror focus. No epileptogenic activities in the first month (3–1); focal spikes in the second (4–22); dependent mirror focus in the third (5–3); independent and autonomous mirror focus in the fourth (6–30)

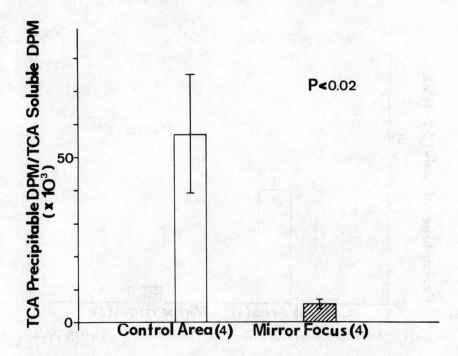

Figure 21.2.   Pool-corrected incorporation of [³H]-uridine into RNA after 1 h pulse (TCA-pre-
cipitable DPM: TCA soluble DPM)

RESULTS

The epileptised animals developed sufficiently homogeneous EEG patterns (figure
21.1) which had shown virtually no epileptogenic activity during the first month
after alumina cream application.

During the second month epileptic activities showed up in the primary lesion
area and in the third month synchronous epileptic activities appeared in the primary
lesion and mirror areas. Finally, during the fourth month autonomous epileptic
activity was registered in the mirror focus.

At this stage [³H] uridine was given to the mirror focus area. The pool-corrected
incorporation of labelled uridine into RNA in the mirror focus was found about ten-
fold reduced in comparison with the control area (figure 21.2).

The proportion of poly(A)-associated, putative, messenger RNA within newly
labelled RNA appeared to be decreased by about eight-fold in comparison with the
control areas in the normal animals (figure 21.3).

In other words the mRNA population appears to be the most involved in the
decrease of synthesis.

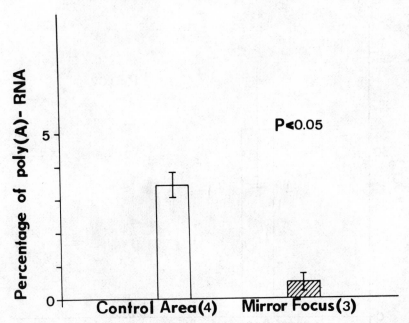

Figure 21.3. Percentage of poly(A)-associated RNA in labelled RNA after 1 h [³H]-uridine pulse

DISCUSSION

The present study confirms the previous experimental observations about the phenomenon of mirror focus formation. The secondary cortical foci we produced in the present experiments corresponded to the theoretical mirror focus definition in two important respects:

(1) They were contralateral and homotopic in respect to the primary lesion by alumina cream.

(2) After a certain time they became autonomous and displayed epileptogenic activity independently of the primary lesion.

Assuming that the pool-corrected incorporation is a measure of the rate of RNA synthesis, the reduced incorporation of labelled uridine into RNA in the mirror focus reflects a remarkable decrease in RNA synthesis rate.

Taking into account also that the proportion of labelled poly(A)-associated messenger RNA is considerably reduced, the decrease in RNA synthesis appears to involve more specifically messenger RNA.

The data we describe indicate a gross derangement of RNA metabolism in the nerve cells of the mirror focus and, taking into account the fundamental biological role of this class of macromolecules, a gross derangement in the cell metabolism.

These biochemical data might be related to ultrastructural studies which showed that neurons of mirror foci in rat brain cortex appeared to be damaged with reduction of RNA components, vacuolisation of the cytoplasm and glial cell proliferation (Bogopolev and Pushkin, 1975). It appears then that the mirror focus nerve cells are seriously damaged from both the biochemical and ultrastructural points of view.

At this stage it is not possible to establish whether in the mirror focus nerve cells the biochemical events determine the structural ones or the contrary. Nevertheless, it seems interesting to consider the fact that the reduction in RNA synthesis is accompanied by a decrease almost of the same order of magnitude of the poly(A)-associated RNA proportion within newly labelled RNA.

A possible explanation for these results might be found in the fact that both total RNA synthesis rate and the proportion of poly(A) RNA within newly synthesized total RNA depend rather strictly on nerve cell ATP concentration. If we assume that in the mirror focus nerve cell ATP concentration falls to values below that of normal controls, we might explain the findings reported above.

A large reduction in the ATP concentration seems to be in line with the results of Bogopolev and Pushkin (1975) who described disappearance of mitochondria in the neurons of cortical mirror foci in the rat.

From this standpoint, a general picture of a fully established mirror focus might be that of a population of rather severely damaged neurons presenting both structural damages and biochemical derangements.

This picture is, in our opinion, hard to reconcile with the hypothesis of the mirror focus as a learning model (Barondes, 1969).

REFERENCES

Barondes, S. H. (1969). The mirror focus and long-term memory storage. In *Basic Mechanisms of the Epilepsies* (H. H. Jasper, A. A. Ward and A. Pope eds.). Little, Brown and Co., Boston

Bogopolev, N. N. and Pushkin, A. S. (1975). Submicroscopic changes of cortex nerve cells in chronic mirror epileptic focus in rat. *Brain Res., 94*, 173–85

Dewar, A. J., Dow, R. C. and McQueen, J. K. (1972). RNA and protein metabolism in cobalt induced epileptogenic lesions in rat brain, *Epilepsia, 13*, 552–60

Engel, J. and Morrell, F. (1970). Turnover of RNA in normal and secondary epileptogenic rabbit cortex. *Expl Neurol., 26*, 221–38

Hydén, H. and Egyhazi, E. (1962). Nuclear RNA changes of nerve cells during a learning experiment in rats. *Proc. natn. Acad. Sci. U.S.A., 48*, 1366–73

Hydén, H. and Egyhazi, E. (1964). Changes in RNA content and base composition in cortical neurons of rats in a learning experiment involving transfer of handedness. *Proc. natn. Acad. Sci. U.S.A., 52*, 1030–35

Morrell, F. (1959). Experimental focal epilepsy in animals. *Arch. Neurol., 1*, 141–47

Morrell, F. (1964). Modification of RNA as a result of neural activity. In *Brain Function: II. RNA and Brain Function, Memory and Learning* (M. A. B. Brazier, ed University of California Press, Los Angeles, pp. 183-202

Westmoreland, B. F., Hanna, G. R. and Bass, N. H. (1972). Cortical alterations in zones of secondary epileptogenesis. A neurophysiologic, morphologic and microchemical correlation study in the albino rat. *Brain Res., 43*, 485-99

22
THE PHARMACOLOGY OF CALLOSAL TRANSMISSION: A GENERAL SURVEY

C. E. GIURGEA and F. MOYERSOONS

INTRODUCTION

The study of interhemispheric relationships, the functions of the cerebral commissures and their role with respect to memory and learning is in active progress. The neuropharmacologist has a double task in this field: first, a fundamental one, contributing to the elucidation of the nature of interhemispheric transmission, by using drugs, and secondly, an applied one, producing drugs that either selectively enhance the efficiency of interhemispheric transmission or that act to compensate eventual deficits in this field.

GENERAL SURVEY

Since the 1974 Lyons symposium, when we made a short survey of the then available pharmacological studies (Giurgea and Moyersoons, 1974), little is to be added, in spite of a computer-oriented bibliographical research. Table 22.1 summarises the pharmacological studies that we have been able to find up to now.

Special comments are to be made concerning two other papers. Levitt and O'Hearn (1972) implanted cannulae in several cerebral structures, including the corpus callosum, in the rat. When carbachol (a cholinomimetic drug) was injected via a cannula into the corpus callosum, drinking was elicited, whereas the injection of eserine (a cholinesterase inhibitor and thus enhancing local brain levels of acetylcholine) had no effect. The authors draw attention to the fact that a steep versus a gradual rise in brain acetylcholine level leads to different effects.

A paper by Marrazi (1974) gives a summary of his views in this field. Marrazi advocates that, all over the CNS, neurotransmitters exert the same postsynaptic effects, so that for instance acetylcholine is always excitatory, whereas catecholamines and serotonin are always inhibitory. It is interesting to recall in this respect the well-known data that Feldberg obtained in cats: intraventricular administration of andrenaline and serotonin invariably produces sleep, whereas that of acetylcholine produce behavioural stimulation up to myoclonic jerks or even convulsions (Feld-

Table 22.1

Transcallosal response—the effect of drugs

Compounds	Doses (mg/kg)	Effect of drug on response	Animal	Administration	Stimulated area	References
Acetylcholine	0.001	↑				
Adrenaline	0.01	↓				
Noradrenaline	0.15	↓				
Mescaline	2.5	↓	cat lightly anaesthetised	l. carotid stimulated side	lateral gyrus (optic cortex)	Marrazi (1957)
Serotonin	0.01	↓				
Bufotenine	0.005	↓				
Adrenochrome	2	↓				
LSD 25	0.075	○				
Chlorpromazine	0.05	○				
Reserpine	0.1	○				
Azacyclonol	1	○				
GABOB	1 ml-5%	↓ / ○	cat anaesthetised / cat curarised	i.v.	suprasylvian gyrus	Minobe (1963)
Pipradrol	?	↓	rabbit curarised	i.v.	cortex	Smirnov and Vinogradova (1968)
Amphetamine	?	↓				
5-HT	0.003–0.05	↓	cat anaesthetised	l. carotid recording side	anterior suprasylvian gyrus	Bond and Guth (1968)
LSD	0.006–0.1	↓				
Thiopental	35	↑ amplitude / ↑ duration	rabbit curarised	i.v.	parietal cortex	Zakuzov and Ostrovskaja (1971)

Drug	Dose	Effect	Condition	Route	Location	Reference
γ-Oxybutyrate	750	↑ amplitude ↑ duration				
Chlorpromazine	5	○ / ↓	rabbit curarised	i.v. slow / i.v. rapid	l. carotid / corpus callosum	Giurgea and Moyersoons (1972)
Thiopental	5	↑ inj. side ○ other side	rabbit curarised			
Dexedrine	10–20	↓				
Caffeine	5–10	(↑)				
Phenobarbital	30–100	↑ pattern change				
Chlorpromazine	10	slight pattern change				
Chlordiazepoxide	10–30	pattern change	cat curarised	i.v.	med. suprasylvian gyrus	
Piracetam	10–500	↑				
Centrophenoxine	30–100	○				
Pyrithioxine	33	○				
Ether		↓			med. suprasylvian gyrus	Plekhotkina and Golovchinskii (1973)
Halothane		↓		inhalation		
Cyclopropane		↓	cat curarised			
Methoxyflurane		(↑)		i.v.		
Thialbarbital	?	(↑)			med. suprasylvian gyrus	
Propanidide	?	↑				
Physostigmine	0.1	↓	rabbit curarised			
L-Dopa	25	↓				
Perimethazine	0.1–5	↑		i.v.	corpus callosum	Ikeda and Murayama (1975)
Chlorpromazine	1–2	↑				
Pentobarbital	5–20	↑				

↑ Amplitude increase; ↓ amplitude decrease; ○ no effect; (↑) slight amplitude increase.

berg, 1963). Regarding unit recording of the TCR, Marrazi found that serotonin by ipsilateral carotid artery injection produced inhibition in 24 units and in none of them excitation, whereas acetylcholine produced excitation in seven units and in none of them inhibition.

The study of antagonists or blockers (also given by close arterial injection) gives Marrazi additional evidence for his theories concerning the neuropharmacology of callosal transmission. Indeed, chlorpromazine prevents catecholamine- and serotonin-induced amplitude decrease of TCR by blocking specific receptors, while atropine prevents its cholinergic enhancement.

Obviously, this point of view is against a specific cholinergic callosal transmission as several authors, such as Levitt and O'Hearn (1972) and Ikeda and Murayama (1975), consider. It merely emphasises that when a drug is affecting the central excitability tonus, its effect on TCR might then well be an indirect, not necessarily a specific, callosal one.

Indeed, central tonus is always the result of a balance between different antagonistic functional systems like the cholinergic–adrenergic one. During arousal, the balance inclines towards adrenergic predominance, whereas during relaxation and sleep the reverse is seen.

It therefore makes sense that, in spite of different experimental conditions, most authors agree that neuroleptics or barbiturates, in appropriate dosages, usually enhance callosal-evoked potentials, whereas stimulants decrease them. This is also in agreement with Baldissera et al. (1965), who have shown that in cats TCR is greater during light sleep periods than during arousal.

NEW EXPERIMENTAL DATA

Our own approach to the pharmacology of callosal transmission is a pragmatic one, aimed at finding drugs that might selectively enhance the efficiency of interhemispheric communication. Studies on neurotransmitters and/or their precursors are to be considered in the light of this purpose of applied pharmacology.

Material and methods

As experimental details were described elsewhere (Giurgea and Moyersoons, 1970, 1972), only a summary will be given here.

In curarised cats we stimulate intracortically the median suprasylvian gyrus. The stimulation voltage is adjusted to obtain a near-maximal TCR. Recording of TCR on the contralateral homotopic cortex is made by an active and a passive electrode. The obtained TCR is usually the one classically described: a positive, negative wave followed by some slow after-potentials, perhaps of extracallosal origin (Rutledge, 1963; Rutledge and Kennedy, 1960). The TCR being relatively stable during 3–4 h is averaged 20–60 times every 10–30 min. Drugs are given by the intravenous or oral route and eventual changes are followed for 2–3 h.

RESULTS

(1) Cholinergic effect

Dimethylamino-ethanol, a cholinomimetic drug, was injected intravenously in seven cats (see table 22.2 and figure 22.1).

Comment: DMAE mainly increases TCR amplitude without affecting its morphology.

TRANSCALLOSAL RESPONSE

Stim. g. suprasylv. 10V 0,2 ms

Control tracing : 60 resp. averaged (20 + 20 + 20)

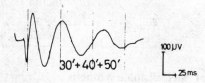

30′+40′+50′

100 μV

25 ms

DMAE 28,1 mg/kg I.V.

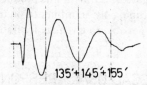

135′+145′+155′

Figure 22.1. The augmenting effect of DMAE on TCR is clearly visible in this figure. In this and all following TCR figures negativity is upwards. The first tracing is the control one and is the average of 60 responses (3 ×20 evoked potentials at 10 min intervals). The second is recorded after the injection of the drug, at a moment when the effect is most pronounced

Table 22.2
Dimethylamino-ethanol

Doses (mg/kg, i.v.)	No. treated animals	Effect on TCR	
		amplitude	morphology
8, 9	3	Increase 30–40% in 2 animals	No effect (3 anim.)
		No effect in 1	
29	4	Increase 20–30% in 2 animals	No effect (4 anim.)
		No effect in 2	

(2) Adrenergic interferences

In earlier tests with dexamphetamine we observed an amplitude decrease of the response. New results with methamphetamine *in vitro* are given in table 22.3.

Comment: methamphetamine, like dexamphetamine, decreases TCR amplitude without influencing its general pattern.

Table 22.3
Methamphetamine

Doses (mg/kg, i.v.)	*No. treated* *animals*	*Effect on TCR* amplitude	morphology
1	4	Decrease 15–20% in 3 animals No effect in 1	No effect (4 anim.)
3	2	Decrease 30–45% in 2 animals	No effect (2 anim.)

(3) Inhibition of catecholamine synthesis

α-Methyl-*meta*-tyrosine, which inhibits dopa-decarboxylase, was studied in this respect (table 22.4 and figure 22.2). With this product we did not obtain the expected increase of TCR amplitude; only an influence on morphology of the response was observed. We are not yet able to given an accurate interpretation of this pattern change.

TRANSCALLOSAL RESPONSE

Stim. g. suprasylv. med.   15 V   0,2 ms

Control tracing: 60 resp. averaged (20 + 20 + 20)

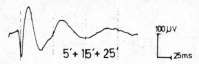

5′+ 15′+ 25′   100 μV   25ms

∝ _ methyl _ meta _ tyrosine 10 mg/kg I.V.

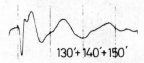

130′+ 140′+ 150′

Figure 22.2.   A typical example of changes in the pattern of the negative phase of the TCR provoked by α-methyl-*meta*-tyrosine

Table 22.4
α-Methy-*meta*-tyrosine

Doses (mg/kg, i.v.)	No. treated animals	Effect on TCR amplitude	morphology
5	1*	No effect	Change (1 anim.)
10	5	No effect (5 animals)	Changes (3 anim.) No effect (2 anim.)

*This animal received 25 mg/kg afterwards, which induced a morphology change.

(4) Serotonergic interferences

(a) Inhibition of serotonin synthesis

p-Chlorophenylalanine depletes brain serotonin by inhibition of tryptophan-hydroxylase. The drug was given orally (table 22.5 and figure 22.3).

Conclusion: increase in amplitude and/or change in morphology. This morphology change is the same as that observed with α-methyl-*meta*-tyrosine.

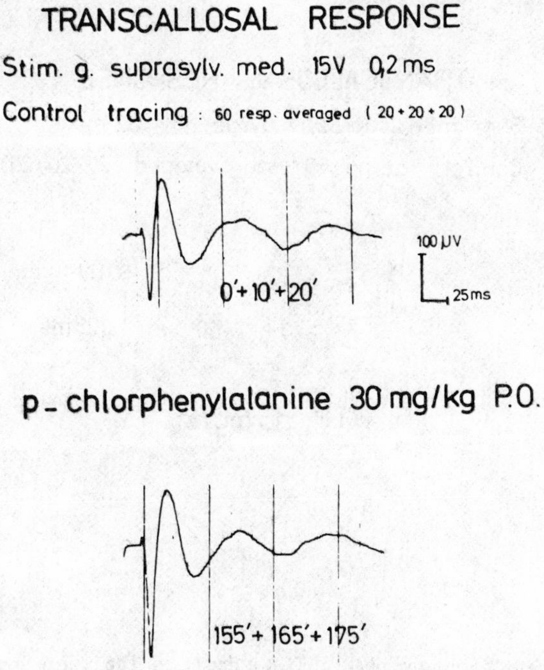

TRANSCALLOSAL RESPONSE

Stim. g. suprasylv. med. 15V 0,2 ms

Control tracing : 60 resp. averaged (20 + 20 + 20)

0' + 10' + 20'

100 µV

25 ms

p - chlorphenylalanine 30 mg/kg P.O.

155' + 165' + 175'

Figure 22.3. A typical example of amplitude increase, $2\frac{1}{2}$ h after oral administration of the drug

Table 22.5
p-Chlorophenylalanine

Doses (mg/kg, p.o.)	*No. treated animals*	*Effect on TCR* amplitude	morphology
30	5	Increase 15–35% (3 animals) at about 3 h after ingestion 2 animals: change in morphology only	Change in 3 animals (2 of them without amplitude increase)
50	1	Increase 35%	No change

(b) 5-HTP

Table 22.6 summarises the effect of this precursor of serotonin (see also figure 22.4). The most important effect of 5-HTP on TCR is its effect on morphology of the response; in most of the animals the positive wave, as measured by respect to the baseline, is increased while the negative wave is decreased. The increase of amplitude in two animals was observed 2–3 h after injection.

TRANSCALLOSAL RESPONSE

Stim. med. suprasylv. gyrus 15v 0,2 ms

Control tracing : 60 resp. averaged (20'+20'+20')

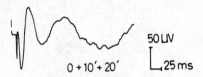

0 + 10'+ 20'   50 µV   25 ms

5 HTP 15 mg/kg I.V.

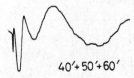

40'+ 50'+ 60'

Figure 22.4. Here the negative phase of TCR is decreased. The change in morphology is evident, as shown by the shorter duration of the negative phase and the increase of the first slow wave

Table 22.6
5-HTP

Doses (mg/kg, i.v.)	No. treated animals	Effect on TCR amplitude	morphology
10	1*	No effect	Change
15	4	Increase in 2 (20–40%) 1 no change 1 decrease	Change in 4 anim.
20*	1* after 10 mg/kg	No effect	Change

*Same animal.

(5) GABA-ergic interferences

(a) Inhibition of GABA-transaminase

Gamma-aminobutyric acid in the brain can be increased indirectly by injecting inhibitors of GABA-transaminase, as for instance amino-oxyacetic acid (table 22.7 and figure 22.5).

Conclusion: decrease of amplitude of the negative phase.

TRANSCALLOSAL RESPONSE

Stim. g. suprasylv. med. 15V 0,2ms

Control tracing: 60 resp. averaged (20 + 20 + 20)

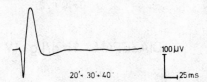

20'+ 30'+ 40'   100 μV   25 ms

Amino ₋ oxy ₋ acetic ₋ acid 10mg/kg I.V.

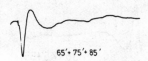

65'+ 75'+ 85'

Figure 22.5. Example of an evident decrease by the amino-oxyacetic acid of the negative phase of TCR

Table 22.7
Amino-oxyacetic acid

Doses (mg/kg, i.v.)	No. treated animals	Effect on TCR amplitude	morphology
1	1	No effect	No effect
5	1	Decrease of negative phase	See effect on amplitude
10	3	Decrease of negative phase (3 animals)	See effect on amplitude

(b) Diazepam

Diazepam, as other benzodiazepines, is supposed to have a GABA-ergic activity (Costa *et al.*, 1975; Fuxe *et al.*, 1975). In view of this modern concept about the mode of action of benzodiazepines we have recently investigated the effect of diazepam on TCR (table 22.8 and figure 22.6).

TRANSCALLOSAL RESPONSE

Stim. med. suprasylv. gyrus 20v 0,2 ms

Control tracing : 60 resp. averaged (20 + 20 + 20)

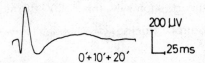

DIAZEPAM 1 mg/kg I.V.

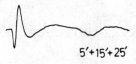

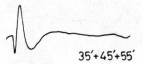

Figure 22.6. Effect of diazepam at 1 mg/kg, i.v.: decrease in amplitude (especially of the negative phase) during the 30 min following the injection. Note the return to normal afterwards

Table 22.8
Diazepam

Doses (mg/kg, i.v.)	No. treated animals	Effect on TCR amplitude	morphology
1	4	Decrease in 3 animals normal at ± 60 min; increase in 2 animals afterwards	Change

The decrease in amplitude seen in three animals during the 60 min following the injection was rather small (10–15%). However, taking into account that the amplitude returns to normal after 1 h, this decrease may be considered to be drug induced. The morphology changes observed are inconsistent and differ from animal to animal.

(6) Piracetam

Some years ago we described a drug (2-oxo-pyrolidinone acetamide) which enhanced rather selectively the amplitude of the transcallosal response (TCR). Selectivity on TCR was claimed in cats, mainly due to lack of any activity, in the same experimental preparation upon the polysynaptic evoked potential on the gyrus sigmoideus posterior at electrical stimulation of the contralateral sciatic nerve (Giurgea and Moyersoons, 1972).

Piracetam has been investigated extensively in animals and in human pharmaco-clinical and therapeutic studies (see the review by Giurgea, 1976). The reasons we are briefly reporting here about this drug are: (a) that on behalf of new threshold studies we can further support the direct, non-reticular mediated nature of the piracetam effect on TCR; and (b) that correlations are now available between the previous electrophysiological findings and some animal and human studies on noetic functions.

Threshold studies

When, in our experimental conditions, we are using several voltage levels to stimulate the suprasylvian gyrus there is a remarkable reproducibility of the voltage-related amplitude of the TCR, including the minimal amount of stimulation to produce a definite response (threshold). Figure 22.7 shows a typical example, in which it can be seen that, after an ascending schedule of stimulations to obtain a maximal TCR, we can reproduce it several times with similar results. Now if, in the given situation, we inject piracetam we see that the 'threshold' remains unchanged, whereas the amplitude of the sub-maximal TCR is enhanced (see figure 22.8).

Whatever the intimate mechanism of action of piracetam might be, the above experiment contributes to the general nootropic concept. Indeed a subcortical, let us

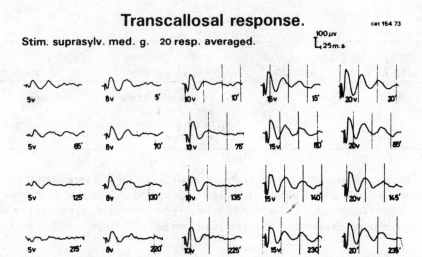

Transcallosal response.

cat 154 73

Stim. suprasylv. med. g.   20 resp. averaged.

100 µv
25 m.s

Figure 22.7.   The TCR average, resulting from a series of 20 stimulations at different voltages (5, 8, 10, 15 and 20 V), is followed during 4 h. Note the stability of voltage-dependent responses throughout the experiment

TRANSCALLOSAL RESPONSE

Stim. g. suprasylv. med.

Control   tracings : 20 resp averaged

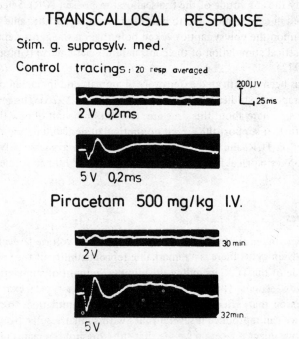

200µV
25 ms

2 V 0,2 ms

5 V 0,2 ms

Piracetam 500 mg/kg I.V.

2 V — 30 min

5 V — 32 min

Figure 22.8.   Control tracing: TCR at sub-threshold and suprathreshold stimulation, before injection. Note the increase in amplitude at suprathreshold stimulation, after piracetam; at sub-threshold the virtual absence of TCR is unchanged by the drug

say reticular, activation would most probably have interfered with threshold values. The fact that piracetam enhances amplitude of a TCR only for supraliminar stimulations, gives further support to the hypothesis of a direct, relatively selective telencephalic impact of the drug.

Noetic (animal and human) correlations with the drug-induced electrophysiological enhancement of commissural efficiency.

Burešová and Bureš (1976) found that piracetam facilitated formation of an efficient, callosal-mediated, secondary engram. In rats submitted to visual discriminative learning, the authors used several models to interfere with callosal mechanisms, based essentially on combining monocular learning with functional, reversible hemidecortication, produced by spreading depression.

To illustrate this approach we shall give here only one example. It will be seen in figure 22.9 that monocular learning results, in saline-treated animals, in a strong, primary engram and a weaker, callosal-mediated, secondary one. Piracetam-treated rats learn monocularly the given task somehow quicker, but the most striking effect is that in the retention test both engrams appear to be equally efficient. Piracetam, therefore, strongly enhances efficiency of this kind of callosal interhemispheric transfer of information.

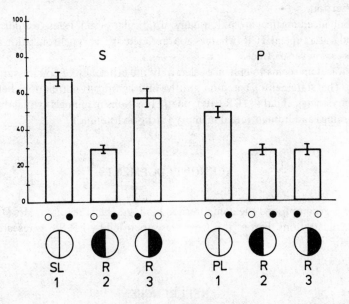

Figure 22.9. Effect of piracetam on monocular pattern discrimination learning (L) and on strength of resulting primary and secondary engrams revealed by hemidecorticate relearning (R). Brain diagrams indicate conditions of experiment on days 1–3 (occluded eye and depressed hemisphere black). P = piracetam-treated rats, S = saline-treated rats. Ordinate: average number of trials to criterion. Vertical bars: s.e.m. values. (Courtesy Burešová and Bureš, 1976)

In young healthy human volunteers, Dimond and Brouwers (1976), showed that piracetam (3 × 400 mg/day, orally, and for 14 days), significantly and rather selectively improved efficiency of verbal memory. Moreover, based on our animal TCR studies, Dimond used dichotic listening memory tests to study an eventual correlation with interhemispheric transfer in man (Dimond, 1975). He found, even after only a week of administration, that: (a) verbal memory for dichotic listening increased by at least 15% (which in those conditions is a highly significant result); and (b) that the change could in the largest measure be attributed to increased response to information presented to the left ear.

Dimond (1975, p.109) concludes that the drug-enhancing callosal efficiency 'would therefore promote the connection of the right hemisphere message to the speech system and thus acts to enhance performance on the left ear'.

CONCLUSIONS

(1) Pharmacology of callosal transmission is still relatively undeveloped. It seems, however, that the concept of a specific cholinergic pathway is not large enough for the available amount of information on drugs. Selective interferences with different synaptic transmitters and postsynaptic receptors give further support to the previous assertion.

(2) Enhanced cortical arousal, usually of reticular origin, leads to a decrease in the amplitude of a typical TCR, whereas appropriate cortical synchronisation has, in most cases, a reverse effect.

(3) Piracetam seems to enhance selectively the efficiency of commissural transmission. This statement is based on positive and significant correlations between electrophysiological data (TCR cats), noetic functions in animals (visual discrimination learning) and human verbal memory (dichotic listening).

ACKNOWLEDGEMENTS

Mrs Figeys accomplished the computerised bibliographical research. Mrs D. Wauthy drew the illustrations. Part of this work was supported by I.R.S.I.A. research grant No. 2583.

REFERENCES

Baldissera, F., Cesa-Bianchi, M. G. and Mancia, M. (1965). Transcallosal, extracallosal and geniculo-cortical responses during physiological sleep and wakefulness. *Experientia*, **21**, 1–4

Bond, H. W. and Guth, P. S. (1968). Interaction of 5-hydroxytryptamine and d-lysergic acid diethylamide in the transcallosal response. *Life Sci.,* **7**, 249-58

Burešová, O. and Bureš, J. (1976). Piracetam induced facilitation of interhemispheric transfer of visual information in rats. *Psychopharmacol. (Berl.),* **46**, 93-102

Costa, E., Guidotti, A. and Mao, C. C. (1975). Evidence for involvement of GABA in the action of benzodiazepines: studies on rat cerebellum. In *Mechanism of Action of Benzodiazepines* (E. Costa and P. Greengard, eds.), Advances in Biochemical Psychopharmacology, vol. 14, Raven Press, New York, pp. 113-30

Dimond, S. J. (1975). Use of a nootropic substance to increase the capacity for verbal learning and memory in normal man. Proc. Symp. Nooanaleptic and Nootropic Drugs, 3rd Congr Internat. College of Psychosomatic Medicine (Agnoli, ed.), Rome, 17 September, pp. 107-110

Dimond, S. J. and Brouwers, E. Y. M. (1976). Increase in the power of human memory in normal man through the use of drugs. *Psychopharmacology,* **49**, 307-.309

Feldberg, W. (1963). *A Pharmacological Approach to the Brain, from its Inner and Outer Surface,* Edward Arnold, London

Fuxe, K., Agnati, L. F., Bolme, P., Hökfelt, T., Lidbrink, P., Ljungdahl, Å, Perez, de la Mora M., Ögren, S. O., (1975). The possible involvement of GABA mechanisms in the action of benzodiazepines on central catecholamine neurons. In *Mechanism of Action of Benzodiazepines* (E. Costa and P, Greengard eds.), Advances in Biochemical Psychopharmacology, vol. 14, Raven Press, New York, pp. 45-61

Giurgea, C. (1976). Piracetam: nootropic pharmacology of neurointegrative activity In *Current Developments in Psychopharmacology,* vol. 3 (W. B. Essmann and Valzelli eds.), Spectrum, New York, pp. 223-73

Giurgea, C. and Moyersoons, F. (1970). Differential pharmacological reactivity of three types of cortical evoked potentials. *Arch. Int. Pharmacodyn.,* **188**, 401-404

Giurgea, C. and Moyersoons, F. (1972). On the pharmacology of cortical evoked potentials. *Arch. Int. Pharmacodyn.,* **199**, 67-78

Giurgea, C. and Moyersoons, F. (1974). Contribution á l'étude électrophysiologique et pharmacologique de la transmission calleuse. In *Les syndromes de disconnexion calleuse chez l'homme* (F. Michel and B. Schott, eds.), Colloque international de Lyon, pp. 53-72

Ikeda, S. and Murayama, S. (1975). Effects of perimetazine and chlorpromazine on the transcallosal response in rabbits. *Jap. J. Pharmac.,* **25**, 74-75P

Levitt, R. A. and O'Hearn, J. Y. (1972). Drinking elicited by cholinergic stimulation of CNS fibers *Physiol. Behav.,* **8**, 641-44

Marrazi, A. S. (1957). The effect of drugs on neurons and synapses In *Brain Mechanisms and Drug Action* (W. S. Fields ed.), Charles C. Thomas, Springfield, pp. 45-70

Marrazi, A. S. (1974). Exploring with drugs: the way of a neuropharmacologist. In *Legacies in the Study of Behavior* (J. W. Cullen, ed.), Charles C. Thomas, Springfield, 96-132

Minobe, K. (1963). The effect of β-hydroxy-γ-aminobutyric acid on cerebral electrical activity. *Folia Psychiat. Neurol. Jap.,* **17**, 71-79

Plekhotkina, S. I. and Golovchinskii, V. B., (1973). Effect of general anaesthetics of various types on transcallosal responses in the association and somatosensory areas of the cat cortex. *Bull. exp. Biol. Med.*, **76**, 1059–64

Rutledge, L. T. (1963). Interactions of peripherally and centrally originating input to association cortex. *EEG clin. Neurophysiol.*, **15**, 958–68

Rutledge, L. T. and Kennedy, T. T. (1960). Extracallosal delayed responses to cortical stimulation in chloralosed cat. *J. Neurophysiol.*, **23**, 188–96

Smirnov, G. D. and Vinogradova, V. M. (1968). Action of catecholamines (Pipradrol and amphetamine) on some cortical synaptic systems. *Byul. Eksp. Biol. Med.*, **64**, 1163–66

Zakusov, V. V. and Ostrovskaja, R. U. (1971). The influence of hypnotics and tranquillizers on some evoked cortical potentials. *Neuropharmacology*, **10**, 1–6

23
PATHWAYS OF INTEROCULAR TRANSFER IN SIAMESE CATS

C. A. MARZI, M. DI STEFANO and A. SIMONI

INTRODUCTION

Siamese cats share with other albino mutants of numerous mammalian species a profound abnormality of their visual systems (see Guillery *et al.*, 1974 for review). In addition to the lack of pigment in the eye and the frequent but by no means constant presence of strabismus (Rengstorff, 1976), their visual pathways are almost totally crossed. Exaggerating a trend already present in ordinary cats (Kirk *et al.*, 1976) fibres from the centremost 20–25 degrees of temporal retina, with the exclusion of a small medial normal segment (Guillery *et al.*, 1974; Shatz, 1977a), instead of projecting ipsilaterally, cross at the optic chiasm and terminate in the contralateral visual centres. The presence of such an extra portion of contralateral visual pathways can be precisely documented both anatomically and electrophysiologically (Guillery and Kaas, 1971; Kalil *et al.*, 1971; Shatz, 1977a) at the level of the lateral geniculate nucleus (LGN). Also, in the optic tectum there is consistent anatomical and electrophysiological evidence for an almost totally contralateral visual input (Berman and Cynader, 1972; Kalil *et al.*, 1971; Lane *et al.*, 1974; Weber and Hartig, 1976).

Furthermore, at the cortical level, the way the aberrant input is dealt with enables Siamese cats to be subdivided into two types. In one, called the Boston type (Hubel and Wiesel, 1971), the extra input is housed at the boundary between visual cortical areas 17 and 18, where in ordinary cats there is a representation of the vertical meridian. In the other, the Midwestern type (Kaas and Guillery, 1973), the input from both the normally and abnormally routed temporal retina is suppressed. Both arrangements seem to serve the purpose of avoiding the disruption of an ordered topographical representation of the visual space in the visual cortex. A further difference between the two types of Siamese cat has recently been described by Shatz (1977a). It concerns the extent of the normal medial segment of temporal retina which is much smaller in Boston than in Midwestern cats. However, notwithstanding such a different cortical and subcortical organisation, both types share a major consequence of the increased optic pathways decussation, namely that nearly all neurons in the visual cortex, instead of being binocularly innervated as in ordinary cats are driven by the contralateral eye alone (Cool and Crawford, 1972; Hubel and Wiesel, 1971; Kaas and Guillery, 1973).

BEHAVIOURAL CORRELATES OF THE SIAMESE CAT'S ABNORMALITIES

Obviously, it might be expected that the above-mentioned abnormalities in the Siamese cat's visual centres would be correlated with specific alterations in visually guided behaviour. Thus, the functional cortical suppression of the input from the entire temporal retina which occurs in Midwestern cats has been shown to have a behavioural counterpart, in that these animals have monocular vision restricted to the temporal portion of the visual field (Elekessy *et al.*, 1973). On the contrary, as it might be expected (Guillery *et al.*, 1974), Boston-type cats have full monocular as well as binocular visual fields (Simoni and Sprague, 1976).

Moreover, the lack of binocularly driven neurons in the Siamese cat's visual cortex has been shown to result in a lack of stereoscopic vision which instead is present in ordinary cats (Packwood and Gordon, 1975).

Contrast sensitivity has also been shown to be somewhat abnormal in Siamese cats, although the nature of such a deficit is by no means settled (Blake and Antoinetti, 1976).

Unfortunately, both the Packwood and Gordon and the Blake and Antoinetti studies have employed strabismic Siamese cats and one might expect stereopsis (Hohmann and Creutzfeld, 1975; Movshon *et al.*, 1972) and visual resolution (Ikeda and Wright, 1976) to be impaired in strabismic subjects anyway.

We have been interested in testing whether the lack of binocular neurons in the Siamese cat's visual cortex is compatible with a normal interocular transfer (IOT) of visual form discriminations. As is well known, cats with surgically induced abolition

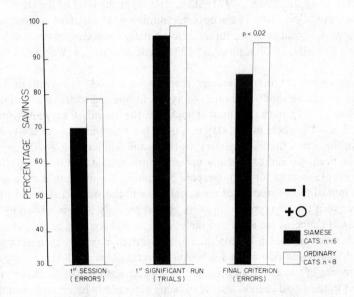

Figure 23.1.   Interocular transfer scores for intact Siamese and ordinary cats. The two pairs of discriminanda used are shown on the right-hand side

of binocular interaction on to visual cortical neurons do not show IOT of visual form discriminations (Myers, 1962). Similarly, mammals whose visual pathways are predominantly crossed show a reduced IOT (Cowey and Parkinson, 1973; Sheridan, 1965; van Hof, 1970), although contrasting findings have been reported probably due to procedural factors (see also chapter 13).

We thought that the use of intact, orthophoric Siamese cats offers a great advant- age for the study of the relationships existing between central binocular coding and IOT, in that it enables the difficulties inherent in using either brain-damaged ani- mals (i.e. split-brain cats) or species whose visual systems have not been as thoroughl studied as the cat's to be overcome. Thus we decided to compare, in Siamese and ordinary cats, the IOT of visual form discriminations that previous experiments in our laboratory (Berlucchi et al., 1978) have shown not to transfer from one eye to the other in split-brain ordinary cats. If binocular convergence at the primary visual cortex level is fundamental for a successful IOT, as it has been proposed for the human visual system (Hohmann and Creutzfeldt, 1975; Mitchell and Ware, 1974; Movshon et al., 1972), then one would predict that Siamese cats, as opposed to ordinary cats, would show an absent or reduced IOT.

INTEROCULAR TRANSFER IN INTACT SIAMESE AND ORDINARY CATS

Following extensive pretraining to accustom the animals to monocular vision with either eye and to the scleral occluder, eight ordinary cats and six Siamese cats were tested in a discrimination box (whose detailed description has appeared in Berlucchi and Marzi, 1970) for IOT of two form discriminations. Part of the results described below have been published elsewhere (Marzi et al., 1976).

IOT was assessed on the basis of percentage of savings, which were calculated as (first eye errors — second eye errors/first eye errors + second eye errors) × 100. Three measures of IOT were used. Percentage of savings for the number of errors made in the first session (one session consisted of 40 trials); percentage of savings for the number of trials taken to perform the first significant run at $P < 0.05$, allow- ing two errors (see Bogartz, 1965); and finally, percentage of savings for the number of errors to final learning criterion (two consecutive sessions with at least 90% cor- rect responses). These three measures allow sampling of IOT at an initial, intermedi- ate and final level, respectively. Five overtraining sessions were given between first and second eye testing.

Figure 23.1 shows the mean percent savings scores in the three measure of IOT for ordinary and Siamese cats. It can be seen that in two of the three measures of IOT there is no difference between ordinary and Siamese cats. A small, although statistically significant (Mann–Whitney U test two-tailed), difference indicating a slight impairment of the Siamese group, shows up only in the more stringent final criterion measure of IOT. No difference was found between the two groups in learning rate with the eye trained first.

Thus, the main finding of this experiment is that Siamese cats have a remarkably good IOT which is nearly indistinguishable from that of ordinary cats.

ELECTROPHYSIOLOGICAL RECORDINGS

Given the unexpectedly good IOT of Siamese cats, we decided to verify whether the particular individuals employed in the study were indeed pure-bred cats with predominance of monocularly driven neurons in their visual cortices. Moreover, we were interested to find out whether our cats were of the Boston or Midwestern type. To accomplish that, at the end of the first series of discriminations brief single-unit recordings were obtained from the visual cortex of the Siamese cats, which were then kept alive for further behavioural testing. Recordings were obtained from some of the ordinary cats as well. Figure 23.2 shows the number of binocular and monocular cells recorded in area 17 and 18 of each Siamese cat tested, including one cat (S11) which participated only in a behavioural experiment to be described later.

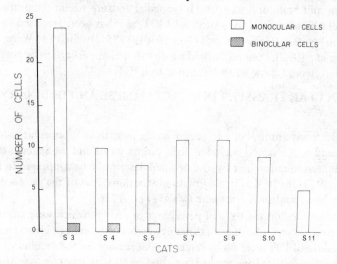

Figure 23.2. Number of monocularly and binocularly activated neurons recorded from the visual cortex of the Siamese cats used in the behavioural experiments reported in the present chapter. A cell was classified as monocular only when no response whatsoever was obtained through visual stimulation of the ipsilateral eye

In accord with previous reports (Cool and Crawford, 1972; Hubel and Wiesel, 1971; Kaas and Guillery, 1973) the vast majority of the recorded cells were driven exclusively from the contralateral eye. Moreover, the pattern of cortical topography was essentially similar to that described by Hubel and Wiesel in Boston Siamese cats. Cells situated at the boundary between area 17 and 18 had their receptive fields in the ipsilateral part of the visual field. The distances of the ipsilateral receptive field centres from the vertical meridian ranged from 1 to 18 degrees of visual angle.

No Midwestern-type cats were found; however we found that three cats, even though they displayed the typical Siamese cat eye and fur coloration, showed no abnormality whatsoever in their visual cortices. The behavioural results of these animals, which probably were not pure bred, are not reported in the present chapter.

WHAT PATHWAYS SUBSERVE IOT IN SIAMESE CATS?

How then can we explain the surprisingly good IOT found in our Siamese cats, given that they indeed lacked binocular neurons in areas 17 and 18? One possibility is that the forebrain commissures might compensate for the nearly total crossing of the visual pathways by permitting some binocular convergence on to neurons in visual areas other than the primary visual cortex. Two recent findings give some support to such a possibility. First, anatomical and electrophysiological work by Shatz (1977b, 1977c) have shown that the callosal connections of Boston Siamese cats are highly abnormal and that unusually widespread regions of cortex are concerned with commissural function. Secondly, lesion studies by Berlucchi *et al.* (1979) indicate that visual areas in the suprasylvian gyrus are more involved in the interhemispheric transfer of visual form discrimination learning than are lesions in the primary visual areas.

These findings are in agreement with recent monkey work (Gross and Mishkin, 1977) demonstrating that a visual area remote from the striate cortex, such as the inferotemporal cortex, is critically involved in the interhemispheric transfer of visual habits. If the widespread callosal connections found in Boston Siamese cats, and our cats turned out to be of the Boston type (see above), could ensure an efficient binocular coding in the suprasylvian areas, then the successful IOT of Siamese cats would be explained.

However, the possibility should also be taken into account that the sparse un-crossed fibres originating from the normal routed patches of temporal retina might be sufficient for relaying visual information to the ipsilateral visual centres during monocular visual discrimination learning. Interestingly enough, although compatible with the Boston-type cortical organisation, such a possibility would not apply to Midwestern-type cats, where the input from the entire temporal retina is supposed to be centrally suppressed (Guillery *et al.,* 1974). To check such a hypothesis it would be quite important to test IOT in cats with electrophysiologically document-ed Midwestern-type cortical organisation.

ROLE OF FOREBRAIN COMMISSURES IN THE SIAMESE CAT'S IOT

In order to verify the first hypothesis mentioned above, namely that successful IOT in Siamese cats is sustained by an unusual pattern of visual commissural connections, we tested intact and commissurotomised Siamese cats for IOT of three additional, more difficult pattern dicriminations.

If the callosal compensation hypothesis were correct, sectioning the forebrain commissures ought to abolish or reduce IOT in Siamese cats but not in ordinary cats. In the latter, the presence of a partial chiasma decussation would permit a bihemi-spheric visual input during monocular vision, even in the absence of the corpus cal-losum and the other forebrain commissures.

Two Siamese cats (S4 and S5) underwent section of the entire corpus callosum, as well as of the hippocampal and anterior commissures, following the surgical procedure described by Trevarthen (1972). In one additional Siamese cat (S3) the rostral one-third of the corpus callosum and the anterior commissure were intentionally spared. Three other Siamese cats (S7, S9 and S10) served as unoperated controls. Two further control groups were formed by intact ordinary cats ($n = 2$) and commissurotomised ordinary cats ($n = 3$). One of the latter ordinary cats received the same extent of sub-total commissurotomy as S3. The completeness of the surgical lesions was histologically confirmed.

Figure 23.3 shows the mean percent IOT saving scores for intact and split Siamese cats. There were no significant differences in IOT in any of the measures of transfer. As one would have expected, no difference was found between intact and split ordinary cats. Also, no difference was evident between the animals with complete and sub-total commissurotomies. Thus, it can be concluded that IOT in Siamese cats cannot be accounted for by the forebrain commissures compensating for the abnormal visual pathways decussation.

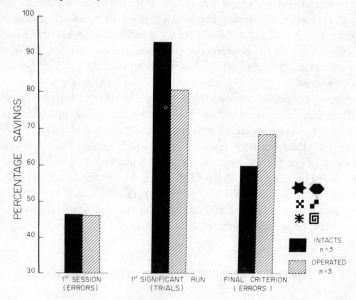

Figure 23.3.   Interocular transfer scores for intact and commissurotomised Siamese cats. The three pairs of discriminanda used are shown on the right-hand side

EFFECT OF DIFFICULTY OF DISCRIMINATIONS

As there was no effect whatsoever of the commissural section both on Siamese and ordinary cats, the scores of intact and split Siamese cats were pooled and compared

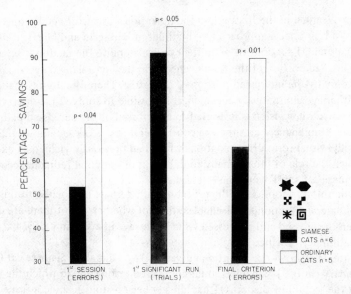

Figure 23.4. Interocular transfer scores for split plus intact Siamese cats and split plus intact ordinary cats on the series of more difficult discrimination problems

with those of intact plus split ordinary cats. Such a procedure allows the study of IOT with more demanding visual discriminations.

Figure 23.4 shows that the Siamese group is now impaired on all the three measures of IOT. All the same, these results indicate again that even though an imperfection of the Siamese cat's IOT can be revealed by using more difficult discriminations, IOT is still largely successful. That the problems used in this second series were more difficult than in the previous series was evident from a comparison of the mean number of errors made by all cats during training with the first eye in the two series of discriminations. As in the first series of discriminations, there were no statistically significant differences in overall learning ability between Siamese and ordinary cats, although there was now some trend toward a slightly inferior performance of the Siamese group.

The IOT of Siamese cats, although significantly impaired, was on difficult discrimination problems still considerably better than one would have expected from the aberrant visual pathways. Accordingly we proceeded to test the second possibility mentioned above, namely that IOT may be subserved by the uncrossed ipsilateral projections originating from the normally routed patches of temporal retina.

ROLE OF THE UNCROSSED PATHWAYS

To check such a possibility we tested some of the intact Siamese and ordinary cats in the retention after unilateral optic tract (OT) section of the two discrimination problems learned in the first series. The operation was performed by open surgery through a transbuccal approach (see methods in Berlucchi and Marzi, 1970). Following unilateral OT section, vision in the eye ipsilateral to the section is subserved only by the crossed portion of the retina, whereas in the contralateral eye vision is subserved only by the uncrossed portion of the retina. Therefore, by testing the animals with either eye alternatively occluded, it is possible to study visual discrimination performance when vision is restricted to the crossed or the uncrossed pathways, respectively. If in Siamese cats the eye contralateral to the OT section would be able to master the visual form discriminations which had previously yielded an excellent IOT, then the role of the normally routed areas of temporal retina in accounting for the Siamese cat's IOT would be established.

Furthermore, adoption of the procedure of alternate monocular testing in cats with unilaterally sectioned OT enables study of whether or not there are differences between the crossed and uncrossed visual pathways in efficiency of visual form discrimination performance in ordinary cats.

Figure 23.5 shows the retention curves for two animals, a Siamese cat (S9) and an ordinary cat (C9) which has so far completed testing and in which the completeness of the section of the left OT has already been histologically confirmed.

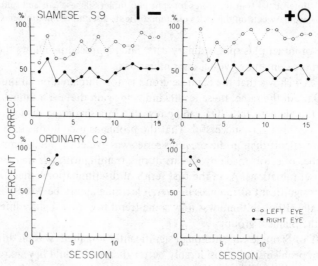

Figure 23.5. Monocular retention curves for one Siamese cat and one ordinary cat following unilateral left optic tract section. Testing was terminated either after each eye had attained criterion (at least 18 correct responses in a 20-trials session) or after a total of 300 trials with each eye

It is evident from inspection of figure 23.5 that, in S9, performance was almost immediately above chance when vision was restricted to the crossed pathways, but that it never rose above chance level when vision was restricted to the uncrossed pathways. On the contrary, the ordinary cat's performance was very good with both eyes.

The difference in the overall performance between S9 and C9 is most likely accounted for by the disturbing effect on the good eye's (ipsilateral to OT section) performance of the trials performed with the bad eye (contralateral to OT section) tested first. This resulted in a marked order effect of eye testing. That vision was indeed very poor, or absent at all, in the eye contralateral to the OT section in S9, as well as in the other Siamese cats still under study, was confirmed by extensive visual perimetry testing (see chapter 20).

Although there may be variations between individual Siamese cats in the amount of aberrant temporal retinal fibres (Guillery *et al.*, 1974), and hence in the extent to which section of the OT affects the contralateral eye, nevertheless the present results and work still in progress indicate that visual input from the uncrossed retinal fibres cannot account for the positive IOT found in Siamese cats. This result is not entirely unexpected considering that in Boston Siamese cats the normal patch of temporal retina subserves vision in the very periphery of the monocular visual field and that the very small normal medial segment is not likely to give a substantial contribution (Shatz, 1977a).

CONCLUSION

Summing up, neither the forebrain commissures nor the uncrossed visual pathways can be responsible for the surprisingly good IOT found in Siamese cats.

Therefore, a third possibility comes into mind, namely that in Siamese cats IOT of form discriminations can occur through a subcortical interhemispheric exchange of visual information.

It is tempting to speculate that a possible candidate pathway for a subcortical convergence of information from the two eyes could be represented by the bilateral corticotectal projection recently described by Powell (1976) in both ordinary and Siamese cats. Such a speculation could be submitted to a direct test by studying IOT after the tectal commissures have been severed in addition to or independently of the forebrain commissures.

REFERENCES

Berlucchi, G. and Marzi, C. A. (1970). Veridical interocular transfer of lateral mirror-image discriminations in split-brain cats. *J. comp. physiol. Psychol.,* **72** (1), 1-7

Berlucchi, G., Sprague, J. M., Levy, J. and Di Berardino, A. (1972). The pretectum and superior colliculus in visually guided behavior and in flux and form discrimination in the cat. *J. comp. physiol. Psychol. Monogr.,* **78**, 123-72

Berlucchi, G., Buchtel, E., Marzi, C. A., Mascetti, G. G. and Simoni, A. (1978). Effects of experience on interocular transfer of pattern discriminations in split-chiasm and split-brain cats. *J. comp. physiol. Psychol.,* **92**, 532-43

Berlucchi, G., Sprague, J. M., Antonini, A. and Simoni, A. (1979). Visual discrimination learning and interhemispheric transfer following suprasylvian lesions in the cat. *Expl Brain Res.*, (in press).

Berman, N. and Cynader, M. (1972). Comparison of receptive-field organization of the superior colliculus in Siamese and normal cats. *J. Physiol., Lond.*, **224**, 363-89

Blake, R. and Antoinetti, D. N. (1976). Abnormal visual resolution in the Siamese cat. *Science*, **194**, 109-10

Bogartz, R. S. (1965). The criterion method: some analyses and remarks. *Psychol. Bull.*, **64**, 1-14

Cool, S. J. and Crawford, M. L. J. (1972). Absence of binocular coding in striate cortex units of Siamese cats. *Vision Res.*, **12**, 1809-14

Cowey, A. and Parkinson, A. M. (1973). Effects of sectioning the corpus callosum on interocular transfer in hooded rats. *Expl Brain Res.*, **18**, 433-45

Elekessy, E. I., Campion, J. E. and Henry, G. H. (1973). Differences between the visual fields of Siamese and common cats. *Vision Res.*, **13**, 2533-43

Gross, C. G. and Mishkin, M. R. (1977). The neural basis of stimulus equivalence across retinal translation. In *Lateralization in the Nervous System* (S. Harnad *et al.*, eds.), Academic Press, New York, pp. 109-22

Guillery, R. W. and Kaas, J. H. (1971). A study of normal and congenitally abnormal retino-geniculate projections in cats. *J. comp. Neurol.*, **143**, 73-99

Guillery, R. W., Casagrande, V. A. and Oberdorfer, M. D. (1974). Congenitally abnormal vision in Siamese cats. *Nature, (Lond.)*, **252**, 195-99

Hohmann, A. Creutzfeldt, O. D. (1975). Squint and the development of binocularity in humans. *Nature (Lond.)*, **254**, 613-14

Hubel, D. and Wiesel, T. (1971). Aberrant visual projections in the Siamese cat. *J. Physiol., Lond.*, **218**, 33-62

Ikeda, H. and Wright, M. J. (1976). Properties of LGN cells in kittens reared with convergent squint. A neurophysiological demonstration of amblyopia. *Expl Brain Res.*, **25**, 63-77

Kaas, J. H. and Guillery, R. W. (1973). The transfer of abnormal visual field representations from the dorsal lateral geniculate nucleus to the visual cortex in Siamese cats. *Brain Res.*, **59**, 61-95

Kalil, R., Jhaveri, S. and Richard, W. R. (1971). Anomalous retinal pathways in the Siamese cat: an inadequate substrate for normal binocular vision. *Science*, **174**, 302-305

Kirk, D. C., Levick, W. R. and Cleland, B. G. (1976). The crossed or uncrossed destination of axons of sluggish-concentric and non-concentric cat retinal ganglion cells, with an overall synthesis of the visual field representation, *Vision Res.*, **16**, 233-36

Lane, R. H., Kaas, J. H. and Allman, J. M. (1974). Visuotopic organisation of the superior colliculus in normal and Siamese cats. *Brain Res.*, **70**, 413-30

Marzi, C. A., Simoni, A. and Di Stefano, M. (1976). Lack of binocularly driven neurones in the Siamese cat's visual cortex does not prevent successful interocular transfer of visual form discriminations. *Brain Res.*, **105**, 353-57

Mitchell, D. E. and Ware, C. (1974). Interocular transfer of a visual after-effect in normal and stereoblind humans. *J. Physiol., Lond.*, **236**, 707-21

Movshon, J. A., Chambers, B. E. and Blakemore, C. (1972). Interocular transfer in normal humans and those who lack stereopsis. *Perception*, **1**, 483-90

Myers, R. E. (1962). Transmission of visual information within and between the hemispheres: a behavioral study. In *Interhemispheric Relations and Cerebral Dominance* (V. B. Mountcastle, ed.), Johns Hopkins Press, Baltimore

Packwood, J. and Gordon, B. (1975). Stereopsis in normal domestic cat, Siamese cat, and cat raised with alternating monocular occlusion. *J. Neurophysiol.*, **38**, 1485-99

Powell, T. P. S. (1976). Bilateral cortico-tectal projection from the visual cortex in the cat. *Nature, (Lond.)*, **260**, 526-27

Rengstorff, R. H. (1976). Strabismus measurements in the Siamese cat. *Am J. Opt. Physiol. Optics*, **53**, 643-46

Shatz, C. (1977a). A comparison of visual pathways in Boston and Midwestern Siamese cats. *J. comp. Neurol.*, **171**, 205-28

Shatz, C. (1977b). Abnormal interhemispheric connections in the visual system of Boston Siamese cats. A physiological study. *J. comp. Neurol.*, **171**, 229-46

Shatz, C. (1977c). Anatomy of interhemispheric connections in the visual system of Boston Siamese and ordinary cats. *J. comp. Neurol.*, **173**, 497-518

Sheridan, C. L. (1965). Interocular transfer of brightness and pattern discriminations in normal and corpus callosum-sectioned rats. *J. comp. physiol. Psychol.*, **59**, 292-94

Simoni, A. and Sprague, J. M. (1976). Perimetric analysis of binocular and monocular visual fields in Siamese cats. *Brain Res.*, **111**, 189-96

Trevarthen, C. (1972). Specialized lesions: the split-brain technique. In *Methods in Psychobiology*, vol. II, (R. D. Myers, ed.), Academic Press, London

Van Hof, M. W. (1970). Interocular transfer in the rabbit. *Expl Neurol.*, **26**, 103-108

Weber, J. T. and Hartig, J. K. (1976). Comparison of retino-tectal pathways in normal and Siamese cats: an autoradiographic analysis. *Neurosci. Abstr.*, **2**, 1098

24
CUTANEOUS AND PROPRIOCEPTIVE INPUT TO THE CORPUS CALLOSUM IN THE CAT

T. MANZONI, G. SPIDALIERI and R. CAMINITI

The callosal interhemispheric transfer enables animals to solve with the untrained paw somaesthetic discriminations involving the use of tactile or proprioceptive cues, at a level of performance as high as that reached by the trained paw. At least for cats, there is well-documented evidence that the interhemispheric transfer of somaesthetic discrimination learning takes place at the level of the somatosensory receiving areas (Teitelbaum et al., 1968). It was shown in fact, in callosum-intact cats, that the occurrence of the somaesthetic transfer is precluded either by the ablation of the first (SI) or of the second (SII) somatosensory area of the trained hemisphere and also by the ablation of SII, but not of SI, of the untrained hemisphere.

From these results it appears that, the homotopic SII-SII and the heterotopic SI-SH callosal projections (Jones and Powell, 1968; Caminiti et al., 1977) are both necessary for inducing the transfer from the trained towards the untrained hemisphere. As is known, the two cortical areas receive information from the periphery through the lemniscal projection paths, whose functional properties are unanimously regarded as the most suitable for preservation of all the features, qualities and spatiotemporal patterns of peripheral stimuli up to the cortical level (Mountcastle, 1974). The ability of the untrained hemisphere to operate at a high level of performance might be ensured by a transfer mechanism subserved by callosal fibres carrying sensory messages which preserve their original specificity and informative contents as faithfully as possible.

In the past few years we have carried out electrophysiological experiments aimed at studying the modes of the callosal transfer of somaesthetic information (Caminiti et al., 1976; Innocenti et al., 1972, 1973, 1974; Manzoni et al., 1975). By means of both macro- and microelectrode recordings from the corpus callosum of cats, we identified in its rostral portion (henceforth called somaesthetic callosal region, SCR; Innocenti et al., 1974) a band of fibres through which the efferent cells of SI and SII send information of peripheral origin to the other hemisphere. We would like to present briefly, in this chapter, part of the results obtained showing that the callosal somaesthetic fibres indeed maintain many of the specific properties which are typical of the lemniscal system.

Some of the findings most relevant to the understanding of the callosal transfer of *exteroceptive information* were obtained from studying (Caminiti et al., 1976;

Manzoni *et al.*, 1975) the functional relationships between the responses recorded from SI and SII, from the corpus callosum and the appropriate spinal dorsal roots after stimulation of superficial nerves of the forelimb (superficial radial and median nerves). The aim was to ascertain whether the behaviour of the callosal responses to peripheral stimuli of increasing strength might parallel the well-known behaviour of the cortical responses (Mark and Steiner, 1958; Oscarsson and Rosén, 1963, 1966).

Employing the averaging technique to detect the smallest potentials, it was found that the Group II fibres of the cutaneous nerves heavily project within the SCR portion where the forelimb is respresented (Innocenti *et al.*, 1974) and that the threshold for both callosal and cortical potentials are almost identical (figure 24.1). Both responses often appeared simultaneously before any potential was detectable in the electroneurograms, thus suggesting that activity restricted to very few of the lowest threshold Group II fibres of cutaneous nerves is sufficient to provoke not only cortical (Oscarsson and Rosén, 1963) but also callosal responses. The input-output curves of cortical and callosal responses (response amplitude versus stimulus strength) were similar in shape, both showing the typical steep rise upon increasing intensity of stimulation. Their full amplitude development was also attained almost simultaneously, well before the maximal development of the Group II elevation in the electroneurograms and even before the engagement of Group III fibres (figure 24.1).

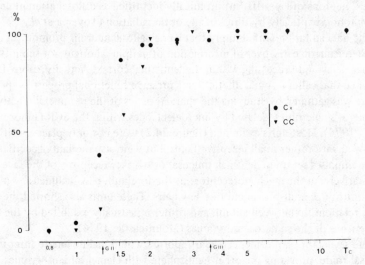

Figure 24.1. Amplitude of cortical and callosal responses as a function of increasing strength of superficial radial nerve stimulation. Amplitude of the positive phase of cortical (SII area; dots) and callosal (triangles) responses, expressed as a percent of its maximum, are plotted as a function of stimulus intensity relative to threshold for cortical potentials (Tc; semilogarithmic plotting). Each plot represents the value obtained from 50 averaged potentials. Appearance in the electroneurograms (recorded from the distal end of a cut dorsal rootlet of C_8) of the potentials due to activation of Group II (GII) and Group III (GIII) fibres of the superficial radial nerve is indicated by arrows in the abscissa. (From Caminiti *et al.*, 1976a)

For cortical responses, this behaviour was regarded by Mark and Steiner (1958) as one of the most compelling testimonies of the powerful nature of the synaptic transfer of impulses at any level of the ascending projection pathways. According to our results, the synaptic input feeding the pool of callosal neurons would also operate at a similar level of efficiency and security. It is relevant, in this connection, that the thalamic afferents might impinge monosynaptically on some callosal neurons. Indeed, according to the measurements of the delay between the onset of the cortical responses to the skin or to the superficial radial nerve stimulation and the transit of callosal impulses at interhemispheric midline (Innocenti *et al.*, 1974), and to the analysis of the thalamocallosal, thalamocortical and corticocallosal conduction time (Innocenti *et al.*, 1976), the fastest callosal impulses elicited by peripheral stimulation could be relayed monosynaptically at the level of the somatosensory areas. Morphological data are now available which would provide the basis for such a possibility.

It was recently shown (Caminiti *et al.*, 1977) that in the somatosensory areas callosal efferent neurons have the shape of pyramidal cells and occur overwhelmingly in layer III. Although thalamocortical afferents terminate mainly on stellate cells of layer IV in the somatic as well as in other sensory areas, some terminals were also found in the adjacent parts of layer III, contacting dendritic spines probably of pyramidal cells (Jones and Powell, 1970). It might also be recalled that in the visual cortex, neurons of layer III, antidromically identified as callosal efferent cells were fired monosynaptically by fibres of the optic radiation (Toyama *et al.*, 1974).

The data so far presented imply that some callosal neurons promote an immediate interhemispheric carry-over of information of peripheral origin not submitted to further delay and processing within the 'emitting' cortex. Actually, more direct evidence that callosal somaesthetic fibres preserve functional properties specific in nature was gathered by studying the characteristics of the peripheral reactivity of a sample of single fibres isolated by microelectrodes within the SCR (Innocenti *et al.*, 1972, 1974). Most units examined (figure 24.2) were not only place-specific and endowed with rather small receptive fields, but were also modality-specific, responding to impulses set up in dentinal, mucosal or whisker receptors of the face or, alternatively, in the mechanoreceptors of the forelimb, paw included, by means of light touchings or displacement of a few hairs. These units also showed the same strict relationship between stimuli and firing, as is usually exhibited by the lemniscal neurons of the somatosensory areas (Mountcastle, 1974).

The several lines of evidence so far reported would incline one to infer that the callosal route, providing the other hemisphere with elemental sensory cues, operates as an extension of the lemniscal paths beyond the sensory receiving areas. The sensory nature of the callosal projections is also suggested by the behavioural evidence, showing that the stimulation of some parts of the corpus callosum in conscious human subjects (Schaltenbrand *et al.*, 1970) provokes subjective paraesthesias in arm and leg similar to those provoked by stimulation of the somaesthetic cortex. One might speculate that the processing of the simple sensory information transmitted by callosal fibres takes place in the 'receiving' hemisphere, and probably within the SII

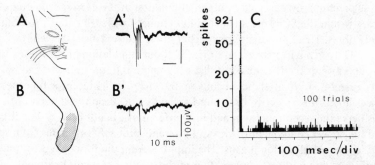

Figure 24.2. Interhemispheric transfer of somatosensory information through single callosal fibres. Examples of the peripheral receptive fields of two callosal fibres reactive to whisker displacements (A) or to light touchings of the dorsal surface of the forepaw (B). The discharges elicited in these fibres by single-shock stimulation of the centre zone of the respective receptive field are shown in A' and B', respectively. In C is shown the post-stimulus time histogram obtained (100 trials; integration time: 3 ms) from the same unit shown in A–A' during 1 per second peripheral stimulation. (After Innocenti *et al.*, 1972, 1974)

area, according to experiments both behavioural (Teitelbaum *et al.*, 1968) and electrophysiological (Innocenti *et al.*, 1973; Robinson, 1973). Actually, several studies in animals showed that during unilateral training the memory trace can be laid down in both hemispheres (Ebner and Myers, 1962; R. W. Doty, personal communication), although the engrams indirectly induced via the corpus callosum seem less efficient than the primary mnemonic system.

In the single unit analysis mentioned above (Innocenti *et al.*, 1974) no fibre was found specifically reactive to stimulation of deep receptors. However, evidence that also the interhemispheric transfer of *proprioceptive information* actually occurs within the SCR came forth from subsequent experiments carried out with a different technique (Caminiti *et al.*, 1976; Manzoni *et al.*, 1975). In these experiments, several deep nerves of the forelimb have been stimulated with graded intensities in order to activate selectively different groups of fibres, and records were simultaneously taken from the appropriate spinal dorsal roots, from the SCR, from area 3a (Oscarsson and Rosén, 1963, 1966) and, on some occasions, from SI or SII as well. It was shown that deep afferents from the forelimb heavily project within the SCR, although the deep projection is less substantial than that from cutaneous nerves. In fact, the potentials elicited by stimulation of the former nerves were, in all the callosal foci explored, remarkably lower in amplitude than those provoked by the impulses of superficial origin.

However, the main distinguishing feature of the callosal transfer of deep afferents is not related to the amount of the information transferred but rather to the types of deep receptors projecting to the corpus callosum. Actually, according to the evidence obtained upon selective stimulation of different groups of fibres of pure muscular, articular and deep mixed nerves of the forelimb, the callosal output appears to result from some kind of 'filtering' action operated by the somatosensory areas on the corticopetal input from deep receptors.

It was preliminarily observed that the stimulation of the deep radial nerve elicited responses within the SCR, provided stimulus strength was high enough to excite the Group II fibres. These responses grew higher upon additional engagement of Group III fibres. Only in a narrow portion of the SCR did stimulation of the lowest theshold Group I afferents elicit small but distinct responses in the averaged callosal records (figure 24.3). No inferences could be drawn about the receptor types feeding the few callosal fibres reactive to Group I volleys of the deep radial nerve. Athough for this nerve the receptor system and their afferents have not been systematically studied, its largest component of Group I afferents probably originates from spindle primary endings and tendon organs. The impulses from the former type of muscle receptors are known to reach several foci of the cerebral cortex (Oscarsson and Rosén, 1963, 1966; Rosén, 1972; Silfvenius, 1970b) and from there part of these impulses might be retransmitted to the corpus callosum. However, we considered that the callosal projections from Group I afferents, if coming from primary endings of muscle spindles, were too scarce to be functionally meaningful and much too scarce if compared with the wide cortical projection from muscle spindles.

It has been reported (Giaquinto *et al.*, 1963; Oscarsson and Rosén, 1963) that the central effects obtained upon stimulation of the deep radial nerve differ from those obtained from other deep nerves of the forelimb, probably because its spectrum of large fibres could be contaminated by afferents from its distal portion which also distributes to the interosseous membrane and carpal joints (Giaquinto *et al.*, 1963; Oscarsson and Rosén, 1963). As is known (Matthews, 1972; Silfvenius, 1970a), some joint receptors might have afferent fibres falling within the Group I range. It was proposed that the callosal responses evoked by low threshold afferents of the deep radial nerve might be of extramuscular origin. In order to test this possibility, a series of experiments was undertaken in which pure muscular and articular nerves have been stimulated separately. According to the results obtained, in spite of large potentials evoked in area 3a, no responses could be evoked within the whole SCR either upon activation of Group I or upon additional engagement of Group II afferent fibres of pure muscular branches of the median nerve (the branch to the palmaris longus, the flexor carpi radialis and I-III heads of the flexor digitorum profundus and the branch to the IV-V heads of the flexor digitorum profundus and pronator quadratus).

Since the corticopetal afferents of Groups I and II from such branches originate from muscle spindle primary and secondary endings (Matthews, 1972), respectively, it follows that the whole cortical input from fusal receptors might have no access to the corpus callosum. Only muscular impulses elicited in fibres of Group III were effective in provoking callosal responses (figure 24.3). In these experiments it was observed that the callosal responses appeared almost simultaneously with small evoked potentials in SI and SII. As is known (Matthews, 1972; Oscarsson and Rosén, 1963, 1966; Rosén, 1972), the high threshold muscle afferents, together with other deep afferents from extramuscular structures, project to these areas, from which impulses could be relayed to the SCR. Indeed, in a current study (R. Caminiti,

G. M. Innocenti and T. Manzoni 1977) in which the technique of the retrograde axonal transport of horseradish peroxidase has been associated with electrophysiological recording methods, several SI neurons labelled with the enzyme injected in the contralateral SII (thus identified as callosal efferent neurons) were found to lie in cortical columns from which both single and multi-unit firing was recorded in response to afferent impulses elicited by manipulations of deep tissues of the forepaw.

The same callosal foci, unreactive to Groups I and II afferent volleys from muscles, exhibited small but definite mass responses upon activation of the lowest threshold fibres of the interosseous branch of the median nerve (figure 24.3). It is worth recalling that the receptor system and the size of the related afferent fibres of this branch have been extensively studied. A high proportion of them, morphologically and functionally identified, pertain to Group I and originate mainly from extramuscular Pacinian corpuscles, from tap and tension receptors and, in a very small proportion, from muscle spindles (Silfvenius, 1970a). The largest fibres of extrafusal origin of this nerve project to cortical foci overlapping those of Group I muscle projection (Silfvenius, 1970b).

However, it was shown that the muscle spindle input and the lowest threshold articular input activate separate pools of cortical neurons (Silfvenius, 1972). Only those cells receiving the impulses from the latter afferents might send fibres to the SCR. Additional evidence was gathered explaining the central effects obtained upon stimulation of the deep radial nerve described above. Selective stimulation of its muscular branch to the extensor carpi radialis yielded the same results as those observed upon activation of the two muscular branches of the median nerve and thus did not activate the SCR, whereas clear-cut potentials were recorded from this callosal region in response to afferent volleys carried by the lowest threshold Group I and/or Group II fibres of its distal portion containing, as reported above, the fibres from the interosseous membrane and carpal joints (figure 24.3).

According to the evidence presented, it is quite likely that the main bulk of deep information involved in the interhemispheric callosal transfer originates from the thin myelinated fibres deriving from muscles and from a wide spectrum of fibres arising from structures which, in a general sense, might be defined as articular in nature, whereas such pieces of information originating from muscle spindles do not participate in the transfer. Of course, because of this 'filtering' of deep information operated by the cortex, the relationships between cortical and callosal responses described for the cutaneous input do not hold for the deep input but, nevertheless, the results obtained emphasise the sensory function of the callosal route interconnecting the somatosensory areas discussed above. It should be recalled in fact that, contrary to the deep afferents of extrafusal origin, the afferent fibres from muscle spindles seem to be inappropriate to elicit conscious sensory experience. Indeed, it has been clearly shown in the cat that the stimulation of such fibres does not produce EEG changes or orienting reactions (Giaquinto et al., 1963; Pompeiano and Sweet, 1962) and neither does it promote discriminative processes (Sweet and Bourassa, 1967).

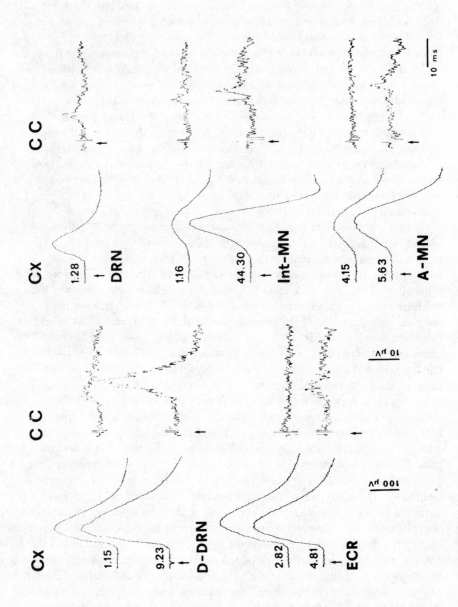

Figure 24.3. Responses recorded from the cerebral cortex and the corpus callosum upon stimulation of several deep nerves of the forelimb. Each pair of averaged responses (50 trials) has been recorded simultaneously from the cortical area 3a (Cx) of the right hemisphere and from the somaesthetic callosal region (CC), following single-shock stimulation (arrows) of deep nerves of the left forelimb, as indicated. D-DRN, distal portion of the deep radial nerve isolated at wrist level; ECR, the muscular branch of this nerve, supplying the extensor carpi radialis; DRN, deep radial nerve isolated above elbow; Int-MN the interosseous branch of the median nerve; A-MN, the muscular branch of this nerve supplying the palmaris longus, the flexor carpi radialis and I–III heads of the flexor digitorum profundus. Responses evoked by D-DRN and ECR, and those elicited by DRN, Int-MN and A-MN, have been obtained from two different animals. Strength of stimuli, for each pair of records, is indicated as a multiple of threshold for cortical responses (After Manzoni *et al.*, 1975)

ACKNOWLEDGEMENT

This work was supported in part by funds granted by Consiglio Nazionale delle Ricerche.

REFERENCES

Caminiti, R., Manzoni, T., Michelini, S. and Spidalieri, G (1976). Callosal transfer of impulses originated from superficial and deep nerves of the cat forelimb. *Arch. Ital. Biol.*, **114**, 155–77

Caminiti, R., Innocenti, G. M. and Manzoni, T. (1977). The 'callosal zone' in the first and second somatosensory areas of the cat. *Neurosci. Abstr.*, **3**, 66

Ebner, F. F. and Myers, R. E. (1962). Direct and transcallosal induction of touch memories in the monkey. *Science*, **138**, 51–52

Giaquinto, S., Pompeiano, O. and Sweet, J. E. (1963). EEG and behavioural effects of fore- and hindlimb muscular afferent volleys in unrestrained cats. *Arch. Ital. Biol.*, **101**, 133–68

Innocenti, G. M., Manzoni, T. and Spidalieri, G. (1972). Risposte topiche callosali a stimoli cutanei. *Atti Accad. Naz. Lincei, Cl. Sci. Fis., Mat. Nat.*, ser. VIII, **52**, 952–59

Innocenti, G. M., Manzoni, T. and Spidalieri, G. (1973). Relevance of the callosal transfer in defining the peripheral reactivity of somaesthetic cortical neurones. *Arch. Ital. Biol.*, **111**, 187–221

Innocenti, G. M., Manzoni, T. and Spidalieri, G. (1974). Patterns of the somaesthetic messages transferred through the corpus callosum. *Expl Brain Res.*, **19**, 447–66

Jones, E. C. and Powell, T. P. S. (1968). The commissural connections of the somatic sensory cortex in the cat. *J. Anat.*, **103**, 433–55

Jones, E. G. and Powell, T. P. S. (1970). An electron microscopic study of the laminar pattern and mode of termination of afferent fibre pathways in the somatic sensory cortex of the cat. *Phil. Trans. R. Soc., B.* **257**, 45–62

Manzoni, T., Michelini, S. and Spidalieri, G. (1975). Transfer callosale di impulsi profondi di diversa origine recettoriale. *Atti Accad. Naz. Lincei, Cl. Sci. Fis., Mat. Nat.,* ser. VIII, **58**, 656–61

Mark, R. F. and Steiner, J. (1958). Cortical projection of impulses in myelinated cutaneous afferent nerve fibres of the cat. *J. Physiol., Lond.,* **142**, 544–62

Matthews, P. B. C. (1972). *Mammalian Muscle Receptors and their Central Actions,* Edward Arnold, London

Mountcastle, V. B. (1974). Neural mechanisms in somaesthesia. In *Medical Physiology,* vol. I (V. B. Mountcastle, ed.), Mosby, St Louis, pp. 307–47

Oscarsson, O. and Rosén, I. (1963). Projections to cerebral cortex of large muscle-spindle afferents in forelimb nerves of the cat. *J. Physiol., Lond.,* **169**, 924–45

Oscarsson, O. and Rosén, I. (1966). Short-latency projections to the cat's cerebral cortex from skin and muscle afferents in the contralateral forelimb. *J. Physiol., Lond.,* **182**, 164–84

Pompeiano, O. and Sweet, J. E. (1962). Identification of cutaneous and muscular afferent fibres producing EEG synchronization and arousal in normal cats. *Arch. Ital. Biol.,* **100**, 343–80

Robinson, D. L. (1973). Electrophysiological analysis of interhemispheric relations in the second somatosensory cortex of the cat. *Expl Brain Res.,* **18**, 131–44

Rosén, I. (1972). Projection of forelimb Group I muscle afferents to the cat cerebral cortex. *Int. Rev. Neurobiol.,* **15**, 1–25

Schaltenbrand, G., Spuler, H. and Wahren, W. (1970). Electroanatomy of the corpus callosum radiation according to the facts of stereotaxic stimulation in man. *Z. Neurol.,* **198**, 79–92

Silfvenius, H. (1970a). Characteristics of receptors and afferent fibres of the fore-limb interosseous nerve of the cat. *Acta physiol. scand.,* **79**, 6–23

Silvenius, H. (1970b). Projections to the cerebral cortex from afferents of the inter-osseous nerve of the cat. *Acta physiol. scand.,* **80**, 196–214

Silfvenius, H. (1972). Properties of cortical Group I neurones located in the lower bank of the anterior suprasylvian sulcus of the cat. *Acta physiol. scand.,* **84**, 555–76

Sweet, J. E. and Bourassa, C. M. (1967). Comparison of sensory discrimination threshold with muscle and cutaneous nerve volleys in the cat. *J. Neurophysiol.,* **30**, 530–45

Teitelbaum, H., Sharpless, S. K. and Byck, R. (1968). Role of somatosensory cor-tex in interhemispheric transfer of tactile habits. *J. comp. physiol. Psychol.,* **66**, 623–32

Toyama, K., Matsunami, K., Ohno, T. and Tokashiki, S. (1974). An intracellular study of neuronal organization in the visual cortex. *Expl Brain. Res.,* **21**, 45–66

25
COMMISSURAL CONNECTIONS BETWEEN THE VESTIBULAR NUCLEI STUDIED WITH THE METHOD OF RETROGRADE TRANSPORT OF HORSERADISH PEROXIDASE

O. POMPEIANO, T. MERGNER and N. CORVAJA

INTRODUCTION

Labyrinthine impulses, originating from semicircular canal receptors and macular receptors of both sides, act on motoneurons innervating the extrinsic eye muscles and the body musculature via the vestibulo-ocular and the vestibulospinal reflex arcs. A close co-operation between the vestibular systems of both sides is required to produce changes in the motor output which results either in conjugated eye movements or in reciprocal patterns of responses of neck and limb extensors during the labyrinthine reflexes. There are several possibilities through which the labyrinthine input of one side may produce reciprocal changes in firing rate of contralateral vestibular neurons. However, the most likely one is that the labyrinthine input of one side is transmitted to the contralateral vestibular nuclei by commissural connections.

The presence of such connections has been demonstrated following lesions involving different parts of the vestibular complex (Carpenter, 1960; Ferraro *et al.*, 1940; Gray, 1926; McMasters *et al.*, 1966). In particular, commissural connections were described between the two superior nuclei (Gray, 1926; McMasters *et al.*, 1966), as well as the two lateral nuclei (Carpenter, 1960). More recently, Ladpli and Brodal (1968) studied the distribution of degenerating fibres with the Nauta method following lesions restricted to individual vestibular nuclei in cats (cf. Brodal, 1972). They found that the two superior vestibular nuclei (SVN) and the two descending vestibular nuclei (DVN) greatly contributed to the commissural pathways. In particular, each of these two nuclei apparently projected to all four contralateral main nuclei. However, while the commissural fibres from the SVN supplied the entire contralateral SVN, all other commissural contingents terminated only in the ventralmost part of the contralateral nuclei. The lateral vestibular nucleus of Deiters (LVN) gave

319

rise to some commissural fibres mainly to the LVN and the DVN of the other side. As to the medial vestibular nucleus (MVN), it was claimed that this structure had clear connections with its counterpart on the other side. However, the precise area of termination of commissural fibres from the MVN could not be determined, since lesions of this nucleus interrupted commissural fibres from the DVN. Finally, no information could be obtained concerning the origin of possible commissural connections from the small cell-groups of the vestibular complex. In a study of efferent fibres from the vestibular nuclei in monkeys, Tarlov (1969) observed terminations of commissural fibres which agreed with the previous findings in the cat.

Although previous studies gave specific information about the terminal sites of possible commissural fibres, no definite conclusion could be drawn about the site of origin of the degenerating fibres, since any vestibular lesion may interrupt non-vestibular fibres, as well as fibres originating from other vestibular nuclei than the damaged one. In the present study we used the method of retrograde axonal transport of horseradish peroxidase (HRP) injected in the vestibular nuclei of one side, to identify contralateral vestibular neurons giving rise to commissural projections.

METHODS

The experiments were performed in 19 adult cats, anaesthetised with pentobarbital sodium (Nembutal, 35 mg/kg), and placed in a stereotaxic head holder. In some instances, extensive injection of HRP (Sigma, type VI) was made by using the hydraulic method. In this case 0.2–0.6 μl of 30% HRP dissolved in 0.9% saline solution was injected, during a period of 15–20 min. The injection was made through a glass micropipette with a tip opening of 30–60 μm, connected to the needle of a 10 μl Hamilton syringe. Smaller injections were achieved by a combined iontophoretic (Graybiel and Devor, 1974) and mechanical method. Details of the method have been described in a previous study (Mergner et al., 1977).

Briefly, a glass micropipette with a tip of 10–20 μm was filled with 5% HRP in a Tris-HCl buffer at pH 8.6 and positioned at the appropriate sterotaxic co-ordinates with a micromanipulator. Positive dc current of 2 μA was passed through the electrode in 500 ms pulses at 1 per second, for 60 min. While passing the current a sharpened tungsten wire, which fitted the tip of the electrode, was slowly driven into the pipette with the help of a second micromanipulator, in order to facilitate injection of the fluid. Towards the end of the injection time, the wire reached the tip of the pipette, thus blocking further ejection of HRP. After the survival period of 48 h, the animals were again anaesthetised, and then perfused with warm saline followed by the appropriate fixative. The brain stem was then removed and prepared according to the method of Graham and Karnowsky (1966). In one experiment the animal was treated as above, but no HRP was injected in the vestibular nuclei; this experiment served as normal control.

RESULTS

Preliminary information about the possible origin of the commissural fibres originating from the vestibular nuclei of one side was obtained in one experiment in which the injection site involved half of the medulla, from the rostral to the caudal part of the vestibular complex. In this experiment the brown reaction, due to spread of HRP solution, was visible over the entire vestibular complex as well as the underlying medullary reticular formation (RF) extending from the trigeminal nuclear complex to the medial longitudinal fasciculus (MLF) close to the midline.

On the contralateral side numerous labelled cells of all sizes were found within the peripheral zone of the SVN, particularly in its ventromedial aspect, within the whole MVN and the ventromedial part of the DVN, particularly at caudal level. Labelled cells were also found in the interstitial nucleus of the vestibular nerve (N.i.n. VIII) (Cajal, 1909–1911), the group y, a small cell-group situated dorsocaudal to the restiform body (Brodal and Pompeiano, 1957), and the group f, an aggregation of rather densely packed, relatively large cells located in the caudal part of the DVN (Brodal and Pompeiano, 1957). Moreover, positive cells were observed in the perihypoglossal nuclei, i.e. in the nucleus praepositus hypoglossi (p.h.), particularly in its peripheral zone, the nucleus intercalatus of Staderini (i.c.) and the nucleus of Roller (R). On the contrary, no labelled cells were found within the central, magnocellular region of the SVN, the whole LVN, the dorsolateral part of the DVN, particularly at rostral level, the central region of the p.h. and the groups x and z (Brodal and Pompeiano, 1957). These negative results indicate that no commissural fibres originate from these regions. However, the labelled neurons observed in the remaining areas of the vestibular complex do not necessarily send commissural fibres to the contralateral vestibular nuclei, since they could represent either vestibuloreticular neurons or secondary vestibular neurons contributing to the contralateral MLF.

Detailed information concerning the possible contribution of the individual components of the vestibular complex to the commissural connections was obtained following selective injections of HRP within the vestibular nuclei. Figure 25.1 illustrates results obtained in one experiment in which the HRP was injected within the SVN, the LVN and the group y. In this case the brown reaction, indicating spread of the HRP solution, invaded also the extreme rostral part of the DVN at dorsal level. Labelled neurons on the contralateral side were observed within the peripheral zone of the SVN, particularly in its dorsomedial aspect, the rostral part of the MVN at dorsal level, and the group y. Only a few scattered cells were found within the rostral part of the DVN and the p.h., as well as in the N.i.n. VIII. On the other hand, no labelled neurons were observed in the central region of the SVN, in any part of the LVN, in most of the DVN including group f, and in the main part of the p.h., nor were any observed in the remaining perihypoglossal nuclei.

Similar results were also obtained in other experiments, in which the HRP was injected within the SVN, the LVN, the rostral part of both DVN and MVN and the group y. However, in addition to the findings reported above, a discrete number of labelled neurons were found, not only in the dorsal but also in the ventral part of the MVN, particularly at rostral level.

In conclusion, it appears from this group of experiments that most of the commissural neurons labelled within the peripheral zone of the SVN, the rostral part of the MVN and the group y project to the contralateral SVN, DVN and probably also to the group y. The possibility that some of these commissural neurons project also to ventralmost aspects of the contralateral LVN (Ladpli and Brodal, 1968) could not be ascertained, since similarly located labelled neurons were also observed in cases in which the injection of HRP did not affect the ventralmost part of this nucleus. In addition to these findings, it appears that the rostroventral part of the MVN projects to the corresponding structure of the contralateral side.

The exact location of the commissural neurons projecting to the DVN and MVN was studied in appropriate experiments. In one case, in which a small injection was

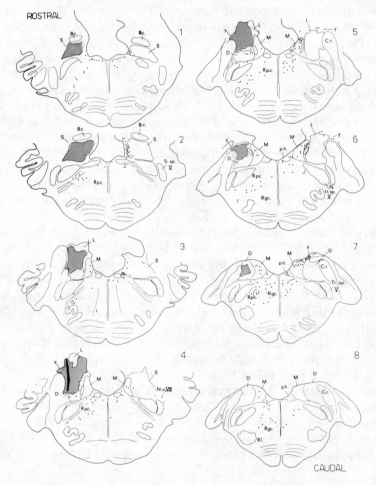

strictly located within the DVN rostral to the group f, a few labelled neurons were observed in the contralateral MVN and DVN particularly close to the borderline between these two nuclei and also in the p.h. It appears, therefore, that these neurons project exclusively to the contralateral DVN. No labelled cells, however, were observed in the remaining vestibular nuclei, the small cell groups of the vestibular complex including group f, and the remaining perihypoglossal nuclei (i.c. and R).

A comparison between the results obtained in this as well as in previous experiments in which the group f was not invaded by the HRP, and those obtained in the preliminary case in which the injection involved the whole vestibular complex including the group f, suggests that the two groups f are reciprocally interconnected.

The commissural connections terminating within the MVN were studied in experiments in which the injection site was limited to this nucleus. Figure 25.2 illustrates such an experiment, in which the brown reaction product did not invade the surrounding DVN or p.h., nor the neighbouring RF. The exact localisation of the neurons labelled in this experiment by the HRP is illustrated in figure 25.3. On the contralateral side numerous labelled neurons were found within the peripheral zone of the SVN, including both the dorsomedial and the ventrolateral borders of this uncleus, and also within the whole extent of the MVN and DVN. Numerous labelled neurons were also found within the group y, the peripheral zone of the p.h., the i.c. and the R nuclei, whereas only a few positive neurons were observed in the N.i.n. VIII. Therefore, all these nuclei of the vestibular complex project to the contralateral MVN. It should be noted, however, that the HRP might have labelled commissural axons located within the MVN in their course to other vestibular nuclei.

No labelled cells were found within the central region of the SVN, any part of

---

Figure 25.1. Distribution of labelled neurons in different medullary structures of both sides, following injection of HRP within the SVN, LVN, rostralmost part of the DVN and the group y. In this figure, as well as in figure 25.3, the black regions correspond to the injection site, whereas the hatched areas indicate the brown reaction due to spread of the HRP solution within the adjacent regions. The drawings of transverse sections through the medulla were taken at regular intervals of 500 μm from rostral to caudal levels. Labelled neurons are indicated by dots. Positive cells on each drawing are taken from 2 out of 10 serial sections, 50 μm thick. Abbreviations used in all figures: B.c., brachium conjunctivum; C.r., restiform body; D, descending (inferior) vestibular nucleus; f, cell group f in the descending vestibular nucleus (Brodal and Pompeiano); i.c., nucleus intercalatus (Staderini); L, lateral vestibular nucleus (Deiters); M, medial vestibular nucleus (Schwalbe); N.cu.e., external (accessory) cuneate nucleus; N.i.n. VIII, interstitial nucleus of vestibular nerve (Cajal); N.r.l., lateral reticular nucleus (nucleus of lateral funiculus); N.tr.s., nucleus of solitary tract; N.tr.sp.V, nucleus of spinal tract of trigeminal nerve; N.VIII, cranial nerve VIII; p.h., nucleus praepositus hypoglossi; R. gc., nucleus reticularis gigantocellularis; R.l., nucleus reticularis lateralis (Meessen and Olszewski); R. pc., nucleus reticularis parvicellularis; R.p.c., nucleus reticularis pontis caudalis; R.v., nucleus reticularis ventralis; S., superior vestibular nucleus (Bechterew); Tr.s., solitary tract; Tr.sp.V, spinal tract of trigeminal nerve; x, cell group lateral to the descending vestibular nucleus (Brodal and Pompeiano); y, cell group dorsal to the restiform body (Brodal and Pompeiano); VI, VII, X, XII, motor cranial nerve nuclei

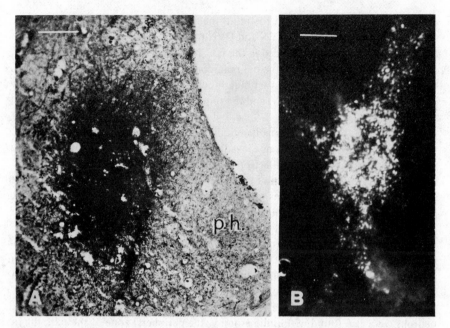

Figure 25.2.   Photomicrographs illustrating one representative case of HRP injection (bright field) and a corresponding example of retrogradely labelled neuron (dark field). (A) The injection is located within the left MVN (same experiment as in figure 25.3); p.h., nucleus praepositus hypoglossi. Magnification scale, 2 mm. (B) A labelled neuron within the contralateral MVN. Magnification scale, 10 μm

the LVN, the dorsomedial part of the MVN at caudal level, the dorsolateral part of the DVN at rostral level, nor in group f.

In all the experiments in which the HRP was injected within the vestibular nuclei of one side, labelled neurons were also observed in the ipsilateral ganglion of the VIII nerve (see figure 25.3 section 1). Moreover, in addition to the contralateral vestibular nuclei, labelled neurons were also found within the ipsilateral structures, indicating the possible existence of internuclear connections within the vestibular complex of one side. These findings, together with the observation that positive cells appeared also within the RF, due to labelling of crossed and uncrossed reticulo-vestibular neurons (see figures 25.1 and 25.3), will be discussed elsewhere.

In summary, the four main vestibular nuclei differ markedly with regard to their contribution to the commissural projections. These originate from the peripheral zone of the SVN, and from large areas of the MVN and DVN, possibly including the group f. On the other hand, no commissural projections originate from the central region of the SVN, the whole LVN, the dorsomedial part of the caudal MVN and the dorsolateral part of the rostral DVN. Commissural projections to the vestibular nuclei originate also from the N.i.n. VIII and the group y, as well as from the peripheral zone of the p.h., the i.c. and the R nuclei. On the other hand, no commissural fibres originated from the central region of the p.h. and the small groups x and z.

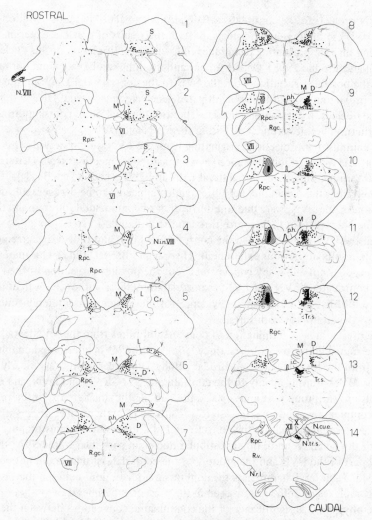

Figure 25.3. Distribution of labelled neurons in different medullary structures of both sides, following a small injection of HRP within the MVN. Drawings of transverse sections through the medulla taken at regular intervals of 500 μm from rostral to caudal levels. Labelled neurons are indicated by dots, whereas labelled axons are indicated by wavy lines. Positive cells on each drawing are taken from 2 out of 10 serial sections, 50 μm thick. Abbreviations explained in caption to figure 25.1

DISCUSSION

If we consider the commissural projections originating from the individual components of the vestibular complex, as studied by the retrograde transport of HRP injected within the different vestibular nuclei, it appears that the peripheral zone of the SVN projects to the contralateral SVN, MVN and DVN and possibly also to the group y. These findings are in agreement with the results of previous experiments, involving silver-impregnating techniques following selective lesion of this nucleus (Ladpli and Brodal, 1968). On the other hand, nothing can be said from our material about the possible projection from the SVN to the contralateral LVN and the group f. This projection can hardly be investigated, since any injection of HRP within Deiters' nucleus, for instance, may also label commissural fibres coursing through this structure, before terminating within the MVN and DVN.

No commissural projections originating from the LVN were observed. This finding conflicts with previous evidence for commissural connections from Deiters' nucleus terminating in the contralateral LVN and DVN (Ladpli and Brodal, 1968). It is likely that these commissural fibres, which appeared to be degenerated following lesion of the LVN, were due to interruption of commissural fibres originating from the N.i.n. VIII in their course through the ipsilateral LVN.

That the DVN sends fibres to the contralateral MVN and DVN is in agreement with the results of previous experiments (Ladpli and Brodal, 1968). Our material, however, does not allow any conclusion about the possible projection of the DVN to the contralateral SVN and LVN, as postulated by these authors, as well as to the group y. Finally, there is no direct evidence for the existence of interconnections between the group f of both sides.

The precise area of termination of commissural fibres from the MVN could not be determined in previous studies, since lesions of the MVN interrupted commissural fibres from the DVN (Ladpli and Brodal, 1968). Our experiments have clearly shown that the MVN projects mainly to the contralateral SVN, MVN and DVN, and possibly also to the group y. It appears also that among the small groups of the vestibular complex, the group y gives rise to a relatively discrete number of commissural fibres, terminating within the contralateral MVN. Possible commissural projections of this small group to other vestibular nuclei, in particular to the SVN, the rostral part of the DVN and the group y of the contralateral side, could not be excluded. Table 25.1 summarises the commissural projections between the vestibular complexes of both sides, as seen in the present experiments.

The physiological significance of the commissural connections between the vestibular complex of both sides should now be considered. There is evidence that some of the main vestibular nuclei, namely the MVN and the group y, which give rise to commissural fibres, receive primary vestibular afferents (cf. Brodal et al., 1962; Walberg, 1972) and contribute efferent projections to the vestibulo-ocular pathways (cf. Brodal et al., 1962; Brodal, 1974; Cohen, 1974). Moreover, physiological experiments have shown that the commissural system in the cat has an inhibitory function acting on the contralateral secondary vestibular neurons in the semicircular canal system (Kasahara and Uchino, 1971, 1974; Kasahara et al., 1968; Mano et al., 1968; Markham, 1968; cf. Shimazu, 1972; Shimazu and Precht, 1966; Wilson et al., 1968). It appears, therefore, that the commissural system is involved in the crossed labyrinthine control of the vestibulo-ocular reflex arc.

It should be mentioned, however, that the nuclear regions giving rise to com-

Table 25.1.

Summary of distribution of the commissural projections originating from the vestibular complex

Nuclei of origin	*Nuclei of termination*						
	SVN	LVN	MVN	DVN	group f	group y	p.h.
SVN peripheral part	++	?	+++	+	?	?	
central part	–	–	–	–	–	–	–
LVN	–	–	–	–	–	–	–
MVN	+	?	+++	++	?	?	
DVN dorsolateral and rostral part	–	–	–	–	–	–	–
ventromedial and caudal part (except group f)	?	?	++	+	?	?	
Group f	–	–	–	?	?		
Group y	?	?	++	?	?	?	
p.h.	?	?	++	+	?	?	
i.c. and R	–	–	++	?	?		–

The number of plus signs indicates the amount of the commissural projections as detected by the density of the corresponding labelled neurons. Absence of commissural projections is indicated by a minus sign. Question marks indicate regions which may receive commissural projections, but whose real existence could not be ascertained. No HRP injection within the p.h. was made in our study (blanks). Abbreviations as in the text

missural projections do not necessarily coincide with those receiving primary vestibular afferents and projecting to motoneurons innervating the extrinsic eye muscles, as shown for both the peripheral zone of the SVN and the ventralmost part of the MVN and DVN. These nuclear regions actually receive afferent projections from the cerebellum, namely from the fastigial nucleus (cf. Brodal, 1974; Brodal *et al.,* 1962; Walberg *et al.,* 1962) and may in turn project to the cerebellum as shown for the ventrolateral parts of the caudal MVN and DVN, including the group f (cf. Brodal, 1974; Brodal and Torvik, 1957; Brodal *et al.,* 1962). These findings indicate that the cerebellum may influence the vestibulo-ocular neurons via the commissural vestibular system (Furuya *et al.,* 1976; Shimazu and Smith, 1971); in addition, we propose that the commissural vestibular system may also be involved in the labyrinthine control of the vestibulocerebellar pathways.

Closely related to the commissural projections originating from the vestibular nuclei are those which originate from the perihypoglossal nuclei. In particular, we found that the peripheral zone of the p.h. nucleus projects to the contralateral MVN and DVN, with very few, if any, projections to the contralateral SVN and the group y. On the other hand the i.c. and R nuclei seem to have an exclusive projection to the contralateral MVN. The perihypoglossal nuclei, which may be reciprocally interconnected (Mergner *et al.,* 1977), receive afferent input from the cerebellum (Allen,

1927; Angaut and Brodal, 1967; cf. Baker and Berthoz, 1975; Brodal, 1952; Thomas et al., 1956; Walberg, 1961) as well as from the vestibular system of both sides (Fuse, 1914; Mergner et al., 1977; Moffie, 1942; Tagaki, 1925). Moreover, the same nuclei project to the cerebellum (Alley et al., 1974; Brodal, 1952; Torvik and Brodal, 1954; cf. Baker and Berthoz, 1975), and also contribute with their efferent projections to the oculomotor system. This last finding, demonstrated in both anatomical (Graybiel and Hartwieg, 1974) and physiological studies (Baker and Berthoz, 1975; Baker et al., 1976; Gresty and Baker, 1976), suggests that the perihypoglossal nuclei intervene in the vestibulocerebellar control of the eye movements.

In contrast with these findings, the LVN does not contribute to these commissural projections, although it may receive crossed vestibular afferents. It is well known that the LVN receives a primary vestibular input, particularly from the macular receptors, and projects monosynaptically, as well as polysynaptically, to motoneurons innervating the ipsilateral extensor muscles (cf. Pompeiano, 1975a). The absence of any commissural connection between the LVN of both sides does not exclude the possibility of reciprocal interactions between these two nuclei. Recent experiments have shown that natural stimulation of macular labyrinthine receptors may modify the activity of ascending spinoreticular and reticulocerebellar neurons (Coulter et al., 1976; Ghelarducci et al., 1974; cf. Pompeiano, 1975b), due to vestibulospinal volleys acting monosynaptically on neurons of the crossed ascending spinoreticular pathway (cf. Pompeiano and Hoshino, 1977). This pathway may then activate the contralateral vermal cortex of the cerebellar anterior lobe, thus inhibiting Deiters' nucleus of the corresponding side.

The failure by Shimazu and Smith (1971) to find inhibition of Deiters' neurons by stimulation of the contralateral vestibular nerve, could be attributed to the fact that the medial part of the cerebellum was removed in their experiments. It appears, therefore, that the absence of an inhibitory commissural projection between the LVN of both sides is compensated by the existence of a long-loop reflex arc, through which the macular labyrinthine input of one side may inhibit the contralateral LVN. This crossed inhibitory mechanism may contribute to the reciprocal pattern of response of limb extensors which occurs during the tonic labyrinthine reflexes (Lindsay et al., 1976; cf. Pompeiano, 1975b), as well as to the postural asymmetries produced either by unilateral section of the VIII nerve or by unilateral lesion of cerebellar (Moruzzi and Pompeiano, 1957) and precerebellar structures (Corvaja et al., 1977).

SUMMARY

The method of the retrograde axonal transport of horseradish peroxidase (HRP) injected in the vestibular nuclei of one side has been used to identify the contralateral vestibular neurons giving rise to commissural projections, apparently more specifically organised than previously known. Commissural projections originate from the peripheral zone of the SVN, and from distinct regions of the MVN and

DVN. On the other hand, no commissural projections originate from the central magnocellular region of the SVN, any of the LVN, the dorsomedial part of the caudal MVN, nor the dorsolateral part of the rostral DVN. Commissural neurons were also found within the N.i.n. VIII, the group y, the peripheral zone of p.h., the i.c. and the R nuclei. Negative results, however, were obtained from the central region of the p.h. and the small groups x and z.

The interconnections between the different components of the vestibular complex of both sides have been described in detail. Distinct regions of the vestibular complex, which give rise to commissural projections, may also receive afferents from the ipsilateral labyrinthine receptors and from the cerebellum. They may also project to the oculomotor system, as well as to the cerebellum. Although there is no complete overlapping of the nuclear regions contributing to these various afferent and efferent projections, the physiological evidence suggests that these commissural pathways exert an important role in the labyrinthine and the cerebellar control of the reciprocal mechanisms involving the vestibulo-ocular systems of both sides.

ACKNOWLEDGEMENTS

This investigation was supported by the Public Health Service Research Grant NS 07685-09 from the National Institute of Neurological and Communicative Disorders and Stroke, N.I.H., U.S.A. and by a research grant from the Consiglio Nazionale delle Ricerche, Italy. Dr T. Mergner is a post-doctoral fellow of the Scuola Normale Superiore, Pisa.

REFERENCES

Allen, W. F. (1927). Experimental–anatomical studies on the visceral bulbo-spinal pathway in the cat and guniea-pig. *J. comp. Neurol.*, **42**, *393–456*

Alley, K., Baker, R. and Simpson, J. I. (1974). Brain stem afferents to the vestibulo-cerebellum as mapped with horseradish peroxidase tracers. *Soc. Neurosci., IVth Annual Meeting*, 116

Angaut, P. and Brodal, A. (1967). The projection of the 'vestibulo-cerebellum' onto the vestibular nuclei in the cat. *Arch. Ital. Biol.*, **105**, 441–79

Baker, R. and Berthoz, A. (1975). Is the prepositus hypoglossi nucleus the source of another vestibulo-ocular pathway? *Brain Res.*, **86**, 121–27

Baker, R., Gresty, M. and Berthoz, A. (1976). Neuronal activity in the prepositus hypoglossi nucleus correlated with vertical and horizontal eye movement in the cat. *Brain Res.*, **101**, 366–71

Brodal, A. (1952). Experimental demonstration of cerebellar connexions from the peri-hypoglossal nuclei (nucleus intercalatus, nucleus praepositus hypoglossi and nucleus of Roller) in the cat. *J. Anat.*, **86**, 110–29

Brodal, A. (1972). Organization of the commissural connections: anatomy. In *Basic Aspects of Central Vestibular Mechanisms, Progress in Brain Research*, vol. 37. (A. Brodal and O. Pompeiano, eds.), Elsevier, Amsterdam, pp. 167–76

Brodal, A. (1974). Anatomy of the vestibular nuclei and their connections. In Vestibular System, Part 1: Basic Mechanisms, *Handbook of Sensory Physiology*, vol. VI/1 (H. H. Kornhuber, ed.), Springer-Verlag, New York, pp. 239-352

Brodal, A. and Pompeiano, O. (1957). The vestibular nuclei in the cat. *J. Anat.*, **91**, 438-54

Brodal, A., Pompeiano, O. and Walberg, F. (1962). *The Vestibular Nuclei and their Connections. Anatomy and Functional Correlations.* Oliver and Boyd, Edinburgh

Brodal, A. and Torvik, A. (1957). Über den Ursprung der sekundären vestibulo-cerebellaren Fasern bei der Katze. Eine experimentell anatomische Studie. *Arch. Psychiat. Nervenkr.*, **195**, 550-67

Cajal, S. R. y (1909-1911). *Histologie dy Système Nerveux de l'Homme et des Vertébrés.* Maloine, Paris

Carpenter, M. B. (1960). Fiber projections from the descending and lateral vestibular nuclei in the cat. *Am. J. Anat.*, **107**, 1-22

Cohen, B. (1974). The vestibulo-ocular reflex arc. In Vestibular System, Part 1: Basic Mechanisms, *Handbook of Sensory Physiology*, vol. VI/1 (H. H. Kornhuber, ed.), Springer-Verlag, New York, pp, 477-540

Corvaja, N., Grofová, I., Pompeiano, O. and Walberg, F. (1977). The lateral reticular nucleus in the cat. II. Effects of lateral reticular lesions on posture and reflex movements. *Neurosci.*, **2**, 929-43

Coulter, J. D., Mergner, T. and Pompeiano, O. (1976). Effects of static tilt on cervical spinoreticular tract neurons. *J. Neurophys.*, **39**, 45-62

Ferraro, A., Pacella, B. L. and Barrera, S. E. (1940). Effects of lesions of the medial vestibular nucleus. An anatomical and physiological study in Macacus Rhesus monkeys. *J. comp. Neurol.*, **73**, 7-36

Furuya, N., Kawano, K. and Shimazu, H. (1976). Transcerebellar inhibitory interaction between the bilateral vestibular nuclei and its modulation by cerebello-cortical activity. *Expl Brain Res.*, **25**, 447-63

Fuse, G. (1914). Beiträge zur Anatomie des Bodens des IV. Ventrikels. *Arb. Hirnanat. Inst., Zürich*, **8**, 213-31

Ghelarducci, B., Pompeiano, O. and Spyer, K. M. (1974). Activity of precerebeller reticular neurones as a function of head position. *Arch. Ital. Biol.*, **112**, 98-125

Graham, R. C. and Karnowsky, M. Y. (1966). The early stages of absorption of injected horseradish peroxidase in the proximal tubules of mouse kidney: ultrastructural cytochemistry by a new technique. *J. Histochem. Cytochem.*, **14**, 291-302

Gray, L. P. (1926). Some experimental evidence on the connections of vestibular mechanism in the cat. *J. comp. Neurol.*, **41**, 319-64

Graybiel, A. M. and Devor, M. (1974). A microelectrophoretic delivery technique for use with horseradish peroxidase. *Brain Res.*, **68**, 167-73

Graybiel, A. M. and Hartwieg, E. A. (1974). Some afferent connections of the oculomotor complex in the cat: an experimental study with tracer techniques. *Brain Res.*, **81**, 543-51

Gresty, M. and Baker, R. (1976). Neurons with visual receptive field, eye movement and neck displacement sensitivity within and around the nucleus prepositus hypoglossi in the alert cat. *Expl Brain Res.*, **24**, 429-33

Kasahara, N., Mano, N., Oshima, T., Ozawa, S. and Shimazu, H. (1968). Contralateral short latency inhibition of central vestibular neurons in the horizontal canal system. *Brain Res.*, **8**, 376–78

Kasahara, M. and Uchino, Y. (1971). Selective mode of commissural inhibition induced by semicircular canal afferents on secondary vestibular neurons in the cat. *Brain Res.*, **34**, 366–69

Kasahara, M. and Uchino, Y. (1974). Bilateral semicircular canal inputs to neurons in cat vestibular nuclei. *Expl Brain Res.*, **20**, 285–96

Ladpli, R. and Brodal, A. (1968). Experimental studies of commissural and reticular formation projections from the vestibular nuclei in the cat. *Brain Res.*, **8**, 65–96

Lindsay, K. M., Roberts, T. D. M. and Rosenberg, J. R. (1976). Asymmetric tonic labyrinth reflexes and their interaction with neck reflexes in the decerebrate cat. *J. Physiol. Lond.*, **261**, 583–601

Mano, N., Oshima, T. and Shimazu, H. (1968). Inhibitory commissural fibers interconnecting the bilateral vestibular nuclei. *Brain Res.*, **8**, 378–82

Markham, C. H. (1968). Midbrain and contralateral labyrinth influences on brain stem vestibular neurons in the cat. *Brain Res.*, **9**, 312–33

McMasters, R. E. Weiss, A. H. and Carpenter, M. B. (1966). Vestibular projections to the nuclei of the extraocular muscles. Degeneration resulting from discrete partial lesions of the vestibular nuclei in the monkey. *Am. J. Anat.*, **118**, 163–94

Mergner, T., Pompeiano, O. and Corvaja, N. (1977). Vestibular projections to the nucleus intercalatus of Staderini mapped by retrograde transport of horseradish peroxidase. *Neurosci. Lett.*, **5**, 309–13

Moffie, D. (1942). *The Comparative Anatomy of the Nucleus Intercalatus (Staderini) and Adjacent Structures*, Van Gorcum Co., Assen

Moruzzi, G. and Pompeiano, O. (1957). Inhibitory mechanisms underlying the collapse of decerebrate rigidity after unilateral fastigial lesions. *J. comp. Neurol.*, **107**, 1–26

Pompeiano, O. (1975a). Vestibulo-spinal relationship. In *The Vestibular System* (R. F. Naunton, ed.), Academic Press, New York, pp. 147–84

Pompeiano, O. (1975b). Macular input to neurons of the spinoreticulocerebellar pathway. *Brain Res.*, **95**, 351–68

Pompeiano, O. and Hoshino, K. (1977). Responses to static tilts of lateral reticular neurons mediated by contralateral labyrinthine receptors. *Arch. Ital. Biol.*, **115**, 211–36

Shimazu, H. (1972). Organization of the commissural connections: physiology. In *Basic Aspects of Central Vestibular Mechanisms*, *Progress in Brain Research*, vol. 37 (A. Brodal and O. Pompeiano, eds.), Elsevier, Amsterdam, pp. 177–90

Shimazu, H. and Precht, W. (1966). Inhibition of central vestibular neurons from the contralateral labyrinth and its mediating pathway. *J. Neurophysiol.*, **29**, 467–92

Shimazu, H. and Smith, C. M. (1971). Cerebellar and labyrinthine influences on single vestibular neurons identified by natural stimuli. *J. Neurophysiol.*, **34**, 493–508

Tagaki, J. (1925). Studien zur vergleichenden Anatomie des Nucleus vestibularis triangularis. II. Vergleichend anatomische Untersuchungen über den Nucleus intercalatus and Nucleus praepositus, das dorsale Langsbündel von Schütz und das Triangularis–Intercalatus–Bündel von Fuse. *Arb. Neurol. Inst. Univ., Wien*, **27**, 235–82

Tarlov, E. (1969). The rostral projections of the primate vestibular nuclei. An experimental study in macaque, baboon and chimpazee. *J. comp. Neurol.*, **135**, 27-56

Thomas, D. M., Kaufman, R. P., Sprague, J. M. and Chambers, W. W. (1956). Experimental studies of the vermal cerebellar projections in the brain stem of the cat (fastigiobulbar tract). *J. Anat.*, **90**, 371-85

Torvik, A. and Brodal, A. (1954). The cerebellar projection of the peri-hypoglossal nuclei (nucleus intercalatus, nucleus praepositus hypoglossi and nucleus of Roller) in the cat. *J. Neuropathol. exp. Neurol.*, **13**, 515-27

Walberg, F. (1961). Fastigiofugal fibers to the perihypoglossal nuclei in the cat. *Expl Neurol.*, **3**, 525-41

Walberg, F. (1972). Light and electron microscopical data on the distribution and termination of primary vestibular fibers. In Basic Aspects of Central Vestibular Mechanisms, *Progress in Brain Research*, vol. 37 (A. Brodal and O. Pompeiano, eds.), Elsevier, Amsterdam, pp. 79-88

Walberg, F., Pompeiano, O., Brodal, A. and Jansen, J. (1962). The fastigiovestibular projection in the cat. An experimental study with silver impregnation methods. *J. comp. Neurol.*, **118**, 49-76

Wilson, V. J., Wylie, R. M. and Marco, L. A. (1968). Synaptic inputs to cells in the medial vestibular nucleus. *J. Neurophysiol.*, **31**, 176-85

26
ROLE OF FOREBRAIN COMMISSURES IN HEMISPHERIC SPECIALISATION AND MEMORY IN MACAQUES

ROBERT W. DOTY, WILLIAM H. OVERMAN, Jr and
NUBIO NEGRÃO

INTRODUCTION

The extensive work of Sperry (e.g., 1974) and his colleagues has dramatically emphasised the functional specialisation of the cerebral hemispheres in man, and the fact that interhemispheric integration of these unilaterally concentrated processes is normally achieved via the forebrain commissures. It seems possible, at present, that the initiating basis of this specialisation may somehow derive from the auditory system since: (a) it is the linguistic faculty that is most strikingly lateralised in man (Milner, 1974); (b) there is decisive evidence for equally strong lateralisation of learned song in canaries (Nottebohm, 1977); and (c) the only tentative suggestion of hemispheric specialisation in macaques, when normal bilateral sensory input is employed, is for analyses of auditory signals (Dewson, 1977).

Efforts to demonstrate a comparable degree of specialisation for one versus the other hemisphere for analysis of visual information by macaques have been clearly negative (Hamilton, 1977). We also have preliminary results, using still another paradigm, which confirm this difference between man and macaque. Kolb and Milner (in preparation) asked human subjects to identify which of the faces constructed from a composite photograph of right or left halves of a human face appeared most like the normal photograph of that individual. The right half was chosen > 70% of the time. This indicates statistically a very significant tendency for facial recognition to be weighted by the information first arriving in the right hemisphere. Using this same procedure with a macaque, however, and employing both human and monkey faces, the macaques choose the left face composites equally as often as the right (Overman and Doty, work in progress). In other words, given the same visual test, human subjects evidence a hemispheric specialisation, whereas the macaques tested so far do not.

One can, of course, create hemispheric specialisation by surgical interference. The most famous example of this is the preparation developed by Downer (1961) in which a macaque, lacking the amygdala in one hemisphere and with optic chiasm and forebrain commissures transected, viewed human beings placidly through the eye ipsilateral to the amygdalectomised hemisphere, but reacted aggressively and fearfully to the human presence seen with the other eye and hemisphere. By slightly modifying this approach it is possible to demonstrate that the splenium of the corpus callosum can serve to integrate the activity of the two hemispheres, each of which has been made highly specialised. If an optic tract is cut, that hemisphere becomes blind. The amygdala is then removed from the other, making it 'motivationally' deficient. Such a macaque behaves normally in regard to human beings so long as the splenium is intact (anterior commissure and remainder of callosum cut), but becomes wholly indifferent to them visually the instant the splenium is transected (Doty et al., 1973). The nature or even the direction of the neural traffic across the splenium (and/or psalterium) by which the integration between these artificially 'specialised' hemispheres is achieved is, of course, unknown, but provides a possibly useful paradigm for the design of neurophysiological approaches to this extraordinary question.

UNILATERAL ENGRAMS

We have found it possible to create hemispheric specialisation in macaques in a more subtle way. If the anterior commissur (AC) is transected and the monkey is then trained to respond to electrical excitation of striate cortex, the process necessary to trigger the learned responses to this excitation remain in this initially 'trained' hemisphere. So long as the splenium of the corpus callosum is intact, the monkey responds equally well to excitation at novel test loci in striate cortex of either hemisphere. However, as soon as the hemispheres are disconnected, by pulling a 'snare' previously placed around the splenium (Doty and Negrão, 1973; Doty et al., 1973), stimulation of these new points in striate cortex becomes ineffective on the side contralateral to that used in initial training, while remaining fully effective at new loci ipsilaterally.

This finding of a 'unilateral engram' led us (Doty and Negrão, 1973; Doty et al., 1973; Negrão and Doty, 1969) to hypothesise that the corpus callosum operates in such a manner as to restrict memory storage to a single hemisphere. Since the callosal system normally provides access by one hemisphere to information resident in the other, there is no logical necessity for duplicating the engram in each hemisphere. Indeed, the raison d'être for such a callosal mechanism is clear: it would double the mnemonic storage capacity of the brain.

In addition to our own experiments with electrical excitation of striate cortex, the existence of a callosal mechanism for producing unilateral engrams is suggested by the data of Kaas et al. (1967) on the auditory system of cats; by the bilaterality of the engrams for speech in a case with agenesis of the corpus callosum (Sperry, 1974); and, to some degree, by the experiments of Burešová and Bureš (1973) with monocular visual learning in rats. However, it is clearly contradicted by the observations of Hamilton (1977) and his colleagues that monkeys with bisected optic chiasm and lacking the anterior commissure (AC) nevertheless know with one hemisphere the visual discrimination learned with the other. Among the possible explanations for these seemingly discordant results (see Doty and Overman, 1977; Hamilton, 1977) we have had the opportunity to explore one which, tentatively, appears to be significant. This is the possibility that input via normal sensory channels, as in Hamilton's experiments, may be processed differently than is input which initially bypasses subcortical channels, as is the case with our electrical excitation of the cortex.

Three macaques were thus prepared with AC transected, splenium ensnared and stimulating electrodes implanted in the optic tract. The animals were trained to press a lever for fruit juice when, and only when, excitation was applied to the optic tract on one side. They were then tested without further training to determine whether they responded (stimulus generalisation) to stimulation of the contralateral optic tract, before and after transection of the splenium (by pulling the snare). One monkey failed to respond initially to contralateral stimulation, and it remains to be determined histologically to what degree the splenium may have been damaged by emplacement of the snare. (Indeed, if the outcome of the experiment is as indicated below, it must be shown that the forebrain commissures are essential for the interhemispheric generalisation of a conditional stimulus applied electrically to the optic tract.) In another of the monkeys the 'test' electrodes were in the chiasm so that potentials were evoked in the visual system bilaterally by their stimulation, thus invalidating any conclusions that could be drawn from the fact that this monkey displayed unequivocal stimulus generalisation before and after transecting the splenium. The third macaque, however, provided a more definitive experiment. Although electrodes were again at the level of the chiasm, they were at its very lateral edge so that the electrically recorded responses to stimulation of either optic tract were strictly unilateral. Generalisation to stimulation of the optic tract contralateral to that used for training was, nevertheless, unhesitant both before and after the splenial transection.

Thus, although additional experiments are obviously needed, we feel the hypothesis of the callosal production of unilateral engrams may require an important corollary, at least for the visual system: to wit, that the callosal mechanism is effective primarily for activity initiated from the cortex, as distinct from that arriving at the cortex via normal sensory channels. This would imply that the prominence of unilateral engrams in man (Berlucchi et al., 1974; Fedio and van Buren, 1975; Milner, 1974) arises consequent to the preponderance of human learning being associated with cortically initiated activity.

ANTERIOR COMMISSURE

Downer (1962) discovered that the anterior commissure (AC) is capable of mediating the interhemispheric transfer of visual information in the absence of the corpus callosum in macaques. This fact has now been extensively confirmed (Black and

Myers, 1964; Gazzaniga, 1966; Noble, 1968; Sullivan and Hamilton, 1973; see Doty and Negrão, 1973, for review), and the physiology of these visual processes is under active investigation (Gross and Mishkin, 1977). With electrical excitation of striate cortex as a conditional stimulus, the AC operates distinctly from the corpus callosum. In such circumstance, where the splenium is the only part of the forebrain commissures remaining, the engram is unilateral; whereas with the AC intact, it is bilateral (Doty and Negrão, 1973; Doty et al., 1973).

Thus, the AC can serve to develop a memory trace or engram in a hemisphere which itself does not otherwise receive adequate input of the relevant sensory event. Obviously, it would be interesting to monitor the neural traffic across the AC at the time such a memory trace is formed. However, in the situation where several days of training are required for the monkey to learn the appropriate response, it is by no means certain when the critical transfer might occur, even though, a priori, the times at which conditional and unconditional stimuli are paired would seem to be the most likely. Efforts to block nerve conduction in the AC by cooling it have so far been unsuccessful (Bartlett, Doty and Brust-Carmona, unpublished). The space available around the AC at the midline seems inadequate to achieve the rate of heat exchange required.

Attempts to interfere with transcommissural conduction by tetanising the AC during each training trial led to an unexpected discovery. The monkeys could not learn in such circumstance. Furthermore, during tetanisation (0.6 mA, 0.2 ms pulses at 50 Hz) they did not recognise the significance of a signal to which they had responded correctly hundreds of times, even though they obviously perceived the signal, i.e. they responded to it but not appropriately (Doty and Overman, 1977; Overman and Doty, 1977). The neural system for this effect could be traced along the radiation of the AC, and to the base of the rostral insula, where fibres pass from the temporal lobe into orbitofrontal cortex (Kuypers et al., 1965). Horel and Misantone (1976) have shown that macaques with limited, bilateral incisions interrupting fibres in this area cannot learn visual discriminations.

We have investigated another three macaques in this regard, using a 'delayed matching to sample' procedure and comparing the effects of tetanising AC versus basal ganglia or hippocampus (Overman and Doty, 1977). The corpus callosum was intact in these animals except for about 7-10 mm of the body, transected to permit visual guidance of the electrodes into the AC. The animals faced a set of three 9 x 15 cm opalescent panels, aligned horizontally, on which 35 mm slides were projected to give a vivid, coloured image of various objects, e.g. yellow tennis ball, coffee mug, pair of scissors, book etc. Slides of 100 such objects were available and, at 50 trials per day in random combinations, the pairings among them were essentially unique for each trial. The monkeys were trained to press the centre panel 5-10 times when it was illuminated with one of the slides, and they were rewarded with fruit juice for doing so. The centre panel was then extinguished at the same instant that the lateral panels were illuminated. The animals readily switched to pressing that panel on which was projected the same object as had first appeared on the centre panel, and they were again rewarded. From that point it was relatively sim-

ple to teach the monkeys to perform in the same fashion when there was a delay of
a few seconds to 3 min (Overman and Doty, 1977) between the extinction of the
pressed centre panel and the appearance of stimuli on the lateral panels, one of
which, the 'correct' one, matched that previously seen at the centre.

Tetanisation (0.6 mA, 0.2 ms pulses, 50 Hz for 4 s) was applied through 'bipolar'
platinum–iridium electrodes permanently implanted at 45 loci which have now been
identified histologically. Each locus was tested with tetanisation 25–35 times in the
'sample' period (centre panel illuminated), the 'delay' period and the 'match' period
(lateral panels illuminated). These test trials were given in random order and interspersed among 2000 control trials in each monkey. With the 'trial unique' pairs of
stimuli and only a 5 s delay the monkeys' performance was stable and accurate, 94%
correct for the control trials. Reduction of performance to chance levels, as occurred for tetanisation at a number of loci, thus represents a very substantial effect.

Tetanisation through three sets of electrodes in the otherwise intact AC, either
at the midline or in its lateral projection, consistently reduced performance to
chance levels when applied either during the sample or match period, but had little
or no effect if applied during the delay period. Two other pairs of electrodes in
midline AC were without effect, yet thereby provided important controls for the
possibility that the effects usually cbserved might arise from unintentional stimulation of septum or fornix. One of the ineffective electrodes was well placed in mid
AC, but the commissure had undergone degeneration consequent to severance by
a haemorrhagic electrode track 5 mm lateral to the midline. The other ineffective
electrode pair just barely penetrated the posterior 100 μm of the midline AC.

It might, of course, be considered trivial that the monkeys fail to respond accurately when the AC is tetanised, since they actually do not respond to the stimuli
at all during the tetanisation, i.e. they do not press the centre sample panel; and
they respond in the match period within an average of about 1.5 s after the tetanisation ceases. However, ample control for this unresponsiveness *per se* is provided
by the data for 10 other loci, several of them in caudate nucleus or putamen, where
tetanisation also eliminated responses during the sample period and the first 4 s of
the match period. Despite this, accuracy of response by the latter monkeys in most
instances did not differ from that in the absence of tetanisation.

Tetanisation in the hippocampus and its immediate vicinity (e.g. fusiform gyrus),
on the other hand, in three of six cases reduced the accuracy of responding to chance
levels regardless of when it was applied, i.e. in sample, delay or match period. There
were, however, some puzzling exceptions, e.g. electrodes in cornu Ammonis which
produced no effect in the sample period (two cases) or in the match period (a third
case), while reducing performance to chance levels when applied in the other periods.
The monkeys usually continued to respond during tetanisation of the hippocampus,
even though electrophysiological records often suggested that the intensity of tetanisation employed would induce local after-discharges. It is, of course, possible that
the vagaries noted in the production of amnestic effects from tetanisation of seemingly similar loci in cornu Ammonis depended upon whether or not after-discharges
were produced, and electrical recording was not performed during the behavioural

testing. However, with the deliberate production of hippocampal after-discharges, Chow (1961) failed to find disruption of learning in macaques; and Ommaya and Fedio (1972), with a paradigm similar to ours, found no disruption of memory from presumed hippocampal stimulation in man.

In our experiments, tetanisation in the basal ganglia also commonly evoked electrical after-discharges at a number of the tetanised loci without evidence of mnemonic disturbance. In no case did tetanisation of the AC yield either behavioural or electrophysiological evidence of after-discharge. This is particularly clear in the latency of the response, which did not differ from that on control trials if measured from the moment of cessation of AC tetanisation. With hippocampal stimulation, on the other hand, it commonly took 4–8 s after the cessation before a response was made.

Given the widely held belief that the hippocampus plays a critical role in mnemonic processes, a belief perhaps most substantially founded in the observations of Penfield and Mathieson (1974), the idiosyncrasies in the disturbance of these processes by intrusive, electrical stimulation of the hippocampus (see Kesner and Wilburn, 1974; and Gustafson et al., 1975, for review) are puzzling. As noted, Chow (1961) as well as Ommaya and Fedio (1972) have clearly negative results, while the disturbance noted by Mordvinov (1976) in macaques with a delayed spatial choice was minimal. Data from the rat (Livesey and Meyer, 1975; Shinkman and Kaufman, 1972), do provide evidence for disruption of learning, but not for all individuals, nor for other problems (Gustafson et al., 1975). Thus, in many respects our experiments provide the most robust evidence to date along these lines to implicate the hippocampus in mnemonic events. We are, however, cautious in this regard because of our clear failures to produce disruption of performance from certain hippocampal loci, and because of the possibility that electrical after-discharge may be required for the effect.

Although stimulation of the caudate nucleus in man can produce mnemonic disturbances (Wood et al., 1977), this is not a consistent finding. Of five loci in caudate nucleus and putamen in our study there was only one instance where correctness of performance differed from control levels: 76% correct for stimulation in the delay period. We thus conclude that this unilateral stimulation has negligible mnemonic effect even though it produces motoric arrest as well as localised after-discharge.

It is also of interest that high rates of self-stimulation could be obtained for the two points in the putamen. However, for the experiment as a whole no correlation was apparent between the motivational effects obtained by stimulation at various loci and whether or not the tetanisation there altered the correctness of performance.

The results with tetanisation of the AC are fully concordant with expectations derived from the several studies showing disruption in performance or learning consequent to electrical stimulation of the inferior temporal area in macaques (Chow, 1961; Kovner and Stamm, 1972; Levine et al., 1970). Zeki (1973) demonstrated that the AC projects into the rostral portion of this area and into the parahippocampal gyrus. We have confirmed this by placing a small tube, loaded with horseradish peroxidase, between the cut ends of the AC for 36 h and then identifying the cells of origin by the procedure of LaVail *et al.* (1973). They are almost exclusively pyramidal cells in layer III, constituting a dispersed population in sharply definable areas of rostral temporal cortex. Their seeming sparseness will make them difficult to encounter with microelectrodes; but the data in hand suggest, *prima facie*, that they are somehow intimately concerned with mnemonic events.

It must, of course, be asked whether the particular effectiveness of the AC tetanisation may be attributable merely to the fact that it engages the temporal areas bilaterally, as compared with the unilaterality of effect produced by stimuli applied elsewhere in this and the study by Kovner and Stamm (1972). This may, indeed, account for its ability to be effective in the apparent absence of elicited after-discharge (as contrasted to the procedure of Chow, 1961; Levine *et al.*, 1970; and, probably, Kovner and Stamm,.1972). However, bilaterality, while probably essential, is not sufficient. Tetanisation at four loci in the splenium of the corpus callosum, which should have a bilaterality of effect equal to that of the AC, had no effect on accuracy of response, even though at two of these points additional engagement of the hippocampal commissure was undoubtedly present.

We hypothesise, therefore, that the system converging in the AC forms an essential link in mnemonic processing. When the AC system is momentarily occupied by the strong but meaningless activity engendered by tetanisation, neither storage nor retrieval are possible. Thus, the sample is not registered, and the match is made before the system has fully recovered its precision. Furthermore, during the tetanisation the animal cannot even recognise the significance of the stimuli presented and thus simply ignores them (Doty and Overman, 1977). Recovery from tetanisation is quick, however; being unimpeded by after-discharge and, as noted even with fully developed electroconvulsive seizures (Kesner *et al.,* 1970), there is no erasure of previously recorded events. Thus, tetanisation during the delay period does not delete the trace formed by the sample, and the system has cleared by the time the match is made.

It remains to be seen whether the system identified here is congruent with that which Horel and Misantone (1976) have interrupted surgically to produce severe deficiencies in visual learning; and whether in turn these systems rather than the hippocampus provide the mnemonic substrate which is so dramatically missing in the human surgical case, 'H.M.' (Milner *et al.,* 1968).

SUMMARY

(1) Macaques deprived of optic tract in one hemisphere and the amygdala in the other register normal visual fear of man so long as the splenium of the corpus callosum is intact, but fail to do so after its transection. Thus, extremes of hemispheric specialisation can be produced surgically, and their special effectiveness can be integrated via callosal mechanisms.

(2) Data are presented to support the hypothesis that, while the corpus callosum, as above, may provide access to information in one hemisphere for integration with that in the other, it also acts to limit the development of memory traces to the hemisphere originating the pertinent activity. In other words, the callosal system provides access to unilateral engrams and, for cortically initiated activity, also produces them.

(3) The anterior commissure, on the other hand, is capable of providing information from one hemisphere to produce an engram in the other. Its intimate relation with mnemonic processes is suggested by the inability of macaques to learn or to perform a learned act while the commissure is being tetanised. As identified by horseradish peroxidase, the pyramidal neurons which project across the anterior commissure are scattered in layer III of clearly defined areas of the rostral, inferior temporal area. There is no evidence that electrical after-discharge is associated with this disruption of performance or learning and, indeed, the tetanisation has minimal or no effect when applied during the delay period in a delayed match to sample. In this regard it differs from tetanisation in the hippocampus, which is inconsistent from one locus to another in its disruptive effect, and which commonly produces after-discharge.

ACKNOWLEDGEMENTS

This work was supported by a grant (NS03606) from the National Institute of Neurological and Communication Disorders and Stroke, National Institute of Health.

We are greatly indebted to Dr John R. Bartlett for his patient assistance with the many electronic problems encountered in this study, and for his perceptive contributions in discussions of the interpretation of our observations.

REFERENCES

Berlucchi, G., Brizzolara, D., Marzi, C. A., Rizzolatti, G. and Umiltà, C. (1974). Can lateral asymmetries in attention explain interfield differences in visual perception? *Cortex,* **10**, 177-85

Black, P. and Myers, R. E. (1964). Visual function of the forebrain commissures in the chimpanzee. *Science,* **146**, 799-800

Burešová, O. and Bureš, J. (1973). Mechanisms of interhemispheric transfer of visual information in rats. *Acta Neurobiol. Exp., Warsaw,* **33**, 673-88

Chow, K. L. (1961). Effect of local electrographic after-discharges on visual learning and retention in monkey. *J. Neurophysiol.,* **24**, 391-400

Dewson, J. H., III. (1977). Preliminary evidence of hemispheric asymmetry of auditory function in monkeys. In *Lateralization in the Nervous System* (S. Harnad, R. W. Doty, L. Goldstein, J. Jaynes, and G. Krauthamer, eds.), Academic Press, New York, pp. 63-71

Doty, R. W. and Negrão (1973). Forebrain commissures and vision. In *Handbook of Sensory Physiology,* vol. VII(3B), (R. Jung, ed.), Springer-Verlag, Berlin, pp. 543–82

Doty, R. W. and Overman, W. H., Jr. (1977). Mnemonic role of forebrain commissures in macaques. In *Lateralization in the Nervous System* (S. Harnad, R. W. Doty, L. Goldstein, J. Jaynes and G. Krauthamer, eds.), Academic Press, New York, pp. 75–88

Doty, R. W., Negrão, N. and Yamaga, K. (1973). The unilateral engram. *Acta Neurobiol. Exp., Warsaw,* **33**, 711–28

Downer, J. L. deC. (1961). Changes in visual gnostic functions and emotional behavior following unilateral temporal pole damage in the 'split-brain' monkey. *Nature (Lond.),* **191**, 50–51

Downer, J. L. deC. (1962). Interhemispheric integration in the visual system. In *Interhemispheric Relations and Cerebral Dominance* (V. B. Mountcastle, ed.), Johns Hopkins University Press, Baltimore, pp. 87–100

Fedio, P. and van Buren, J. M. (1975). Memory and perceptual deficits during electrical stimulation in the left and right thalamus and parietal subcortex. *Brain Lang.,* **2**, 78–100

Gazzaniga, M. S. (1966). Interhemispheric communication of visual learning. *Neuropsychologia,* **4**, 183–89

Gross, C. G. and Mishkin, M. (1977). The neural basis of stimulus equivalence across retinal translation. In *Lateralization in the Nervous System* (S. Harnad *et al.,* eds.), Academic Press, New York. pp. 109–21

Gustafson, J. W., Lidsky, T. I. and Schwartzbaum, J. S. (1975). Effects of hippocampal stimulation on acquisition, extinction and generalization of conditioned suppression in the rat. *J. comp. physiol. Psychol.,* **89**, 1136–48

Hamilton, C. R. (1977). Investigations of perceptual and mnemonic lateralization in monkeys. In *Lateralization in the Nervous System* (S. Harnad *et al.,* eds.), Academic Press, New York, pp. 45–62

Horel, J. A. and Misantone, L. J. (1976). Visual discrimination impaired by cutting temporal lobe connections. *Science,* **193**, 336–38

Kaas, J., Axelrod, S. and Diamond, I. T. (1967). An ablation study of the auditory cortex in the cat using binaural tonal patterns. *J. Neurophysiol.,* **30**, 710–24

Kesner, R. P. and Wilburn, Margaret W. (1974). A review of electrical stimulation of the brain in context of learning and retention. *Behav. Biol.,* **10**, 259–93

Kesner, R. P., McDonough, J. H., Jr. and Doty, R. W. (1970). Diminished amnestic effect of a second electroconvulsive seizure. *Expl Neurol.,* **27**, 527–33

Kovner, R. and Stamm, J. S. (1972). Disruption of short-term visual memory by electrical stimulation of inferotemporal cortex in the monkey. *J. comp. physiol. Psychol.,* **81**, 163–72

Kuypers, H. G. J. M., Szwarcbart, Maria K., Mishkin, M. and Rosvold, H. E. (1965). Occipitotemporal corticocortical connections in the rhesus monkey. *Expl Neurol.,* **11**, 245–62

LaVail, J. H., Winston, K. R. and Tish, A. (1973). A method based on retrograde intraaxonal transport of protein for identification of cell bodies of axons terminating within the CNS. *Brain Res.,* **58**, 470–77

Levine, M. S., Goldrich, S. G., Pond, F. J. Livesey, P. and Schwartzbaum, J. S. (1970). Retrograde amnestic effects of inferotemporal and amygdaloid seizures upon conditioned suppression of lever-pressing in monkeys. *Neuropsychologia*, **8**, 431–42

Livesey, P. J. and Meyer, P. (1975). Functional differentiation in the dorsal hippocampus with local electrical stimulation during learning by rats. *Neuropsychologia*, **13**, 431–38

Milner, Brenda (1974). Hemispheric specialization: scope and limits. In *The Neurosciences, Third Study Program* (F. O. Schmitt and F. G. Worden, Ed.), M.I.T. Press, Cambridge, Mass., pp. 75–89

Milner, Brenda, Corkin, Suzanne and Teuber, H.-L. (1968). Further analysis of the hippocampal amnesic syndrome: 14-year follow-up study of H. M. *Neuropsychologia*, **5**, 215–34

Mordvinov, E. F. (1976). Influence of electrical stimulation of premotor cortex and hippocampus on delayed choice in macaques. *Zhurnal visschei nervnoi deyatel' nosti*, **26**, 30–35 (Russian)

Negrão, N. and Doty, R. W. (1969). Laterality of engram in macaques trained to respond to local electrical excitation of area striata. *Fedn Proc.*, **28**, 647

Noble, J. (1968). Paradoxical interocular transfer of mirror-image discriminations in the optic chiasm sectioned monkey. *Brain Res.*, **10**, 127–51

Nottebohm, F. (1977). Asymmetries in neural control of vocalization in the canary. In *Lateralization in the Nervous System* (S. Harnad *et al.*, eds.), Academic Press, New York, pp. 23–44

Ommaya, A. K. and Fedio, P. (1972). The contribution of cingulum and hippocampal structures to memory mechanisms in man. *Confin. Neurol.*, **34**, 398–411 *Abstr Soc. Neurosci.*, **3**

Overman, W. H. Jr. and Doty, R. W. (1977). Mnemonic disturbance in macaques from stimulation of anterior commissure versus limbic system or basal ganglia. *Abstr Soc. Neurosci.*, **3**

Penfield, W. and Mathieson, G. (1974). Autopsy findings and comments on the role of hippocampus in experiential recall. *Archs Neurol.*, **31**, 145–54

Shinkman, P. G. and Kaufman K. P. (1972). Posttrial hippocampal stimulation and CER acquisition in the rat. *J. comp. physiol. Psychol.*, **80**, 283–92

Sperry, R. W. (1974). Lateral specialization in the surgically separated hemispheres. In *The Neurosciences, Third Study Program* (F. O. Schmitt and F. G. Worden, eds.), M.I.T. Press, Cambridge, Mass., pp. 5–19

Sullivan, M. V. and Hamilton, C. R. (1973). Memory establishment via the anterior commissure of monkeys. *Physiol. Behav.*, **11**, 873–79

Wood, J. H., Lake, C. R. Ziegler, M. G. and van Buren, J. M. (1977). Neurophysiological and neurochemical alterations during electrical stimulation of human caudate nucleus. *J. Neurosurg.*, **46**, 361–68

Zeki, S. M. (1973). Comparison of the cortical degeneration in the visual regions of the temporal lobe of the monkey following section of the anterior commissure and the splenium. *J. comp. Neurol.*, **148**, 167–76

27
INTERHEMISPHERIC TRANSFER OF VISUAL INFORMATION VIA THE CORPUS CALLOSUM AND ANTERIOR COMMISSURE IN THE MONKEY

S. R. BUTLER

INTRODUCTION

The experiments of Myers and Sperry, more than 20 years ago (Myers, 1956; Myers and Sperry, 1953), established the classical procedure for demonstrating interhemispheric transfer of visual information. First, the optic chiasma is transected in the midline; as a result each hemisphere receives information only from the hemianopic field of the ipsilateral eye. The animal is then trained monocularly on a visual discrimination and tested for transfer with the second eye. It is found that if the commissures are intact, learning is usually more rapid with the second eye than the first, provided reward contingencies are also held constant. This is taken to indicate that there is an interhemispheric transfer of information describing both the salient features of the cues and their associations with reward. Much of this chapter will be concerned with evidence for transfer obtained with the use of this method, the essential feature of which is *successive* monocular training. Although the method has been criticised by Bremer (1972) as unrepresentative of the demands made upon the commissures in intact animals, we shall later see that evidence of interhemispheric interactions obtained under conditions of *simultaneous* ocular training may be misleading about the capacity of subcortical pathways to handle structured perceptual information.

To return for the moment to the early work of Myers and Sperry on the cat, it was found that transfer of visual pattern information depended on pathways through the posterior corpus callosum (Myers, 1959). These permitted the animal both to tap information stored in one hemisphere and to establish bilateral memories for simple tasks (Myers, 1957). But the callosum is not the only commissure to exchange visual information in higher mammals. The contribution of other pathways depends upon the species, the conditions of motivation, the type of visual information and whether the commissurotomy is performed in stages or in a single operation. A few examples will suffice:

(1) Species differences

With successive ocular training for food reward, transfer of visual pattern is abolished by section of the corpus callosum alone in the cat (Myers, 1957) but not in the
monkey (Downer, 1959; Noble, 1968; Sullivan and Hamilton, 1973a, 1973b) or
chimpanzee (Black and Myers, 1964). In man, section of the corpus callosum alone
is sufficient to produce profound impairment on pattern transfer (Gazzaniga and
Friedman, 1973), although a quantitative assessment of the efficiency of the remaining pathways does not appear to have been made.

(2) Motivation

After callosectomy, cats trained for food reward show no transfer for visual pattern
but do so when trained in a shock avoidance situation (Sechzer, 1964). It is usually
supposed that the anterior commissure, intact in these animals, was capable of mediating the transfer under the more urgent motivation of shock but the experiment to
test this view does not appear to have been performed.

(3) Type of visual information

Section of the callosum abolishes pattern transfer in the cat but brightness transfer
survives (Meikle and Sechzer, 1960). Parallels are sometimes drawn with the monkey,
in whom section of all the forebrain commissures abolishes pattern transfer (Sperry,
1958; Downer, 1959) but perhaps not colour or brightness transfer (Trevarthen,
1962). However, the transfer observed by Trevarthen appears to have emerged under
conditions of simultaneous rather than successive ocular training, a point to which
further consideration will be given later. Other studies have failed to reveal transfer
of brightness and colour after hemispheric disconnection in the monkey (Hamilton
and Gazzaniga, 1964; Yamaguchi and Myers, 1972).

(4) Serial Sections

In an unusual study (Tieman and Hamilton, 1974a) the interhemispheric transfer of
pattern information survived complete forebrain commissurotomy provided the surgery was performed in certain stages, whereafter it was abolished only if the disconnection extended to brain stem levels. The resistance of the forebrain to serial damage has many precedents in the literature of cortical ablation but a curious aspect of
this finding is that one animal in whom transfer was abolished by posterior callosal
section appears to have regained it when the commissurotomy was completed.

   In recent years studies of interhemispheric transfer of visual information in
higher mammals using the method of successive monocular training for food reward
have concentrated on the monkey. A considerable body of evidence has accumulated
concerning the capacity of both the corpus callosum and extracallosal pathways to

support the transfer of different types of visual information and a measure of agreement has emerged.

Transection of both the corpus callosum and the anterior commissure abolishes interhemispheric transfer for pattern (Butler, 1968; Downer, 1958, 1959; Gazzaniga, 1966; Sperry, 1958; Yamaguchi and Myers, 1972), colour (Downer, 1958, 1959; Hamilton and Gazzaniga, 1964; Hara and Myers cited by Myers, 1972; Sperry, 1958), brightness (Hamilton and Gazzaniga, 1964; Hara and Myers cited by Myers, 1972, Sperry, 1958; Yamaguchi and Myers, 1972), size and three-dimensional perception (Sperry, 1958) as well as for the direction of movement (Hamilton and Lund, 1970) and the occurrence of phosphenes elicited by cortical stimulation (Doty and Negrão, 1973).

As might be inferred on anatomical grounds, the part of the callosum important for visual transfer appears to be the splenium (Gazzaniga, 1966). Moreover, Hamilton and his co-workers have found evidence that different parts of the splenium are not equipotential in their capacity to pass visual information. While the posterior splenium will mediate interocular transfer for pattern tested by successive monocular training, the anterior splenium will not (Hamilton and Brody, 1973). However, the anterior splenium does appear to permit the comparison of inputs presented simultaneously to opposite hemispheres (Hamilton and Brody, 1973; Tieman and Hamilton, 1974b).

In the absence of the callosum, transfer of visual information survives if the anterior commissure is intact (Downer, 1959; Noble, 1968; Sullivan and Hamilton, 1973a, 1973b). Sullivan and Hamilton (1973a, 1973b) expressed the view that splenium and anterior commissure were equally proficient both in tapping information acquired by the trained hemisphere and in establishing bilateral memories. Gazzaniga's findings (Gazzaniga, 1966), on the other hand, indicate that pattern transfer depends chiefly on the splenium, in agreement with findings in the chimpanzee (Black and Myers, 1964, 1968).

One might expect considerable differences in the type of information conducted by the two pathways. The splenium connects large areas of occipital, parietal and inferior temporal cortex, whereas the anterior commissure provides the major link between anterior inferior temporal cortices (Pandya, 1975; Zeki, 1973). The splenium includes fibres which define the retinotopic location of visual stimulation within a degree or so, at least for the vertical meridian of the visual field (Berlucchi et al., 1968). Progressing through the visual association areas, receptive fields appear to lose retinotopic precision. Although recordings do not appear to have been made from cells in anterior inferior temporal cortex itself, cells in posterior inferior temporal cortex already have very extensive receptive fields (Gross et al., 1972; Rocha-Miranda et al., 1975). Therefore, it seems likely that the anterior commissure is ill-equipped to convey retinotopically organised information. To test this view, monkeys with selective section of the commissures were tested for transfer of colour, shape, size and orientation discrimination. The distinction between red and green does not depend upon a retinotopic organisation of stimulus features and should therefore transfer effectively through the anterior commissure. On the other hand, distinction between two squares which differ only in the angle they subtend, or between two patterns which differ only in their orientation, clearly depends on reference to the retinotopic map. Without training for learning set, an animal might therefore be expected to distinguish such cues on a relatively primitive sensory basis rather than abstract high order concepts of size and orientation. Transfer of the salient retinotopic features would thus be expected to be poor for size and orientation. Shape discrimination might lend itself more readily to conceptual abstraction and so become independent of the retinotopic map, although it could equally well be solved in terms of more elementary stimulus features. Nevertheless transfer of this modality should be no better than for colour and no worse than for size and orientation.

METHODS

Ten immature rhesus monkeys served as subjects in this experiment. Midline section of the optic chiasma and total or partial forebrain commissurotomy were carried out in separate operations before training began. The chiasma was approached by the transbuccal route; commissurotomy was performed through a right parietofrontal craniotomy. Both operations were conducted under Nembutal anaesthesia. The animals were divided into four surgical groups: (a) splenium spared, animals 2183 and 2199; (b) splenium sectioned, animals 2236 and 2238; (c) corpus callosum sectioned, animals 2188, 2196 and 2191; (d) total forebrain commissurotomy in which both the corpus callosum and anterior commissure were sectioned, animals 2176, 2201 and 2180.

Histological Verification of Surgery

At the completion of the experiment the animals were killed with Nembutal and the brains perfused through the carotid arteries with saline and formol saline. As each brain was removed its optic chiasma was left in the sella turcica. The brains were embedded in celloidin, sectioned at 100 μm and stained in Luxol Fast Blue. The optic chiasma was removed with the supporting sella turcica from the floor of the cranial cavity and the tissue decalcified, embedded in paraffin wax, cut at 7 μm and stained in Luxol Fast Blue. In seven animals the chiasma was found on histological examination to be completely transected. In three cases, 2238, 2196 and 2191, the chiasma was found at post mortem to be completely separated in the midline and the tissue was not processed.

Serial sections through the forebrain revealed all the intended sections to be complete, except in the case of the anterior commissure of 2176 which was damaged in histology and could not be examined. However, it was clearly seen through the stereomicroscope to be sectioned at the time of surgery. In 2183 and 2199, in whom the surgery was designed to spare the splenium, the posterior 33% and 34% of the length of the callosum remained intact, respectively. In 2236 and 2238, in whom the surgery was intended to cut the splenium, the posterior 48% and 41% of the length of the callosum was sectioned, respectively.

Training

The monkeys were trained in an automated test apparatus in which stimuli were rear-projected on to screens 7 cm × 9 cm, set 3.5 cm apart with food wells behind and at the base of the response panels. The animals had to press the panel displaying the positive cue to get at the food-well, into which a banana flavoured whole-diet pellet was delivered automatically. The cues switched between the panels on a Gellerman schedule. Monocular training was effected with a black macrocorneal contact occluder inserted under Amethocaine local anaesthesia each day just prior to training. The animals were not physically restrained during testing but sat in a transport cage from which they were free to reach out to press the response panels. They then viewed the cues at a distance of approximately 25 cm. They were trained on a sequence of five tasks, 40 trials a day, and fed after training on a restricted diet of B41 diet pellets and fruit. The five tasks in order of training were:

(1) Black–white discrimination

The panel comprising the positive cue was illuminated with a 2 in × 2 in square and the animals trained binocularly to a criterion of 90 correct responses in 100 consecutive trials, the criterion used throughout this study. The contact occluder was then introduced and the animals retrained with each eye successively.

This served both to familiarise the animal with the occluder and with working under conditions of hemianopic vision, and to test for any major field defects.

(2) Cross–circle shape discrimination

Images of a cross and circle, matched for surface brightness, were projected on to the panels and choice of the cross rewarded. No binocular training was given. Animals were trained to criterion with each eye successively.

(3) Small and large square discrimination

Images of squares 25 mm × 25 mm and 50 mm × 50 mm matched for total luminous flux were projected on to the panels and choice of the smaller square was rewarded. The animal was again trained monocularly with each eye successively.

(4) Red and green discrimination

The panels were flooded with red and green light, choice of the red panel being rewarded. The panels were matched for subjectively equal brightness to a human eye.

Table 27.1.
Trials to criterion for each animal on each task

task	eye used	Ant. 2/3 corpus callosum + ant. commissure		Splenium only		Corpus callosum			Corpus callosum and anterior commissure		
		2183	2199	2236	2238	2186	2196	2191	2176	2201	2180
white square	Both	261	44	1597	154	273	92	44	105	495	7
vs.	1st	0	0	342	142	148	0	0	378	157	30
black square	2nd	0	29	520	79	142	0	0	0	0	0
cross	1st	94	124	518	258	40	571	146	96	3	121
vs.	2nd	30	0	447	24	52	138	13	442	4	57
circle											
small square	1st	307	0	261	25	216	74	165	552	16	0
vs.	2nd	0	0	547	13	455	24	0	119	157	6
large square											
red panel	1st	21	38	73	78	226	28	50	129	74	12
vs.	2nd	0	0	0	0	90	0	0	46	73	26
green panel											
vertical bars	1st	107	96	174	204	198	93	65	171	202	74
vs.	2nd	0	0	20	40	93	121	189	146	76	348
horizontal bars											

No attempt was made in this study independently to vary the intensity of the colour to prevent animals from attempting to solve the problem in terms of brightness. However, after they had been trained to criterion with each eye separately, two animals were tested with the brightness ratio perturbed and showed immediate retention, indicating choice was based upon colour and not on brightness.

(5) Pattern orientation discrimination

Identical patterns of five bars arranged to form a block 50 mm × 50 mm were displayed on the panels and the animals trained to select horizontal bars and reject vertical ones. Once more the two eyes were trained to criterion successively.

RESULTS

Table 27.1 shows the number of trials taken to reach criterion by each animal on each task. Some monkeys who found the initial binocular white–black discrimination difficult needed further training with one or both eyes when tested monocularly but there is little indication of visual field defect arising from the section of the chiasma. Five monkeys, in addition to the 10 described here, began the study but their performance is not reported since they showed evidence of field defects after surgery. Monkey 2176 required a large number of trials to relearn the white–black discrimination with the first eye but this probably indicates that the other hemisphere dominated the initial learning. It showed immediate retention when the second eye was tested and there is no indication of continuing difficulty with the first eye in the animal's performance on the next task.

The raw scores in the rest of table 27.1 reveal that animals with the splenium intact quickly relearned all tasks with the second eye. High levels of transfer also occurred in the absence of the splenium in animals with the anterior commissure intact but only on the colour discrimination.

Total saving scores are plotted in figure 27.1 for each animal on each task. They are calculated from the formula:

$$\frac{\text{Trials to criterion with first eye} - \text{Trials to criterion with second eye}}{\text{Trials to criterion with first eye} + \text{Trials to criterion with second eye}}$$

A total saving score of 1 thus means perfect transfer when tested with the second eye. A score of 0 means that the animal required the same number of trials to reach criterion with both eyes, i.e. no transfer. Table 27.2 summarises the total saving scores, averaging them by groups. The saving scores reflect the high savings on all tasks by animals with the splenium intact and on the colour discrimination by animals with the anterior commissure intact. Animals with only the splenium sectioned and those with the whole corpus callosum transected have been averaged together in table 27.2, since there is no indication in other studies that the anterior

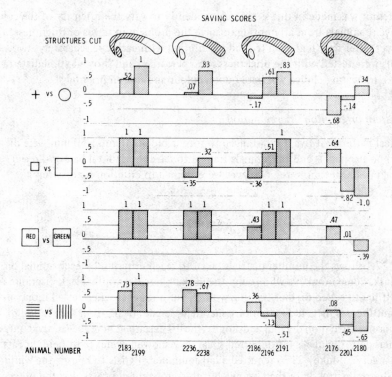

Figure 27.1.   Total savings scores for each animal on each task. The method of computing these scores from trials to criterion is described in the text

Table 27.2.
Mean of total saving scores by groups

Operation group	Splenium spared	Ant. commissure intact with or without ant. callosum	Ant. commissure and corpus callosum transected
Discrimination			
shape	0.76	0.44	−0.15
size	1.00	0.22	−0.39
colour	1.00	0.89	0.02
orientation	0.87	0.24	−0.34

callosum contributes to simple discrimination transfer. Partial transfer occurs for shape, size and orientation in animals with the anterior commissure intact, although reference to figure 27.1 reveals the performance of individual animals to be some-what variable. Animals with both the corpus callosum and anterior commissure transected do not, as a group, show positive transfer on any task. Indeed there is actually evidence of retarded learning by the second hemisphere on the shape, size and orientation tasks.

An alternative index of interhemispheric transfer is provided by the level of performance when the animal is first tested with the second eye. The chief disadvantage with this method is that on easy tasks sufficient learning may occur within the first day's testing to raise the score above chance level without the contribution of interhemispheric transfer. One way round this is to compare the animal's level of performance of the first day, using the first eye, with that on the first day, using the second eye, according to the following formula:

$$\frac{\% \text{ errors first day, first eye} - \% \text{ errors first day, second eye}}{\% \text{ errors first day, first eye} + \% \text{ errors first day, second eye}}$$

Now a score of 1 indicates perfect retention on the first day using the second eye. A score of 0 indicates that the animal performed no better on the first day with the second eye than it did on the first day with the first eye.

Table 27.3.
Mean of initial saving scores by groups

Operation group	Splenium spared	Ant. commissure intact with or without ant. callosum	Ant. commissure and corpus callosum transected
Discrimination			
shape	0.63	0.23	0.07
size	0.84	0.14	0.26 (0.09*)
colour	0.70	0.60	−0.04
orientation	0.74	0.37	−0.09

*Excluding the aberrant performance of 2176 on the first day with the second eye.

Using this index it is again seen (see table 27.3) that animals with the splenium intact show high levels of transfer on all tasks, as do animals with the anterior commissure intact on the colour discrimination. Those with the anterior commissure intact show intermediate levels of transfer on shape, size and orientation, while monkeys with total forebrain commissurotomy show virtually no evidence of transfer on any task. The figure of 0.26 for this last group on the size discrimination is misleading and due to an inordinately high level of performance by 2176 on the first day of testing with the second eye which was not maintained on subsequent days. The indices for the other animals with total forebrain commissurotomy on this task are 0.08 and 0.10 for 2201 and 2180, respectively. Thus, but for the odd performance of 2176 on the first day of transfer on one task, the group showed no evidence of transfer on any task.

DISCUSSION

The present findings indicate that the splenium permits almost perfect transfer of all the dimensions of visual perception tested in the experiment. The anterior commissure is equally effective for the transfer of colour but affords only partial transfer for shape, size and pattern orientation.

These results support and extend the few quantitative reports of effects of partial commissurotomy on interhemispheric transfer of monocularly learned visual discriminations in primates. Previous studies have been confined to work on shape discrimination. The superiority of the splenium for shape transfer may be inferred from the work of Gazzaniga (1966). Transfer was perfect in one animal with only the anterior callosum divided but poor or absent in two animals with the posterior callosum divided. Sullivan and Hamilton (1973a) provide a more detailed assessment of the effectiveness of the anterior commissure in callosum-sectioned monkeys. Four animals showed partial savings on several tests of shape transfer, with a mean savings score of 0.47.

In the present study shape transfer through this commissure varied considerably between animals, though the mean savings score of 0.44 resembles that found by Sullivan and Hamilton. It should be added that these authors offered an alternative and higher figure for savings after excluding an animal whose transfer was poor on this test but who later revealed behaviour signs of remaining fibres in the optic chiasma. Whichever figure is adopted a picture emerges of partial and variable transfer of shape through the anterior commissure. It was argued earlier that animals might solve the shape discrimination either in terms of conceptual abstraction of shapes or by attending to relatively simple features of their retinotopic projections. The variability in transfer on the shape task might reflect the use of different strategies by different animals. Only those who adopted the higher order strategy would handle information in a form sufficiently abstracted from the retinotopic map to permit its transfer through the anterior commissure.

Information about shape crossed the splenium with much greater facility than the anterior commissure. One animal showed perfect transfer while the other needed only a third as many trials to reach criterion with the second eye as with the first. There are few quantitative reports in the literature on primates with which to compare this result, although Black and Myers (1964) found shape to transfer more effectively through the splenium than the anterior commissure in the chimpanzee. The controls used by Sullivan and Hamilton had only the posterior 5 mm of the splenium intact and showed somewhat less efficient transfer than the animals in the present study. In the latter, the posterior 1 cm of the corpus callosum was left at surgery and this proved at post mortem to be the posterior third.

The difference between the splenium and the anterior commissure in their capacity to transfer size and orientation was even greater than it was for shape. Table 27.2 shows that the difference between the two pathways in terms of total savings was greater for size and orientation than for shape. It should perhaps be noted at this point that the 'size' discrimination might not have been treated as such by the monkeys. The squares were equated for total flux and thus could have been discriminated on the basis of surface brightness. Had the surface brightness been held constant, the animals could still have adopted a brightness strategy, this time on the basis of total flux. The variability in the level of transfer shown by different animals on this task may again reflect the adoption of different strategies since a brightness strategy, being indpendent of retinotopic stimulus features, might again facilitate transfer.

The prediction that the anterior commissure would transfer colour more efficiently than size or orientation is supported by both total and initial saving scores. The more proficient transfer of colour cannot be ascribed to the ease of this task. Though it was indeed the easiest, judged by trials to criterion with the first eye across all animals, the rank order of task difficulty does not fit the rank order for transfer by either measure of savings. The position of shape in the hierarchy of transfer proficiency is somewhat equivocal. It transfers much better than size or orientation judged by total saving scores but less well than orientation judged by initial saving scores. The best that can be said is that the outcome of the shape transfer test does not pose any problems for the present hypothesis by surpassing colour transfer or being worse than transfer for size. The present findings thus provide initial support for the idea that the anterior commissure is more proficient at handling information devoid of retinotopic specificity than raw stimulus features. The next stage must be to test whether the anterior commissure can handle conceptual abstractions more effectively than retinotopic features. As a means of assessing the level at which the inferotemporal cortex handles information, this method has the great advantage of not incurring the behavioural disorders which accompany ablation of this area of cortex. While these disorders are themselves of considerable interest in relation to visual learning their significance within the framework of visual information processing has proved difficult to interpret and an approach in terms of the level of abstraction at which information is handled might be enlightening.

On the orientation task, animals in whom the anterior commissure alone was intact showed little or no evidence of transfer. Those in whom the anterior callosum was additionally intact showed good transfer. This might be a chance partition of high saving scores between the groups and be no more than a manifestation of the variability in level of transfer seen in the shape and size tasks. Certainly the previous literature has suggested that the anterior callosum does not contribute to interhemispheric transfer of simple visual discriminations (Gazzaniga, 1966; Noble, 1973). It is conceivable, however, that some form of peripheral cross-cueing occurred in this task as a result of postural reactions to the orientation of the patterns with transfer for the significance of these postures via the anterior callosum.

Total forebrain commissurotomy abolished transfer on all tasks. The initial savings are uniformly close to zero, perturbed only by the performance of 2176 on the size discrimination. This animal's performance subsequently fell back but not to chance levels. It ultimately showed savings scores in trials to criterion. The possibility cannot be ruled out that this animal's anterior commissure was partially intact because it was not available for histological verification, although this should have shown up in other tasks and the section appeared complete at surgery. It is unlikely it succeeded where others failed by adopting a brightness strategy on the size problem. Studies cited in the introduction to this chapter appear to have ruled out the possibility that brightness transfer occurs under successive monocular testing. This animal aside, the chance-level scores on the first day of testing on all tasks are in accord with the many studies also cited earlier which point to the abolition of gnostic transfer for all dimensions of visual perception after complete forebrain disconnection.

However, total saving scores reveal that learning with the second eye was actually retarded in many animals. This was not due to surgical damage to the retracted right hemisphere since the eye trained first differed in different animals of the group. There is a precedent for such negative transfer (Gazzaniga, 1966), and it occurred sporadically among the animals studied by Yamaguchi and Myers (1972) and Sullivan and Hamilton (1973a). It is conceivable that in some animals, or under certain conditions of testing, the trained hemisphere may intervene and interfere in some way with learning by the second hemisphere.

Two possible mechanisms may be considered. If the hands are unrestrained the animal may continue to attempt to respond with the trained hand when tested with the second eye. This could account for the present findings, since there was no restraint on the use of hands. It would not account for the effect in the other studies since these were constrained to use of the contralateral eye–hand combination at all times. An alternative mechanism might operate through some non-specific interaction between the hemispheres surviving forebrain commissurotomy such as that proposed by Gavalas and Sperry (1969). If we consider evidence for interhemispheric interaction under conditions of bilateral visual input it will be seen that such a mechanism may exist.

Although investigations based upon successive monocular training lead uniformly to the view that total forebrain commissurotomy abolishes all dimensions of visual transfer, training with bilateral input reveals some form of interhemispheric interaction which survives hemispheric disconnection. Such interaction has been found effective in colour and brightness discriminations (Trevarthen, 1962) as well as size discriminations (Trevarthen, 1965). Hamilton and Brody (1973) found interhemispheric interactions on a matching to sample task after section of the posterior splenium even though the surgery prevented transfer of a two-choice visual discrimination on successive monocular training. Tieman and Hamilton (1974a) likewise found that section of the posterior splenium, while abolishing transfer on a go/no-go visual discrimination permitted interhemispheric comparison of cue location. Sperry and Green (1964), Gavalas and Sperry (1969) and Butler (1975) found that monkeys could compare the relative position of visual cues seen in the two halves of the visual field after total forebrain commissurotomy. These positive findings have in common that stimulus information was presented simultaneously to the two hemispheres. Indeed, there appears to be only one report that interhemispheric 'comparison' of visual stimuli is abolished by forebrain commissurotomy (Hamilton et al., 1968). Such tasks may be performed successfully with the aid of relatively simple binary signalling between the two hemispheres which might be mediated by the diencephalic or midbrain systems that survive forebrain commissurotomy (Trevarthen, 1968; Diamond and Hall, 1968). This would not require gnostic transfer of structured visual information. Such a mechanism of interaction might also be responsible for the retarded learning of the second hemisphere in the present study. In successive monocular testing, signals reaching the untrained hemisphere from the trained side would not be linked to immediately prevailing stimulus conditions since the trained hemisphere would not have access to structured information about the cues. The signals would thus contribute noise rather than relevant information and so impede rather than facilitate learning by the second hemisphere. The existence and operation of such a mechanism is only speculative as an explanation for the negative savings in the present study. It is however of wider importance. If visual transfer in the absence of forebrain commissures can be ascribed to the operation of elementary cross-cueing signals devoid of structured stimulus information, then conflicts with the classical view that gnostic transfer is mediated solely by corticocortical pathways are removed.

SUMMARY

Interhemispheric transfer of visual information was tested in 10 rhesus monkeys after total or partial forebrain commissurotomy. The animals were trained with each eye successively on shape, size, colour and orientation discrimination.

(1) A high level of interhemispheric transfer occurred on all tasks so long as the splenium was intact.

(2) The anterior commissure permitted a high level of transfer for colour but partial and variable transfer on the remaining tasks. The facility with which transfer occurs via this pathway is not related to task difficulty but may be related to the limited ability of the cells of origin of the anterior commissure (in the inferotemporal cortex) to deal in retinotopic information.

(3) Total forebrain commissurotomy abolished interhemispheric transfer for all the dimensions of visual perception tested in the experiment. There was some evidence that learning by the second eye was retarded. It is suggested that this was due to non-specific interhemispheric interaction via diencephalic or midbrain pathways. It is further suggested that such interaction may be the mechanism responsible for successful interhemispheric 'transfer' under conditions of bilateral hemispheric input.

ACKNOWLEDGEMENTS

This work was supported by the Mental Health Research Fund. The author is grateful to Mrs Andy Peplow, Miss Lorraine Statton and Mr Mike Chinn for their assistance, and to Mrs Jackie Lidstone for typing this manuscript.

REFERENCES

Berlucchi, G., Gazzaniga, M. S. and Rizzolatti, G. (1967). Microelectrode analysis of transfer of visual information by the corpus callosum of cat. *Arch. Ital. Biol.,* **105**, 583–96

Black, P. and Myers, R. E. (1964). Visual functions of the forebrain commissures in the chimpanzee. *Science,* **146**, 799–800

Black, P. and Myers, R. E. (1968). Brain stem mediation of visual perception in a higher primate. *Trans. Am. Neurol. Assoc.,* **93**, 191–93

Black, P. and Myers, R. E. (1969). Behavioural studies in the commissure sectioned chimpanzee. *Proc. 2nd Int. Congr. Primat. Atlanta Ga.,* **3**, 64–67

Bremer, F. (1972). Reflections on the physiological significance of the callosal commissure. In *Cerebral Interhemispheric Relations* (J. Cernacek and F. Podivinsky, eds.), Vydatelstvo Slovenskey Akademie Vied., Bratislava

Butler, C. R. (1968). A memory record for visual discrimination in both hemispheres in monkey when only one hemisphere has received direct visual informaion. *Brain Res.,* **10**, 152–67

Butler, S. R. (1975). The integration of left and right visual hemifields. *J. Physiol., Lond.,* **256**, 113–14P

Diamond, I. T. and Hall, W. C. (1969). Evolution of neocortex. *Science,* **164**, 251–62

Doty, R. W. and Negrão, N. (1973). Forebrain commissures and vision. In *Handbook of Sensory Physiology* vol. 7 (R. Jung, ed.), Springer-Verlag, Berlin

Downer, J. L. (1958). Role of corpus callosum in transfer training in *Maccaca Mulatta. Fedn Proc.,* **17**, 37

Downer, J. L. (1959). Interhemispheric integration in the visual system. In *Interhemispheric Relations and Cerebral Dominance* (V. B. Mountcastle, ed.), Johns Hopkins, Baltimore

Gavalas, R. J. and Sperry, R. W. (1969). Central integration of visual half fields in splitbrain monkeys. *Brain. Res.,* **15**, 97–106

Gazzaniga, M. S. (1966). Interhemispheric communication of visual learning. *Neuropsychologia,* **4**, 183–89

Gazzaniga, M. S. and Friedman, H. (1973). Observations on visual processes after posterior callosal section. *Neurology (Mineap.),* **23**, 1126–30

Gross, C. G., Rocha-Miranda, C. E. and Bender, D. B. (1972). Visual properties of neurons in inferotemporal cortex of the macaque. *J. Neurophysiol.,* **35**, 96–111

Hamilton, C. R. and Brody, B. A. (1973). Separation of visual functions within the corpus callosum of monkeys. *Brain. Res.,* **49**, 185–89

Hamilton, C. R. and Gazzaniga, M. S. (1964). Lateralisation of learning of colour and brightness following brain bisection. *Nature (Lond.),* **201**, 220

Hamilton, C. R. and Lund, J. S. (1970). Visual discrimination of movement: midbrain or forebrain? *Science,* **170**, 1428–30

Hamilton, C. R., Hillyard, S. A. and Sperry, R. W. (1968). Interhemispheric comparison of colour in splitbrain monkeys. *Expl. Neurol.,* **21**, 468–94

Meikle, T. H. and Sechzer, J. A. (1960). Interocular transfer of brightness discrimination in 'split-brain' cats. *Science,* **132**, 734–35

Myers, R. E. (1956). Function of corpus callosum in interocular transfer. *Brain.,* **79**, 358

Myers, R. E. (1957). Corpus callosum and interhemispheric communication: enduring memory effects. *Fedn Proc.*, **16**, 398

Myers, R. E. (1959). Localisation of function in the corpus callosum. *Archs Neurol.*, **1**, 74–77

Myers, R. E. (1972). The forebrain commissures and their functions. In *Cerebral Interhemispheric Relations* (J. Cernacek and F. Podivinsky, eds.), Vydatelstvo Slovenskey Akademie Vied., Bratislava

Myers, R. E. and Sperry, R. W. (1953). Interocular transfer of a visual form discrimination habit in cats after section of the optic chiasma and corpus callosum. *Anat. Rec.*, **115**, 351–52

Noble, J. (1968). Paradoxical interocular transfer of mirror image discriminations in the optic chiasma sectioned monkey. *Brain. Res.*, **10**, 127–151

Noble, J. (1973). Interocular transfer in the monkey: rostral corpus callosum mediates transfer of object learning set but not of single problem learning. *Brain Res.*, **50**, 147–62

Pandya, D. N. (1975). Interhemispheric connections in the primate. In *Les Syndromes de Disconnexion Calleuse chez l'Homme* (F. Michel and B. Schott, eds), Hôpital Neurologique, Lyon

Rocha-Miranda, C. E., Bender, D. B., Gross, C. G. and Mishkin, M. (1975). Visual activation of neurons in inferotemporal cortex depends on striate cortex and forebrain commissures. *J. Neurophysiol.*, **38**, 475–91

Sechzer, J. A. (1964). Successful interocular transfer of pattern discrimination in 'split-brain' cats with shock avoidance motivation. *J. comp. physiol Psychol.*, **58**, 76–83

Sperry, R. W. (1958). Corpus callosum and interhemispheric transfer in the monkey. *Anat. Rec.*, **131**, 297

Sperry, R. W. and Green, S. M. (1964). Corpus callosum and perceptual integration of visual half fields. *Anat. Rec.*, **148**, 339

Sullivan, M. V. and Hamilton, C. R. (1973a). Interocular transfer of reversal and nonreversal discrimination via the anterior commissure in monkeys. *Physiol. Behav.*, **10**, 355–59

Sullivan, M. V. and Hamilton, C. R. (1973b). Memory establishment via the anterior commissure in monkeys. *Physiol. Behav.*, **11**, 873–79

Tieman, S. B. and Hamilton, C. R. (1974a). Interocular transfer in splitbrain monkeys following serial disconnection. *Brain Res.*, **63**, 368–73

Tieman, S. B. and Hamilton, C. R. (1974b). Interhemispheric communication between extra-occipital visual areas in the monkey. *Brain Res.*, **67**, 279–87

Trevarthen, C. B. (1962). Double visual learning in splitbrain monkeys. *Science*, **136**, 258–59

Trevarthen, C. B. (1965). Functional interactions between the hemispheres in the splitbrain monkey. In *Functions of the Corpus Callosum* (G. Ettlinger, ed.), Churchill, London

Trevarthen, C. B. (1968). Two mechanisms of vision in primates. *Psychol. Forsch.*, **31**, 299–337

Yamaguchi, S. and Myers, R. E. (1972). Age effects on forebrain commissure section and interocular transfer. *Expl Brain Res.*, **15**, 225–33

Zeki, S. M. (1973). Comparison of the cortical degeneration in the visual region of the temporal lobe of the monkey following section of the anterior commissure and the splenium. *J. comp. Neurol.*, **148**, 167–75

28
MIRROR-IMAGE TRANSFER IN OPTIC CHIASM SECTIONED MONKEYS

BERYL STARR

INTRODUCTION

In terms of gross anatomy almost all animals are bilaterally symmetrical. Each animal can be divided into a left half and a right half, which are more or less identical except that they are mirror-images of each other. The central nervous system reflects this bilateral symmetry and the primate cerebral cortex has two 'mirror-image' hemispheres. One interesting line of enquiry is whether sensory systems are affected by the bilateral symmetry of the cortex, since information coded spatially appears to be laterally inverted on passing across the cerebral commissures from one hemisphere to the other.

An early study (Ettlinger and Elithorn, 1962) showed mirror-image reversal of tactual information crossing the corpus callosum. Monkeys were trained with one hand to discriminate between a large C shape (positive) and its mirror-image. When the untrained hand was tested the mirror-image shape was preferred.

Most of the experimenters investigating the mirror-image equivalence of the two halves of the brain have studied the visual system. In the first of these (Mello, 1966), pigeons were trained with one eye occluded to peck a response key on which was displayed an oblique line at $45°$ to the horizontal. When the other eye was tested the pigeons preferred a $135°$ oblique line, the exact mirror-image of the original stimulus.

Noble (1966) extended these studies to the optic chiasm sectioned monkey. After this operation each eye is directly connected only to the ipsilateral hemisphere. Monkeys were trained with one eye occluded to discriminate between mirror-image shapes in a Wisconsin General Test Apparatus.

On reaching criterion the occluder was changed to the other eye and the monkey's preference tested by rewarding responses to either shape. When left/right mirror-image shapes were used the monkeys always preferred the incorrect shape, i.e. the mirror-image of the shape chosen by the trained eye. Noble coined the term paradoxical transfer to express the curious nature of this result. On the other hand, tests with up/down mirror-image shapes always gave veridical transfer, i.e. the same shape was chosen with either eye open.

Noble explained his results in terms of the anatomy of the monkey visual system.

358

The pattern of excitation produced by a visual stimulus in one hemisphere should match the pattern of excitation produced by its mirror-image when the information crosses the corpus callosum. He suggested that the contradictory left/right information in each hemisphere might explain the difficulty encountered by many species in distinguishing between stimuli that are left/right mirror-images of each other.

Similar experiments using optic chiasm sectioned cats were performed by Berlucchi and Marzi (1970) and more recently by Hranchuk and Webster (1975). The cats were monocularly trained on left/right discriminations in a two-choice discrimination apparatus or in a suitably modified version of the Wisconsin General Test Apparatus. In every case when the untrained eye was tested transfer was found to be veridical.

Other experiments showed that it was possible to obtain both veridical and paradoxical transfer in the goldfish and in the monkey by altering the size of the stimulus shapes. Ingle (1967) and Campbell (1971) showed that, in goldfish, mirror-image shapes subtending a visual angle at the eye of 15° were transferred paradoxically, whereas shapes subtending a visual angle of 5° were transferred veridically. Starr (1971) found that monkeys in a Wisconsin General Test Apparatus transferred small shapes veridically and large shapes paradoxically. The critical size was somewhere between 3° and 10°. The size could not be specified more exactly, either because of genuine individual differences in the subjects or because of the relative freedom to make head and eye movements in the Wisconsin General Test Apparatus.

An alternative explanation of paradoxical transfer has been proposed which may throw light on these findings. Beale and Corballis (1968) provided evidence that the pigeon with one eye occluded attends to only one-half of the stimulus, i.e. the side nearest the open eye. This enables the pigeon to make a left/right mirror-image discrimination based on cues other than left/right information. When the other eye is open the pigeon attends to the other side of the stimulus and this will result in an apparent reversal of preference.

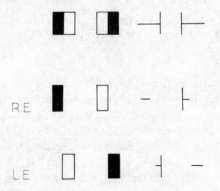

Figure 28.1. Effects of the loss of half of the visual field on the discriminability of two typical left/right mirror-image problems. RE indicates that the right eye is viewing the problems, LE the left eye

This point may be made clearer by considering the visual field of the optic chiasm sectioned monkey. Chiasm section destroys those fibres from the nasal portion of the retina. With one eye open the monkey will lose the half of the visual field normally monitored by the nasal hemiretina. If the animal fixates the centre of each shape whilst discriminating, only one-half of the shape will be observed.

Figure 28.1 shows two typical lateral mirror-image discriminations used to test interhemispheric transfer in monkeys. With the right eye open only the left half of the shapes will be observed and the mirror-image discrimination may be converted into a simple brightness or size discrimination. With the left eye open only the right half of the shapes will be seen and the monkeys will appear to have reversed their preference, i.e. to show paradoxical transfer. This was shown to be so by Hamilton *et al.* (1973) and in the same year by Lehman and Spencer (1973) who found convincing evidence for a bitemporal hemianopia in the optic chiasm sectioned monkey.

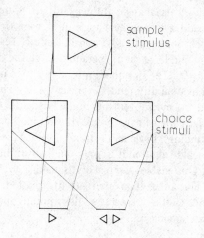

Figure 28.2.   Split-input procedure. Polarising filters are arranged so that the sample stimulus is viewed by one eye and the choice stimuli by the other eye

I also came to the same conclusion from the results of very different experiments. I had decided to investigate interhemispheric transfer using a matching to sample technique. The monkey was presented with a sample stimulus and two choice stimuli. One of the choice stimuli was identical to the sample and the task was to choose this stimulus. Using polarising filters it was possible to restrict the sample stimulus to one eye and the choice stimuli to the other eye, i.e. split-input procedure (figure 28.2). This meant that the 'match' was made using information that had crossed the corpus callosum. It was hoped that this would provide a method for directly assessing the equivalence of mirror-image stimuli in the two hemispheres. Either binocular or monocular experience of the matching to sample problems could be allowed before the critical split-input trials.

METHODS

Subjects

Two optic chiasm sectioned monkeys were used, M25 and M26.

Apparatus

The monkeys worked in a large metal cage 30 in × 20 in × 22 in in size. At one end of the cage were three circular panels of ground glass of 2 in diameter. Stimuli were back-projected on to the panels using a slide projector. In front of the stimulus panels was a black Perspex partition which kept the monkey 6 in from the stimuli. There were two eyeholes and two armholes in the partition. To control which eye was stimulated the stimulus panels and eyeholes were fitted with polarising lenses. The monkey showed that it could discriminate between stimuli by pressing the appropriate panels. A correct response activated a pellet dispenser which delivered one sugar pellet into a food tray situated below the panels.

Procedure

The monkeys were trained with both eyes open to match to sample using colour and patterned stimuli. In all cases the sample stimulus was projected on to the top panel with the two choice stimuli being projected on to the two bottom panels. The sample and choice stimuli were displayed simultaneously. The monkey's task was first to press the sample panel and then the choice panel displaying the stimulus identical to that on the sample panel. A correct choice led to a sugar pellet reward. Each monkey received two training sessions per day. One training session was comprised of 100 matching to sample trials.

The monkeys were then trained to match to sample with both eyes open on a left/right and an up/down mirror-image problem until a low criterion of 80% correct on two consecutive sessions was reached. In the next part of the experiment 50 up/down trials and 50 left/right trials were randomly intermixed in one session.

First, the monkeys underwent four of the intermixed sessions with both eyes open. Then the polarising filters were arranged so that the sample stimulus went to the left eye and the choice stimuli to the right eye for two sessions. These were the 'split-input' sessions when the match had to be made using information that had crossed the corpus callosum. For the left/right problem during split-input sessions a response to either stimulus was rewarded. The monkeys were retrained to criterion with both eyes open and then another two split-input sessions were given, but now the sample stimulus was seen by the right eye and the choice stimuli by the left eye.

Then the two monkeys were trained to match to sample with another left/right and an up/down problem but this time the initial training was monocular. M25 learned with the right eye viewing the stimuli and M26 with the left eye. Otherwise the training programme was exactly the same, monocular matching to sample for four sessions, then two split-input sessions, then retraining to criterion and a further two split-input sessions.

RESULTS

The results when the monkeys were binocularly trained are shown in figure 28.3. During the split-input sessions both monkeys showed veridical matching of up/down and left/right mirror-image shapes. There was no difference when left/right mirror-image stimuli were matched across the corpus callosum from matching performed within one hemisphere.

The results when the monkeys were monocularly trained are shown in figure 28.4. Both animals showed veridical matching of up/down stimuli in all sessions. However, for left/right mirror-images during split-input trials matching was paradoxical. Both animals made an incorrect 'mirror-image' match.

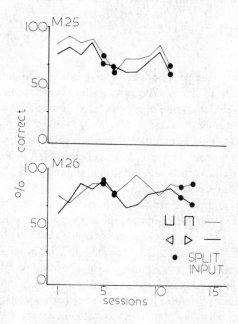

Figure 28.3. Graphs showing the percent correct matches for left/right and up/down mirror-image shapes after binocular training, with both eyes viewing the stimuli and with split-input. M25 and M26 are animal numbers; the thick line shows scores for left/right mirror-images; the thin line shows scores for up/down mirror-images; the discrimination shapes are shown; each point represents the percent correct during 50 matching trials; both eyes view the stimuli except for split-input trials which are marked with large dots

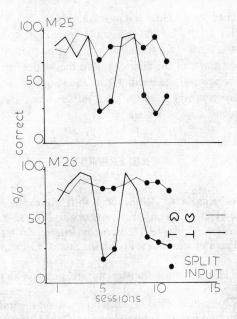

Figure 28.4. Graphs showing the percent correct matches for left/right and up/down mirror-image shapes after monocular training, with one eye only viewing the stimuli and with split-input. The key is as in figure 28.3. Stimuli are viewed with one eye except for split-input trials which are marked with large dots

DISCUSSION

On the split-input sessions I had expected paradoxical matching to the mirror-image shape, as Noble's theory of mirror-image equivalence of the two hemispheres would predict. Yet the results showed that paradoxical matching only occurred when initial training on the left/right problem was monocular. This implies that paradoxical transfer, as suggested by Hamilton *et al.* (1973), is an artefact of the experimental situation, the optic chiasm sectioned monkey attending to only one-half of the shape during monocular training. With binocular training the discrimination is based on the whole shape producing veridical transfer.

It seems that three experimenters have come separately to the same conclusion, i.e. that paradoxical transfer in optic chiasm sectioned monkeys is caused by visual field neglect and not by the mirror-image topography of the two cerebral hemispheres.

This does not directly explain why the size of shapes should be a critical factor in the monkey as to whether veridical or paradoxical transfer is obtained. It may simply be that small shapes are not masked by the missing portion of the visual field and discriminations between them are based on left/right cues. If this is true then the species difference between cat and monkeys is puzzling. The cat does not show paradoxical transfer. It may be that cats, unlike monkeys, do not maintain a steady fixation point in the centre of a stimulus. A further possibility is that this difference is related to the sharpness of the division about the vertical meridian in the retina in cat and monkey, between fibres passing from the temporal retina to the ipsilateral hemisphere and those passing from the nasal retina to the contralateral hemisphere. This question remains to be answered.

REFERENCES

Beale, I. L. and Corballis, M. C. (1968). Beak shift. An explanation for interocular mirror-image reversal in pigeons. *Nature (Lond.)*, **220**, 82–83

Berlucchi, G. and Marzi, C. A. (1970). Veridical interocular transfer of lateral mirror-image discriminations in split-chiasm cats. *J. comp. physiol. Psychol.*, **72**, 1–7

Campbell, A. (1971). Interocular transfer of mirror-images by goldfish. *Brain Res.*, **33**, 486–90

Ettlinger, G. and Elithorn, A. (1962). Transfer between the hands of a mirror-image tactile shape discrimination. *Nature (Lond.)*, **194**, 1101

Hamilton, C. R., Tieman, S. B. and Winter, H. L. (1973). Optic chiasm section affects discriminability of asymmetric patterns by monkeys. *Brain Res.*, **49**, 427–31

Hranchuk, K. B. and Webster, W. G. (1975). Interocular transfer of lateral mirror-image discriminations by cats. *J. comp. physiol. Psychol.*, **88**, 368–72

Ingle, D. (1967). Two visual mechanisms underlying the behaviour of fish. *Psychol. Forschung*, **31**, 44–51

Lehman, R. A. W. and Spencer, D. D. (1973). Mirror-image shape discrimination: interocular reversal of responses in the optic chiasm sectioned monkey. *Brain Res.*, **52**, 233–41

Mello, N. K. (1966). Concerning the interhemispheric transfer of mirror-image patterns in pigeons. *Physiol. Behav.*, **1** 293–300

Noble, J. (1966). Mirror-images and the forebrain commissures of the monkey. *Nature (Lond.)*, **211**, 1263–65

Starr, B. S. (1971). Veridical and paradoxical interocular transfer of left/right mirror-image discriminations. *Brain Res.*, **31**, 377

29
REPORT OF A SEVERE ACCURACY DEFICIT IN THE SPLIT-BRAIN MONKEY PERFORMING A BETWEEN-HAND CHOICE-RT TASK: EVIDENCE FOR A UNILATERAL FUNCTIONING HYPOTHESIS

YVES GUIARD

INTRODUCTION

Perhaps the most significant issue in the animal split-brain studies on perception and learning has been the finding that sensory information delivered to one hemisphere may remain unknown to the other hemisphere (Cuénod, 1972; Myers, 1956; Myers and Sperry, 1953). That some functional independence exists between the two cerebral hemispheres of the split brain was thus clearly demonstrated in studies using the interhemispheric transfer of learning paradigm.

The finding of such independence for both the visual and tactile modalities in commissurotomised cats (e.g. Ebners and Myers, 1962; Glassman, 1970; Myers, 1956; Stamm and Sperry, 1957) and monkeys (e.g. Downer, 1958; Hamilton and Gazzaniga, 1964; Hunter et al., 1975; Sperry, 1958) has been held as strong suggestion that the corpus callosum is the critical integration structure transmitting information continuously from one cortex to the other, and that the two cerebral hemispheres function in a parallel mode for the processing and recall of information (Dimond, 1972; Sperry, 1961; Zangwill, 1976).

As a matter of fact, studies using the transfer paradigm cannot provide any definite evidence for these views. Even though, in a number of tasks, the transfer critically depends on callosal integrity, it has neither been demonstrated in transfer studies that critical information is transmitted through the corpus callosum, nor that both hemispheres of the commissurotomised animal were alert during the learning or the recall of the task.

Direct tests of the parallel functioning hypothesis were performed by Gazzaniga and Sperry (1966) and Gazzaniga and Young (1967) in commissurotomised patients and monkeys. Using dual tasks involving the hemispheres separately, these authors presented evidence for the view that the two halves of the split brain simultaneously process information without interference. But their results were unconvincing, and since then have not been replicated. By contrast, quite clear evidence against the dual functioning hypothesis was gained in split-brain patients performing bilateral motor (Kreuter *et al.*, 1972), visual (Levy *et al.*, 1972) and auditory (Milner *et al.*, 1968; Sparks and Geschwind, 1968; Springer and Gazzaniga, 1975) tasks. These studies clearly showed that a unilateral neglect phenomenon occurs in the split-brain subject when both sides of space require attention, suggesting that after commissurotomy only half of the channel capacity is available for the processing of information.

In the present study, the capacity for the performance of a visual reaction time (RT) task that involved a between-hand choice for the response was examined in split-brain monkeys. With a dual-functioning hypothesis, i.e. both hemispheres ready for the response at the time of occurrence of the signal, one should expect no deficit in the split-brain monkeys, since no interhemispheric transfer of information was required in the task; with a unilateral suppression hypothesis, i.e. only one hemisphere ready for the response at the time of occurrence of the signal, one should expect the split-brain performance to be lower than the performance of the controls, in terms of speed, accuracy, or both.

METHODS

Four baboons (*Papio papio*) were used in this study. Two of them had undergone, prior to training, complete midsagittal section of the neocortical commissures and optic chiasma. The two others, one of which had received the chiasma transection, were used as intact-brain controls. These animals are still alive and are employed in further experiments.

The task was a visual choice-RT involving a choice between a left- and a right-hand response, a quite common task in psychology laboratories but which, to our knowledge, has not been previously used in split-brain research. The monkey was free-moving in a Trevarthen cage (Trevarthen, 1972) and spontaneously started the trials with a bimanual pressure on two levers (see figure 29.1). He had to wait for 1 s with both levers kept down. One visual signal, either left or right at random, was then delivered on the working panel by means of a light-emitting diode, and the monkey was accordingly required to release the lever located at the same side as the signal, and before signal offset. Correct responses were automatically rewarded with a peanut. Errors (the wrong lever released in first order) and any response following signal offset led to no reinforcement. True RTs were obtained by gradually reducing the signal duration down to 400–500 ms.

A polaroid filtering system was used such that each signal could only be perceived by the contralateral eye. Since the hemisphere receiving the visual signal was the one contralateral to the demanded response, no cross-talk between hemispheres was required on any trial (e.g. left signal–right hemisphere–left response).

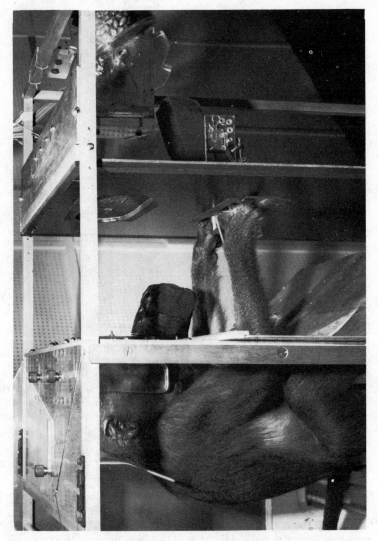

Figure 29.1. Standard working posture of the monkey waiting for a visual signal. While keeping both levers pressed down, the monkey watches the panel through a mask

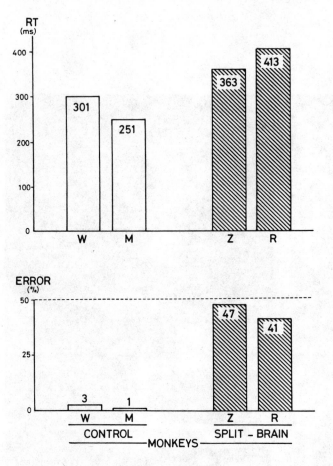

Figure 29.2. Overall mean RT and overall mean error rate for each of the four monkeys. The data for the left and right signals have been collapsed. Each value is representative of about 700 trials for the controls, and 2000 trials for the split-brain monkeys. The horizontal dotted line represents the chance error rate. Monkey M is the control animal with a split chiasma

RESULTS AND DISCUSSION

Figure 29.2 presents the performance plateau, in terms of overall mean RT and overall mean error rate, that was reached by each of the four monkeys in a series of experimental sessions following appropriate training. In spite of much greater amounts of training, it appears that the two split-brain monkeys were practically unable to produce accurate choice-responses, carrying out the task with error rates not far from the chance 50% level. By contrast, the two controls display nearly perfect accuracy scores.

Turning to RT data, results show that the considerable accuracy difference between the two groups cannot be explained in terms of a different speed–accuracy trade-off: in effect, the split-brain group produced consistently slower reactions than the control group.

It may be subsidiarily observed that the chiasma transection alone did not entail any defects: the best accuracy and speed are found in monkey M, the control animal with a split chiasma.

Thus, integrity of the neocommissural bridge appears to be a necessary condition for the performance of a between-hand choice-RT task, which is contrary to the prediction of the dual functioning hypothesis. In further investigations dealing with the two split-brain monkeys Z and R, it was found, first, that their choice inaccuracy was dependent not on the separation of the two signal alternatives between eyes, but on the separation of the two response alternatives between hands. As far as a single-handed choice-response was required under the same input conditions, excellent accuracy scores were observed in these two animals. It was found, secondly, that the scores remained unimproved in a condition where both hemispheres were simultaneously given the relevant information (a positive signal to the one; a negative signal to the other). In view of this result it may be concluded that the split-brain monkeys did not and presumably could not process the parallel information. Therefore it becomes likely that the clear-cut accuracy deficit observed in the two commissurotomised monkeys for the performance of the between-hand choice-RT task was due to their inability to deal with both equiprobable alternatives of the task.

Thus, while militating against the dual functioning hypothesis of the split brain, the present results suggest, in agreement with Kinsbourne (1974), that the corpus callosum may play a role in the dynamical distribution of attentional capacity between the two halves of the functional space.

REFERENCES

Cuénod, M. (1972). In *Structure and Function of Nervous Tissue,* vol. V (G. H. Bourne, ed.), Academic Press, New York

Dimond, S.J. (1972). *The Double Brain*, Churchill Livingstone, London

Downer, J. L. de C. (1958). *Fedn Proc.,* **17**, 37

Ebners, F. E. and Myers, R. E. (1962). *J. Neurophysiol.,* **25**, 380–91

Gazzaniga, M. S. and Sperry, R. W. (1966). *Psychon. Sci.,* **4**, 261–62

Gazzaniga, M. S. and Young, E. D. (1967). *Expl Brain Res.,* **3**, 368–71

Glassman, R. B. (1970). *J. comp. physiol. Psychol.,* **70**, 470–75

Hamilton, C. R. and Gazzaniga, M. S. (1964). *Nature (Lond.),* **201**, 220

Hunter, H., Ettlinger, G. and Maccabe, J. J. (1975). *Brain Res.,* **93**, 223–40

Kinsbourne, M. (1974). In *Hemispheric Disconnection and Cerebral Function* (M. Kinsbourne and W. L. Smith, eds.), Thomas, Springfield

Kreuter, C., Kinsbourne, M. and Trevarthen, C. (1972). *Neuropsychol.,* **10**, 453–61

Levy, J., Trevarthen, C. and Sperry, R. W. (1972). *Brain,* **95**, 61–78
Milner, B., Taylor, L. and Sperry, R. W. (1968). *Science,* **161**, 184–86
Myers, R. E. (1956). *Brain,* **79**, 358–63
Myers, R. E. and Sperry, R. W. (1953). *Anat. Rec.,* **115**, 351–52
Sparks, R. and Geschwind, N. (1968). *Cortex,* **4**, 3–16
Sperry, R. W. (1958). *Anat. Rec.,* **131**, 297
Sperry, R. W. (1961). *Science,* **133**, 1749–57
Springer, S. P. and Gazzaniga, M. S. (1975). *Neuropsychol.,* **13**, 341–46
Stamm, J. S. and Sperry, R. W. (1957). *J. comp. physiol. Psychol.,* **50**, 138–43
Trevarthen, C. (1972). In *Methods in Psychobiology,* (R. D. Myers, ed.), Academic Press, New York
Zangwill, O. (1976). *Br. J. Psychol.,* **67**, 301–14

30
CONTRIBUTION OF POSITIONAL AND MOVEMENT CUES TO VISUOMOTOR REACHING IN SPLIT-BRAIN MONKEY

DANIEL BEAUBATON, ARLETTE GRANGETTO and
JACQUES PAILLARD

INTRODUCTION

Animal studies consistently report that commissurotomy has no effect on the visual guidance of the limb contralateral to the seeing hemisphere. In contrast, there are notable differences of opinion regarding the ipsilateral limb; some authors emphasise dyspraxias following the suppression of interhemispheric connections (Brinkman and Kuypers, 1973; Downer, 1959; Gazzaniga, 1963; Geschwind, 1965; Lund *et al.*, 1970); others describe the motor deficits as transitory and slight, if not totally absent (Black and Myers, 1965; Hamilton, 1967; Myers *et al.*, 1962).

These contradictions may stem from two main factors. The first concerns the nature of the afference or re-afference accessible to the hemisphere involved. It has been suggested that tactile cues may be exploited when visual information is not available to guide the movement of the limb in its final phase (Beaubaton and Chapuis, 1974; Brinkman and Kuypers, 1973; Gazzaniga, 1970). The second factor is related to whether the motor act involves distal or proximal muscle groups, depending on the complexity of the movement, from a simple one to sequences of very elaborate manipulations.

The present study was concerned with pointing to a visual target. This type of response can be analysed in terms of the different kinds of sensory information intervening at the afferent level and the different ways of organising the motor commands on the efferent side. The organisation of visual reaching involves two different components (cf. Paillard and Beaubaton, 1975, 1976, 1977); first, the triggering of a motor programme for the ballistic transport of the hand toward the target, and second the final guiding of the movement to ensure the correct placement of the hand on this target. The execution of the initial motor programme depends on an 'open-loop' operation that requires only the spatial coding of visual information.

In contrast, the steering of the hand close to the target, the visual positioning of the hand grip and the tactile adjustment of the fingers to the shape of the object depend on 'closed-loop' operations. In this case, the motor act is dependent on feedback that enables the movement to be adjusted to the peripheral conditions of its execution. Within this frame of reference, the problem of visuomotor co-ordination has been studied in split-brain monkey. The split-brain method, by sectioning the optic chiasma and the telencephalic commissures, restricts direct visual input to one hemisphere. The question then is to investigate the capacity of the 'seeing' hemisphere to trigger and guide the contralateral and ipsilateral limbs during a visuomotor task.

Previous results suggested that the impairment of performance observed in split-brain monkeys, using an ipsilateral command and monocular vision, may be interpreted in terms of a deficit of the visuomotor correction of the positional errors of the limb in relation to the target at the end of the trajectory (Paillard and Beaubaton, 1976). Compensation for this deficit may occur when the hemisphere that does not receive direct visual information related to the target position has access to other sensory information: tactile cues (Beaubaton and Chapuis, 1974; Brinkman and Kuypers, 1973) or visual information concerning the position of the hand (Beaubaton and Chapuis, 1975).

The present experiment compared the visual open-loop and closed-loop conditions in the split-brain monkey performing the pointing task without tactile information about the position of the target. The main question concerned the role of the visual cues provided by the moving hand and the importance of the hemispheric distribution of such information in guiding the contralateral or ipsilateral limb.

METHOD

Animals

Two adult baboons (*Papio papio*) were used. The first animal received, in addition to midline section of the optic chiasma, a midline section of the corpus callosum and the anterior commissure. The complete section of these structures was confirmed histologically. The second animal was normal and used as control.

Procedure

The animals performed in a cage designed by Trevarthen (1972) in order to standardise the working posture of the animal and restricted performance to one hand. The head was partially restrained by lateral and horizontal sliding panels, in order to maintain its correct position in the mask.

A trial was initiated by depressing a lever situated centrally on a vertical panel, in front of the cage. The monkey was trained to hold the lever pressed until the response signal appeared. This signal was a 5 mm illuminated target on the panel, 2 cm up or down from the horizontal plane of vision. On the appearance of the signal, the animal was required to release the level and touch the target with one finger before the light went off in order to be rewarded with fruit juice directly into the mouth.

The target appeared either 0.5 s or 1.0 s after the lever was pressed. The duration of the target signal was 1.0 s and its position on the panel was randomly varied. The programmed sequences were automatically controlled by an electronic device.

Throughout the experimental sessions the cage was placed in a soundproof room illuminated by a monochromatic green light, and the target consisted of a red electroluminescent diode. Vision of the moving limb was eliminated by fitting the mask with coloured filters that suppressed vision of the hand while preserving vision of the target (open-loop condition). The selective distribution of visual information to each hemisphere was achieved by placing a green and a red filter in front of each eye. Therefore, the hand and the panel illuminated by the green ambient light were only seen by one (contralateral or ipsilateral) hemisphere and the target was perceived by the other.

Experimental design

Six different experimental conditions were arranged (figure 30.1) according to the two visual conditions and the eye-hand combinations. Since the left hand was being used by the two monkeys, it was possible to restrict vision of the moving hand in front of the panel to one eye (right or left) and vision of the target alone to the

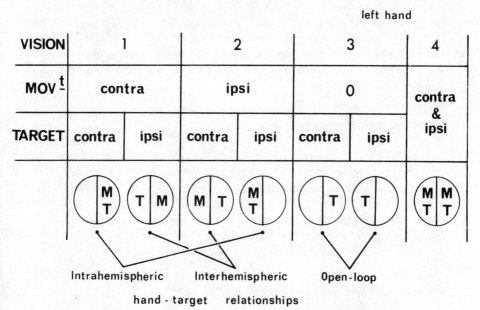

Figure 30.1. Experimental conditions. The seven circles represent the experimental situations with a distribution of the visual information provided by the movement (M), or by the target (T) on the left or the right hemisphere, respectively, ipsilateral or contralateral to the active hand

other eye. In the control condition the vision was normally binocular and without filters, all information being provided to both hemispheres. The experiment consisted of 35 daily sessions, each including about 100 trials, so the six experimental conditions and the control condition were each tested over five sessions.

Analysis of the data

The first contact of the finger with the surface of the panel automatically provided the rectangular co-ordinates of the pointing response (Clottes, 1969). The data were then processed by a PDP 12 computer. The relative errors corresponded to the distance between the spatial positions of the target and the mean point of the distribution. An estimation of the spatial dispersion of the contacts was given by computing the surface of a circle, the radius of which is the standard deviation of the distribution. The statistical significance of error differences in relation to experimental conditions was evaluated by Duncan's multiple range test (see Edwards, 1968).

RESULTS

Binocular versus monocular vision

Comparison of the binocular control situation with the contralateral, monocular condition (table 30.1, figure 30.2) confirmed that, in this type of task, the occlusion of one eye had no effect on the precision of visuomotor performance, either in the split-brain, or in the control subject. The performance was not significantly different for either animal.

Movement cues versus location cues

Figure 30.3 presents the results when visual information related to the movement or to the target was disconnected and distributed to different hemispheres. It will be noted that, in these conditions, the performance of the control subject did not vary significantly. The visuomotor performance of the commissurotomised monkey however was differentially impaired according to whether the contralateral or ipsilateral hemisphere was involved. The impairment was more severe (error = 30 mm) when movement was seen by the eye ipsilateral to the active hand.

Contralateral versus ipsilateral control

Figure 30.4 shows data from the conditions in which the target is seen by the right eye, *contralateral* to the left performing hand. In addition, vision of the moving hand was either restricted to the right hemisphere (target-seeing eye) or to the left eye

Table 30.1.

Results obtained in the split-brain subject and the control one. The different experimental conditions are presented with the hemispheric distribution of the movement cues (M) or the target vision (T) on the left, ipsilateral, hemisphere or the right, contralateral, one. According to Duncan's test, Rg7 represents, for each subject, the shortest significant range for the largest minus the smallest mean. Each difference between pairs of means is significant at a $P = 0.05$ probability threshold, if it exceeds the Rg7 value

Experimental conditions	Hemispheric distribution ipsi./contra.	Split-brain		Control	
		error (mm)	surface (cm²)	error (mm)	surface (cm²)
Closed-loop (binocular)	MT/MT	7	3.9	11	2.5
Closed-loop (monocular)					
contralateral	/MT	8	4.7	11	2.6
ipsilateral	MT/	24	7.2	15	3.1
Open-loop (monocular)					
contralateral	/T	14	5.3	14	3.3
ipsilateral	T/	26	9.7	21	4.1
Dissociated input					
contralateral	M/T	31	4.6	12	2.5
ipsilateral	T/M	14	7.2	13	3.2
		Rg7 = 5.93		Rg7 = 4.12	

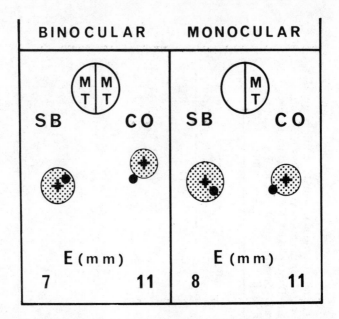

Figure 30.2. Data observed with the split-brain monkey (SB) and the control one (CO) in the binocular condition and the monocular contralateral eye–hand pair. The situations are presented with the same symbols as in figure 30.1. In the centre are presented the averaged distributions of the pointing responses (stippled areas). The mean error (E), given in the lower part, corresponds to the distance between the centre of the pointing surface (cross) and the position of the target (dot)

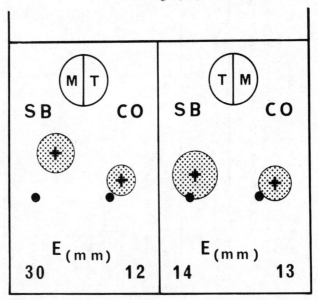

Figure 30.3 Data observed in two situations corresponding with the different hemispheric repartition of visual cues related to the movement (M) or to the target (T). Same presentation as in figure 30.2

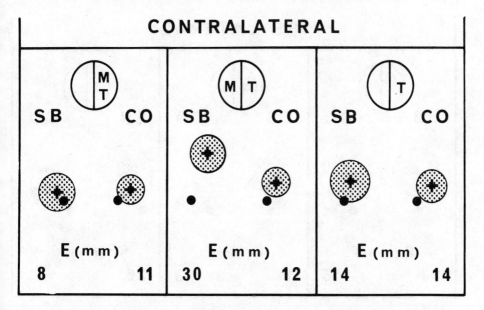

Figure 30.4. Data observed in three cases of distribution of the target (T) on the right, contralateral hemisphere. The movement (M) is either seen by the same hemisphere (left-hand side of the figure) or by the ipsilateral one (centre), or completely suppressed (right). Same presentation as in figure 30.2

only, or completely prevented to both eyes.

Suppression of the vision of the hand resulted in less accurate responses in both monkeys. But, as shown previously, when the ipsilateral hemisphere 'knows' the position of the limb (centre of the figure) the visuomotor performance is much more impaired in the split-brain subject, whereas it was slightly improved in the normal monkey.

The data from the conditions in which the target is seen by the *ipsilateral* hemisphere are presented in figure 30.5. In the three cases the target was seen by the left eye, while the left hand was used. The movement was either seen by the same hemisphere as the target or by the contralateral hemisphere, or it was not accessible to either hemispheres. The data observed in the first, closed-loop condition showed the inaccuracy of the brain-bisected monkey using an ipsilateral eye–hand combination. The mean error (24 mm) may be compared with the mean error (8 mm) obtained in the same closed-loop condition but with a contralateral combination. The standard deviation of the response also increased (table 30.1).

The main focus of these results is the comparison of pointing responses in the split-brain animal with and without vision of the movement. In contrast to the control subject, the responses of the commissurotomised monkey were as inaccurate in the closed-loop as in the open-loop condition. The lack of statistically significant difference between the two conditions (24–26 mm) shows that vision of the move-

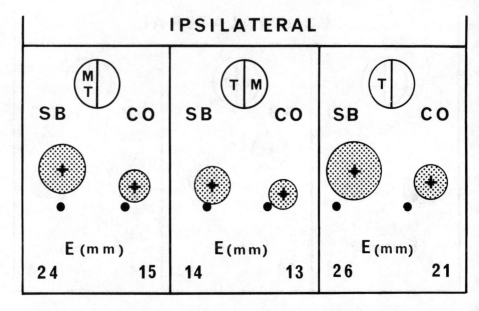

Figure 30.5.   Data observed in three cases of distribution of the target (T) on the left, ipsilateral hemisphere. Same presentation as in the previous figures

ment did not improve precision of performance, when vision of the target was accessible to the ipsilateral eye. The data obtained from ipsilateral presentation of the target and contralateral vision of the movement suggested a partial compensation of the deficit involved by the ipsilateral localisation (figure 30.5, middle part). In this case, the contralateral (right) hemisphere had access to a visual information and seemed able to attempt corrections, in spite of the apparent lack of direct visual information concerning the position of the goal.

DISCUSSION

Hein and Held (1967), investigating the ontogenetic development of the visual placing reaction in the kitten, contrasted two operations—visually elicited extension of the forelimb and visual guidance to ensure a correct positioning of the paws. Paillard and Beaubaton (1975, 1976) suggested that data resulting from pointing performance in split-brain monkeys could be interpreted analogously. The deterioration observed with an ipsilateral eye–hand combination may be attributable to a specific impairment of the mechanisms of final adjustment, whereas the ballistic, visually triggered movement can be correctly performed. Therefore the distinction between a ballistic, open-loop component and an error-correcting closed-loop mechanism led to the prediction that ipsilateral performance after commissurotomy should be equally imprecise in localisation, with or without vision of the movement.

The results obtained in this experiment clearly showed visuomotor impairment in the open-loop condition, so confirming the classical view (Vince, 1948; Woodworth, 1899) according to which, in the absence of visual feedback, the final correction of the movement to ensure correct placement is missing. But the point to be emphasised concerns the responses performed by the split-brain monkey using an ipsilateral eye–hand combination in monocular testing. These responses are consistently impaired whether or not the vision of the moving limb is allowed, in comparison with the accuracy obtained with the contralateral eye–hand combination, or in the control animal during the closed-loop condition. When vision of the target is given to the ipsilateral eye, the brain-bisected subject seems unable to use the visual cues provided by the movement in order to improve the precision of performance. In this case, it could be suggested that the seeing hemisphere is only able to trigger the open-loop aspect of the performance, namely the programme of ballistic transport of the ipsilateral limb, and the deterioration may be due to the lack of corrective mechanisms using visual feedback at the end of the trajectory.

Regarding the performance of the split-brain animal, the problem arises as to whether the bisected brain can connect and use separate visual inputs—directional cues provided by movement detection and positional cues about the location of the target. The data so far obtained show that, in fact, the disconnection may impair visuomotor performance but in different ways depending on the eye–hand combination involved.

When the contralateral eye-hand combination is used with positional cues target available for the right hemisphere and with vision of the moving left hand restricted to the left eye (figure 30.3, left), then performance is still worse than that observed in the complete open-loop condition, namely without visual information about the moving hand. In other words, in that case movement information received by the left hemisphere is not functionally useful.

A different pattern is obtained when the position of the target is accessible to the eye ipsilateral to the moving hand, whereas the hemisphere contralateral to the moving hand only receives information about movement of the limb (figure 30.3, right). In this case, the pointing movements are much more precise than those observed with a simple ipsilateral eye–hand combination. So, in contrast to the preceding condition, movement cues available to the hemisphere contralateral to the moving hand are functionally useful.

Thus, location cues about target position are functionally used in either contralateral or ipsilateral eye–hand combination to trigger the performance of reaching; movement cues (about the movement of the hand), in relation to the spatial frame provided by the work panel, are usefully processed only by the hemisphere contralateral to the moving hand and not in the ipsilateral eye–hand combination. The question then arises as to the mechanisms involved.

Reaching a visual target requires, first, the encoding of parameters related to the direction and amplitude of the movement of the hand directed toward the target. Moreover, it needs for its precise adjustment corrective information and detection of error signals.

The triggering mechanisms of the motor programme of reaching require the use of positional cues about the location of the visual target. The target-localisation processes depend on the direction of gaze resulting from foveal capture of the stimulus. In this operation the contribution of the efferent signal triggering the ocular saccade has been demonstrated (Festinger and Canon, 1965; see also the review of Berthoz, 1974). The control processing of such an ocular, efferent signal has yet to be specified.

Moreover the centring of the head associated with eye positioning probably provides an important additional source of spatial information.

Gazzaniga (1969, 1970) has shown that the steering of the hand by the ipsilateral eye in callosotomised monkeys is greatly impaired when the head is fixed. This effect has also been shown in our laboratory with normal human subjects: fixating the head leads to a significant impairment of the accuracy of pointing. There is the additional evidence of the role played by information about the position of the head in calibrating the trajectory of the limb to reach a target in space (Paillard, 1971, 1974); and the supplementary role of cervical articular receptors in eye–head co-ordination after labyrinthectomy (Dichgans *et al.*, 1973) and the striking visuomotor disorders resulting from a rhizotomy of the cervical dorsal roots in monkeys (Cohen, 1961). It is probable that such proprioceptive information about head position is bilaterally available for both hemispheres even when they are functionally separated by division of callosal commissures. This could explain how positional cues about target location are efficiently used in ipsilateral as well as in contralateral eye–hand combination.

It is worth mentioning here that experimental evidence in support of 'two visual systems' (Held, 1968; Ingle, 1968; Schneider, 1968; Trevarthen, 1968) emphasises the role of subcortical structures in the visual processing of spatial information. It is theoretically conceivable that information supplied by mesencephalic structures can be bilateraly distributed to both hemispheres. Lastly we want to stress the fact that peripheral vision may also be involved in the encoding of location cues through the gathering of information about the spatial frame of reference supplied by the experimental ambient field. It has been shown in man that open-loop pointing at a visual target displayed on a black screen is less accurate than pointing at the same target in a structured field (Conti and Beaubaton, 1977). However, we do not know, as yet, if such peripheral visual information is processed as well in the ipsilateral as in the contralateral eye–hand combination.

Turning now to the feedback corrective mechanisms used to guide the movement once started, and to adjust hand position in the vicinity of the target, we have observed that such mechanisms only operated efficiently in the contralateral eye–hand combination. The impairment of visuomotor co-ordination observed in ipsilateral eye–hand combination has been attributed to loss of visual guidance of fine distal movements, whereas reaching is possible even after destruction of the contralateral sensory motor cortex by Brinkman and Kuypers (1972, 1973). In fact, anatomical considerations suggest that motor control of the ipsilateral limb is restricted to the proximal musculature by way of the ventromedial corticospinal descending pathways (Lawrence and Kuypers, 1968a, 1968b). However, impairment of finger positioning, as observed by Brinkman and Kuypers (1973), could be explained, at least in part, by an inability to set hand and fingers in an appropriate posture. This defect of this 'grip-posture', noticed earlier by Downer (1959). Gazzaniga (1963), Lund *et al.* (1970), does not seem to be related to a lack of direct visual control of finger movement, since an appropriate grip-posture can be observed in the open-loop condition without visual guidance of the hand. In fact, anticipatory mechanisms involved in reaching are responsible for the postural setting of the hand and fingers in relation to the perceived size and weight of the object. In our procedure, the pointing task involves a well-practised postural setting that does not require fine distal adjustment. It is therefore significant that reaching is inaccurate in the ipsilateral eye–hand combination, although the distal posture is the same as that used in the contralateral eye–hand pair. The impairment therefore is probably attributable to the inefficacy of visual correction of hand position in the vicinity of the target and not to the lack of visual guidance of finger movements. This hypothesis could also explain the results reported by Keating (1973): visuomotor deterioration in ipsilateral reaching, even for movements not involving the distal musculature.

Given a specific inability of the hemisphere to guide the ipsilateral hand through the use of visual error signals relating the position of the hand to the target, how can we explain the surprising improvement of performance when the hemisphere contralateral to the moving hand can see the hand moving without have any direct visual information about the location of the target? We are led to suppose that the information about hand movement given by peripheral vision could be matched with some indirect, non-visual information about the target location. As stressed earlier, convergence of both eyes toward the target may give an important cue to the hemisphere able only to see the hand but not the target. Corrective adjustments may be derived from peripheral vision of the limb moving towards the foveal region that is correctly oriented toward the invisible target. Disparity signals could, moreover, provide additional information.

Whatever the explanation, it must be admitted that the exact nature of the neurophysiological mechanisms switched off by section of the telencephalic commissures remains to be clarified. In particular, the relationship between visual information processed by the nervous system as location cues for triggering movement and as error signals in corrective feedback loops has to be specified.

Finally, we conclude from the present experiment that the accuracy of pointing responses performed by a split-brain monkey with an ipsilateral pairing of eye and hand is consistently impaired in contrast with that obtained by the contralateral eye–hand combination, whether or not vision of the moving limb is available. Moreover, the contralateral hemisphere, deprived of direct visual information about the location of the target but informed about limb movement, can contribute to the guidance of the movement and then improve the accuracy of pointing responses. After commissurotomy, the 'target-seeing' hemisphere is therefore able to use positional cues to trigger the programme for the ballistic part of an ipsilateral pointing movement, and the contralateral 'arm-seeing' hemisphere is able to use movement cues to compensate, at least in part, for the deficit of the terminal adjustment.

REFERENCES

Beaubaton, D. and Chapuis, N. (1974). Rôle des informations tactiles dans la pré cision du pointage chez le singe split-brain. *Neuropsychologia,* **12**, 151-55

Beaubaton, D. and Chapuis, N. (1975). Champ visuel monoculaire ou binoculaire et précision du pointage chez le singe split-brain. *Neuropsychologia,* **13**, 369-72

Beaubaton, D., Nysenbaum-Requin, S. and Paillard, J. (1970). Etude du transfert interhémisphérique de l'analyse de la forme ou de la position du signal chez le singe à cerveau dédoublé. *J. Physiol. (Paris),* **62**, 343

Berthoz, A. (1974). Oculomotricité et proprioception. *Rev. Electroenceph. Neurophys. Clin.,* **4**, 569-86

Black, P. and Myers, R. E. (1965). A neurological investigation of eye–hand control in the chimpanzee. In *Function of the Corpus Callosum* (E. G. Ettlinger, ed.), Little, Brown, Boston, pp. 47-59

Brinkman, J. and Kuypers, H. G. J. M. (1972). Split-brain monkeys: central controls of ipsilateral and contralateral arm, hand and finger movements. *Science,* **176**, 536-39

Brinkman, J. and Kuypers, H. G. J. M. (1973). Cerebral control of contralateral and ipsilateral arm, hand and finger movements in the split-brain rhesus monkey. *Brain,* **96**, 653-74

Clottes, A. (1969). Prélèvement des coordonnées X-Y du premier point d'un plan touché du bout du doigt. *Electronique Electromécanique Appl. Physiol.,* **6**, 26-28

Cohen, L. A. (1961). Role of eye and neck proprioceptive mechanisms in body orientation and motor coordination. *J. Neurophysiol.,* **24**, 1-11

Conti, P. and Beaubaton, D. (1976). Utilisation des informations visuelles dans le contrôle du mouvement: étude de la précision des pointages chez l'Homme. *Travail Humain,* **39**, 19-32

Conti, P. and Beaubaton, D. (1977). Structuration of visual field and accuracy of pointing movement, in press.

Dichgans, J., Bizzi, E., Morasso, P. and Tagliasco, V. (1973). Mechanisms underlying recovery of eye–head coordination following bilateral labyrinthectomy in monkeys. *Expl. Brain Res.,* **18**, 548-69

Downer, J. L. de C. (1959). Changes in visually guided behavior following midsagittal division of optic chiasma and corpus callosum in monkeys (*Macaca mulatta*), *Brain,* **82**, 251-59

Edwards, A. L. (1968). *Experimental Design in Psychological Research.* Holt, Rinehart, Winston, New York, 455 pp.

Festinger, L. and Canon, I. K. (1965). Information about spatial location based on knowledge about efference. *Psychol. Rev.,* **72**, 373-84

Gazzaniga, M. S. (1963). Effects of commissurotomy on a preoperatively learned visual discrimination. *Expl Neurol.*, **8** 14–19

Gazzaniga, M. S. (1969). Cross-cueing mechanisms and ipsilateral eye–hand control in split-brain monkeys. *Expl Neurol.*, **23**, 11–17

Gazzaniga, M. S. (1970). *The Bisected Brain.* Appleton Century Crofts, New York, 172 pp.

Geschwind, N. (1965). Disconnexion syndromes in animal and man. *Brain*, **88**, 237

Hamilton, C. R. (1967). Effects of brain bisection on eye–hand coordination in monkeys wearing prisms. *J. comp. physiol. Psychol.*, **64**, 434–43

Hein, A. and Held, R. (1967). Dissociation of the visual placing response into elicited and guided components. *Science*, **158**, 390–92

Held, R. (1968). Dissociation of visual functions by deprivation and rearrangement. *Psychol. Forsch.*, **31** (1–4), 338–48

Ingle, D. (1968). Two visual mechanisms underlying the behavior of fish. *Psychol. Forsch.*, **31** (1–4), 1–51

Keating, E. G. (1973). Loss of visual control of the forelimb after interruption of cortical pathway. *Expl Neurol.*, **41**, 635–48

Lawrence, D. G. and Kuypers, H. G. J. M. (1968a). The functional organization of the motor system in the monkey. I. The effects of bilateral pyramidal lesions. *Brain*, **91**, 1–14

Lawrence, D. G. and Kuypers, H. G. J. M. (1968b). The functional organization of the motor system in the monkey. II. The effect of lesions of the descending brainstem pathways. *Brain*, **91**, 15–36

Lund, J. S., Downer, J. L. de C. and Lumley, J. S. P. (1970). Visual control of limb movement following section of optic chiasma and corpus callosum in the monkey. *Cortex*, **6**, 323–46

Myers, R. E., Sperry, R. W. and McCurdy, N. (1962). Neural mechanisms in visual guidance of limb movements. *Archs Neurol. (Chicago)*, **7**, 195–202

Paillard, J. (1971). Les déterminants moteurs de l'organisation de l'espace. *Cah. Psychol.*, **14**, 261–316

Paillard, J. (1974). Le traitement des données spatiales. In *De l'espace corporel à l'espace écologique.* Symp. Assoc. Psychol. Sci. Langue Français (Bruxelles, 1972). Paris P.U.F., pp 7–54

Paillard, J. and Beaubaton, D. (1975). Problèmes posés par le contrôle visuel de la motricité proximale et distale aprés disconnexion hémisphérique chez le singe. In *Les syndrômes de disconnexion calleuse chez l'homme* (B. Schott and F. Michel, eds.), SPCM/Imprimerie J. J., Lyons, France, pp. 131–71

Paillard, J. and Beaubaton, D. (1976). Triggered and guided components of visual reaching: their dissociation in split-brain studies. In *Motor System: Neuropsychology and Muscle Mechanism* (M. Shahani, ed.), Elsevier, Amsterdam, pp. 333–47

Paillard, J. and Beaubaton, D. (1978). De la coordination visuo-motrice à l'organisation de la saisie manuelle. In *Du contrôle de la motricité à l'organisation du geste* (H. Hecaen, ed.), Masson, Paris, pp. 225–60

Schneider, G. E. (1968). Contrasting visuomotor functions of tectum and cortex in the golden hamster. *Psychol. Forsch.*, **31** (1–4), 51–62

Trevarthen, C. (1968). Two mechanisms of vision in primates. *Psychol. Forsch.*, **31** (1–4), 300–37

Trevarthen, C. (1972). The split-brain technique. In *Methods in Psychobiology* (R. E. Meyers, ed.), Academic Press, London, pp. 251–84

Vince, M. A. (1948). Corrective movements in a pursuit task. *Q. Jl exp. Psychol.*, **1**, 85–103

Woodworth, R. S. (1899). The accuracy of voluntary movement. *Psychol. Rev. Monogr.*, **3**, 54–59

31
INTERHEMISPHERIC TRANSMISSION OF LEARNING AND OF ABNORMAL ELECTRICAL DISCHARGES: WHY SHOULD THERE BE DIFFERENCES?

G. ETTLINGER

INTRODUCTION

We know from several anatomical studies that the left- and right-sided posterior parietal areas (areas 5 and 7 of Brodmann) are richly interconnected through the corpus callosum. It would therefore seem likely that any behavioural function of one posterior parietal area could become accessible to the other, 'corresponding', parietal area through the corpus callosum. On this view, section of the corpus callosum in the midline could prevent the interchange of information relevant to behaviour between the left and right posterior parietal regions. For example, a monkey might fail to transfer tactile learning between the hands after division of the corpus callosum.

Analogously, any electrically abnormal discharging activity in one posterior parietal area could become accessible to the corresponding area through the same commissural pathways. In that case, division of these same pathways might result in the failure of such electrical discharges to be transmitted from one to the other posterior parietal area.

We have done both kinds of investigation in the recent past. Curiously, the outcome is not the same for the behavioural and electrical studies. Here, I would like to consider why this is so.

METHODS

For our work we have used adolescent rhesus monkeys (*Macaca mulatta*), and here we only refer to observations on animals with standard 'deep' commissure sections which involved division of the whole of the corpus callosum, the anterior and posterior commissures and the massa intermedia.

385

BEHAVIOURAL OBSERVATIONS

These observations agree in all essential respects with the work of others. A representative study is that by Hunter *et al.* (1975, 1977). The findings are clear: our deep midline surgery prevents transfer of tactile training from hand to hand irrespective of the precise task, the level of overtraining before transfer testing or the amount of experience in transfer testing before surgery. It should, however, be noted: (1) we have never worked with electrical shock as motivation; (2) the first hand was always trained (as well as the second hand always tested for transfer) after surgery; and (3) no substantial differences in outcome are known to me that can be related to the species of animal studied.

ELECTRICAL OBSERVATIONS

Our own observations on monkeys are contained in the reports of Nie *et al.* (1974), Lowrie *et al.* (1978) and in unpublished work by J. Wilden and G. Ettlinger. As a standard procedure four celluloid caps containing boiled aluminium hydroxide were placed exclusively on to the left posterior parietal cortex immediately after deep commissure section. (However, Wilden and Ettlinger applied penicillin exclusively to the left posterior parietal cortex several months after deep commissure section.) EEG recordings were then routinely taken at monthly intervals for animals with aluminium hydroxide, and continuously or hourly after penicillin for about 2-3 days. These observations indicate unequivocally that interictal abnormalities, both transmitted (i.e. synchronous with primary discharges) and independent (i.e. asynchronous), can be recorded from the hemisphere opposite to that treated with the epileptogenic chemical agent, even after histologically verified deep commissure section. The secondary transmitted discharges tend to survive ablation of the secondary cortex but not ablation of the primary cortex; the secondary independent discharges survive ablation of the primary but not ablation of the secondary cortex (Lowrie *et al.*, 1978). After the application of penicillin, secondary transmitted events but never secondary independent events are seen, although the transmitted events may appear to be asynchronous by up to 10 ms (Wilden and Ettlinger).

It should, however, be noted: (1) our own observations were all made with posterior parietal epileptogenic implants, and a different outcome might have been obtained, even in monkeys, if the aluminium hydroxide had been injected (instead of applied topically), or if another area of cortex (e.g. sensorimotor cortex) had been studied; (2) we have done no control experiments to exclude the remote possibility of the transport of the epileptogenic agent from the primary to the secondary hemisphere; and (3) I am aware of substantial differences in outcome related to species (see Discussion).

DISCUSSION

A major problem posed by these observations is: how do the abnormal electrical discharges reach the secondary (contralateral) cerebral hemisphere after deep commissure section?

Transmitted secondary discharges

In view of the recent findings of Barrett *et al*. (1976) it seems likely that the secondary transmitted discharges observed frequently in our monkeys with deep commissural sections reach the secondary electrodes by passive electrical spread (i.e. volume conduction). This does not, of course, imply that transmitted events are necessarily derived in this way when the commissures are intact. Indeed, there is evidence (Ettlinger *et al.*, 1978; Schwartzkroin *et al.*, 1975) to the contrary.

Independent secondary discharges

(1) There may exist in the monkey a commissural pathway below the diencephalon; this may then permit the abnormal discharges, but not behavioural information, to cross from one hemisphere to the other. However, Walker and Rivera (1964) failed to observe subcortical involvement with parietal (as contrasted with other) foci.

(2) Alternatively, according to a recent immunological hypothesis (Ettlinger and Lowrie, 1976), an antigen could be released by tissue destruction at the primary focus, and the resultant antibodies could be responsible for the development of both primary and secondary discharges. Some evidence for this view is tabulated in Ettlinger (1978).

So far, we have considered only observations derived from the monkey. However, there seem to be species-specific effects in that the cat, like the monkey, can develop independent secondary discharges after commissure section (Majkowski *et al.*, 1976; Wada and Cornelius, 1960), but the rat fails to do so (Cohen and Prosenz, 1971; see also chapter 12). The differences between species could be a consequence of either the existence in the cat and monkey, but not in the rat, of a commissural pathway below the diencephalon; or of a difference between species in their immunological reactivities. In the absence of known differences between the monkey and the rat in their commissural pathways it may be worth while noting that:

(a) the immunological system of the rat is more effective than that of the monkey (i.e. rats are less susceptible to infection);

(b) stronger chemical agents have generally to be used to produce discharges in the rat (e.g. metallic cobalt, which often kills a monkey as a consequence of brain oedema);

(c) in the rat primary and secondary discharges are produced sooner and they are more transient than in the monkey—possibly related to the more rapid formation of antibodies and the more rapid neutralisation of the antigen.

These points do not bear directly on the absence of independent secondary events after commissure section in the rat; rather, they provide a possible framework for species differences in the development of primary and secondary foci. In terms of the immunological hypothesis, the rat may fail to develop secondary discharges after commissure section because:

(i) the surgical procedure (division by tightening a ligature) may have impaired the blood circulation (e.g. divided branching vessels from the anterior cerebral artery); and/or

(ii) the corpus callosum may be tonically more active in the rat than in the monkey (as suggested by other kinds of evidence), and the absence of such tonic excitation may have attenuated the hypothetical action by antibodies on the receptors of synapses; and/or

(iii) the regional specificity of cortical areas may be altered by commissure section in the rat.

CONCLUSIONS

We do not know why deep commissure section prevents intermanual transfer of training in monkeys but often does not prevent the development of secondary epileptic foci. Not all of the observations can at this time be adequately explained. However, the development of secondary foci (as well as of primary foci) may be a consequence of an immunological response; and commissure section would not be expected to influence such an immunological process. Species differences are known to exist not only in the development of abnormal discharges but also for immunological responsiveness; and to some extent there are correspondences between these kinds of species differences.

ACNOWLEDGEMENT

I thank Mrs M. B. Lowrie for helpful comments on this chapter.

REFERENCES

Barrett, G., Blumhardt, L., Halliday, A. M., Halliday, E. and Kriss, A. (1976). A paradox in lateralization of the visual evoked response. *Nature (Lond.)*, **261**, 252-55

Cohen, M. and Prosenz, P. (1971). Antigenicity of epileptic tissue. *Dis. nerv. System*, **32**, 314–15

Ettlinger, G. (1978). Experimental epilepsy in the monkey: some behavioural and electrophysiological observations. Festschrift for Dr E.T. O. Slater. *Br. J. Psychiat., in press*

Ettlinger, G., Holmes, O. and Nie, V. (1977). Unitary activity in temporal epileptic foci in the monkey, *J. Physiol., Lond.*, **270**, 49–50P

Ettlinger, G. and Lowrie, M. B. (1976). An immunological factor in epilepsy. *Lancet*, **i**, 1386

Hunter, M., Ettlinger, G. and Maccabe, J. J. (1975). Intermanual transfer in the monkey as a function of amount of callosal sparing. *Brain Res.*, **93**, 223–40

Hunter, M., Lowrie, M. B., Ettlinger, G. and Maccabe, J. J. (1977). The effect of prolonged pre-operative transfer testing on intermanual transfer of training in the monkey. *Cortex*, **13**, 215–16

Lowrie, M. B., Maccabe, J. J. and Ettlinger, G. (1978). The effects of ablations on primary and secondary epileptic discharges in commissure-sectioned rhesus monkey. *Electroenceph. clin. Neurophysiol.*, **44**, 23–36

Majkowski, J., Sobieszek, A., Bilińska-Nigot, B. and Karliński, A. (1976). EEG and clinical studies of the development of alumina cream epileptic focus in split-brain cats. *Epilepsia*, **17**, 257–69

Nie, B., Maccabe, J. J., Ettlinger, G. and Driver, M. V. (1974). The development of secondary epileptic discharges in the rhesus monkey after commissure section. *Electroenceph. clin. Neurophysiol*, **37** 473–81

Schwartzkroin, P. A., Futamachi, K. J., Noebels, J. L. and Prince, D. A. (1975). Transcallosal effects of a cortical epileptiform focus. *Brain Res.*, **99**, 59–68

Wada, J. A. and Cornelius, L. R. (1960). Functional alteration of deep structures in cats with chronic focal cortical irritative lesions. *Archs Neurol.*, **3** 425–47

Walker, A. E. and Rivera, J. F. (1964). Sub-cortical recording in experimental focal chronic epilepsy, *Trans. Am. Neurol. Ass.*, **89**, 37–39

32
INTERFIELD DIFFERENCES IN REACTION TIMES TO LATERALISED VISUAL STIMULI IN NORMAL SUBJECTS

G. RIZZOLATTI

When a visual stimulus is projected to the right of a fixation point the response with the right hand to that stimulus is faster than the response with the left hand, and similarly, when a stimulus is projected to the left of fixation the response with the left hand is faster than that with the right hand. This advantage of ipsilateral over contralateral responses was first described by Poffenberger at the beginning of the century in experiments in which he measured reaction times to simple light stimuli. Poffenberger (1912) attributed this advantage (which was of about 4 ms in his experiments) to the different lengths of the nervous circuits responsible for the two responses. Thus ispsilateral responses can be executed using central nervous circuits located entirely in one hemisphere, whereas the contralateral responses need pathways which cross the interhemispheric commissures. Since the pathway in this last condition is longer and most likely includes one additional synapse, a response mediated by it requires more time. Poffenberger also calculated, using the few data available on the conduction velocity of nervous fibres, how long the delay should be between ipsilateral and contralateral responses provided his interpretation was correct. He wrote: 'If the speed of transmission of the nerve impulse be taken as 30 m/per second, then in one sigma it would travel 3 cm. Considering the length of these fibers (corpus callosum) to be 6 cm the reaction time would be 2 sigma, which would be constant entity.' (Poffenberger, 1912, p. 68).

Poffenberger's findings have been confirmed in modern times (Anzola *et al.*, 1977; Arutyunova and Blinkov, 1962; Berlucchi *et al.*, 1971; Berlucchi *et al.*, 1977; Jeeves, 1969; Jeeves, 1972). Experiments in which simple reaction times to lateralised visual stimuli were measured have shown that the delay between ipsilateral and contralateral responses is very close to that theoretically predicted (2 ms). Furthermore, now that a better knowledge of the diameters of the corpus callosum fibres has become available (Tomasch, 1954), the theoretical delay calculated by Poffenberger on the basis of rather weak evidence turns out to be quite plausible if the largest fibres are those responsible for the behavioural response (cf.

Berlucchi *et al.*, 1971). As a consequence the anatomical interpretation of the laterality effects first advanced by Poffenberger has been generally accepted.

More recently, however, doubts have been raised as to the validity of this interpretation. First, attempts to measure the transmission time from one side to the other of the brain using paradigms different from that of simple reaction time, have given values much larger than those previously reported (Filbey and Gazzaniga, 1969; McKeever and Gill, 1972; Moscovitch and Catlin, 1970); secondly, other experiments such as that of Wallace (1971) have shown that differences between ipsilateral and contralateral responses could be obtained in conditions in which the anatomical factor can be ruled out as being responsible for the laterality effect. Since this latter criticism is very substantial it will be discussed first.

In the experiment of Wallace, subjects had to discriminate between two visual patterns which were presented one at a time on either the right or the left of a fixation point. The subjects had to respond to one pattern with the right hand and to the other with the left hand. As predicted from previous studies the responses with the right hand were faster when the pattern appeared on the right, and the responses with the left hand were faster when the patterns appeared on the left. However, when the subjects were tested with their hands crossed so that the right hand was positioned on the left side of the body and the left hand on the right, the relation between the faster hand and the side of the stimulus changed. The responses to stimuli coming from the right became faster with the left hand than with the right, and those to stimuli coming from the left were faster with the right hand than with the left. Since it is obvious that crossing the hands cannot modify the fixed anatomical interhemispheric connections, a simple anatomical interpretation such as that proposed by Poffenberger has to be ruled out.

The Wallace results and those of others demonstrating, with slightly different procedures, the same phenomenon (Brebner, 1973; Brebner *et al.*, 1972) were obtained in choice reaction time situations but they challenged also the explanation of the delay between ipsilateral and contralateral responses obtained using simple reaction times (see Broadbent, 1974). It may be, in fact, that the laterality effect observed in simple reaction time reflects, as in the Wallace experiment, some dynamic relationship of contiguity between stimulus and response which favours a given hand according to its position, independently of the fixed anatomical connections. In other words the delay between ipsilateral and contralateral responses in simple reaction time would be a particular case of stimulus response compatibility as defined by Fitts and Seeger (1953) and not at all a measure of interhemispheric transmission time.

This interpretation can be tested experimentally if simple reaction times to lateralised stimuli are measured in subjects whose hands are crossed. If the fixed elementary connections are the main factor in determining the laterality effect in simple reaction times, the right hand, even when it is on the left of the body, should respond faster to stimuli presented to the right of the fixation point, and conversely the left hand should respond faster to stimuli coming from the left than from the right, even when it is placed on the right side of the body. On the contrary, if the compatibility interpretation is true the hand on the same side of the body as the stimulus should be faster even though the anatomical connections are unfavorable.

We recently performed this experiment on 16 subjects (male students). The stimulus, a circle of light subtending less than $\frac{1}{2}°$ of visual angle, was presented for 100 ms, 5° to the right or left of a fixation point. Both eyes were open and a ready signal preceded the stimulus by a variable interval. At the appearance of the light, the subject has to press a microswitch with the thumb of one hand as quickly as possible. There were four randomised conditions: stimulus in the right visual field, response with the right hand; stimulus in the left visual field, response with the left hand; stimulus in the right visual field, response with the left hand; and stimulus in the left visual field, response with the right hand. Each situation was used once in each session. The subjects were divided into two groups: the first group responded with hands in the normal position, the second group with hands crossed. The subjects attended nine sessions, one for practice and eight for data collection. At the end, the overall median reaction times were calculated for each subject in the four conditions.

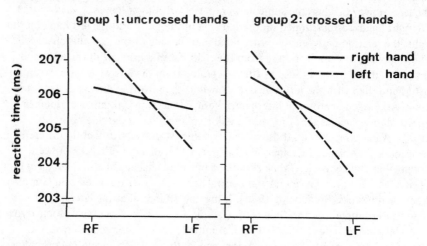

Figure 32.1 Means of median reaction times to stimuli presented to the right visual field (RF) and left visual field (LF). (From Anzola *et al.*, 1977)

The results are shown in figure 32.1. On the left side are shown the data of the group which performed the task with hands in the normal positions; on the right are the data of the subjects which had their hands crossed. One can see that regardless of the hand position the responses with the right hand were faster than with the left hand when the stimuli were presented on the right of fixation, and that responses were faster with the left hand than with the right hand in the opposite condition. Figure 32.2 shows the same data replotted in terms of ipsilateral (anatomically uncrossed) and contralateral (anatomically crossed) reaction

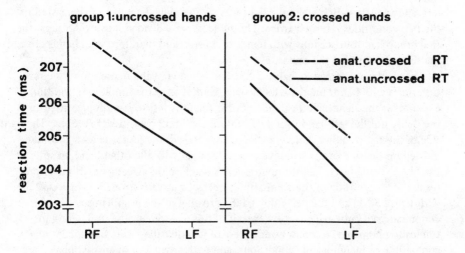

Figure 32.2. Same data as in figure 32.1 but with anatomically crossed and uncrossed responses being connected

times. One can see that for both groups the ipsilateral responses were faster than the contralateral ones. An analysis of variance showed that this difference was highly significant.

Similar data have been independently obtained by Berlucchi *et al.* (1977). In their study the stimuli were presented on the horizontal meridian at 5, 10 and 35° to the right or to the left of fixation. In some sessions, the subjects had to respond with the hands in the normal position, in others with the hands crossed. It was found that the ipsilateral responses were faster than the contralateral responses regardless of hand position and that the advantage of the ipsilateral responses did not change with the different eccentricities of the stimulus.

A point which seems to differentiate the compatibility effects from the laterality effects of simple reaction time experiments is the magnitude of the two phenomena. One finds a delay of only a few milliseconds between ipsilateral and contralateral responses in the simple reaction time paradigm, whereas when compatibility is involved the difference is in tens of milliseconds. However, since the two sets of data have been obtained in different laboratories and under rather different experimental conditions we thought it of some interest to repeat the compatibility experiments using the same experimental set-up employed in the study of simple reaction time described above.

Two lights identical with those of the previous experiment were used, one located 5° to the right and the other 5° to the left of fixation. The order of presentation of the lights was quasi-random. The subjects (eight male students) held two micro-switches, identical with the one used in the previous experiment, one in each hand. In condition A, they were instructed to press the right switch when the light appeared on the right, and to press the left switch when the light appeared on the left; in condition B, they had to press the right switch when the light was on the left, and the left switch when the light was on the right. Each session consisted of the two conditions repeated twice. The subjects were divided into two groups: the first group had four sessions with hands uncrossed and then four with hands crossed: the second group did the opposite.

The results are shown in figure 32.3. The left side of the figure shows the reaction times with hands uncrossed. One can see that as in the simple reaction time experiment the right hand responded faster than the left to stimuli presented to the right, and the left hand responded faster to stimuli presented to the left. The right side of the figure shows that, with the hands crossed, the response with the hand located on the side of the stimulus was faster than with the other hand, in spite of the fact that the latter had the anatomical advantage. In agreement with previous results the magnitude of the compatibility effect was very strong (cf. figure 32.3 with figure 32.1) and the delay due to the crossing of the interhemispheric commissure was not evident. However, if in this experiment the ipsilateral (anatomically uncrossed) responses, regardless of whether they were obtained under compatible or incompatible conditions, and with crossed or uncrossed hands, are compared with the contralateral (anatomically crossed) responses which are pooled in the same way, a prevalence of the ipsilateral responses is still present, although the difference (a few milliseconds) was not significant, very likely because of the large variance due to the variety of conditions mentioned above.

In conclusion, the evidence from these studies permits us to exclude the possibility that in the simple reaction time paradigm, response compatibility is

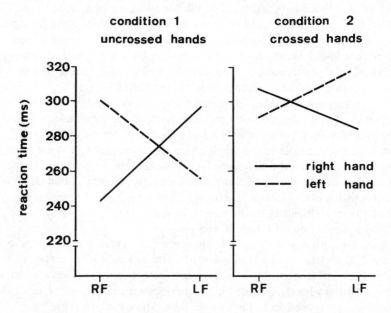

Figure 32.3. Means of median reaction times. Abbreviation as in figure 32.1.(From Anzola *et al.* 1977)

responsible for the laterality effect. In these conditions the main factor determining which hand is faster in responding to a lateralised visual stimulus is the basic organisation of sensory and motor pathways.

The second objection recently raised against the conclusions drawn from simple reaction time experiments concerns the magnitude of the interhemispheric transmission time. In several experiments in which rather complex situations, but not involving stimulus response compatibility, were employed, delays were found between responses involving one or both hemispheres which were much greater than 2 ms (Filbey and Gazzaniga, 1969; McKeever and Gill, 1972; Moscovitch and Catlin, 1970). For example, McKeever and Gill (1972) measured discriminative reaction time to letters tachistoscopically projected on the right or on the left of the fixation point. They found that verbal responses to stimuli presented to the left of the fixation point were about 30 ms longer than those presented to the right. They interpreted this long delay as the time necessary for the visual information to cross the corpus callosum to the language centres of the left hemisphere. Long 'interhemispheric transfer times' were found also by other researchers employing similar procedures (Filbey and Gazzaniga, 1969; Moscovitch and Catlin, 1970; see, however, McKeever et al., 1975).

At this point one may ask whether both the measures of 'interhemispheric transfer' really correspond with the time necessary for nervous impulses to cross the corpus callosum, or whether one of them is incorrect. Since besides the large fibres mentioned before, many small myelinated and unmyelinated fibres are present in the corpus callosum (Tomasch, 1954) neither the delay of 2 ms nor that of 30 ms can be excluded *a priori* on basic anatomical or physiological grounds. In order to solve the discrepancy it has been suggested (see Gazzaniga, 1971) that in the simple reaction time paradigm both the ipsilateral and the contralateral responses are executed under the control of the motor cortical areas ipsilateral to the visual areas receiving the stimulus and that the responses are mediated, in the first case, by the crossed corticospinal pathways and, in the second, by the uncrossed ones. Since the latter are known to be anatomically less developed and functionally less efficient than the former, the 2 ms delay between ipsilateral and contralateral responses would reflect the difference in efficiency between the crossed and uncrossed corticospinal routes, and not the transmission time across the corpus callosum. This explanation appears to be very unlikely. There is good evidence from experimental as well as from clinical neurology that finger movements of the type used in reaction time experiments are controlled exclusively by the contralateral motor areas (Lawrence and Kuypers, 1968; Tower, 1940; Travis, 1955). Therefore, any idea that an inefficient ipsilateral motor control is responsible for the delay seen in simple reaction time lacks experimental support.

An alternative explanation for the discrepancy in the 'interhemispheric transfer times' of simple and discriminative reaction time results, is that in discriminative reaction times the long delay reflects other factors than, or in addition to, the transmission time across the corpus callosum. There exists in fact, a fundamental difference in what is required of the cerebral centres when complex material is used, as in a discriminative reaction time experiment, as opposed to when simple unstructured light stimuli are employed. In this last case, that of the simple reaction time experiment, both hemispheres are virtually equal in their ability to analyse the stimulus; in contrast, in discriminative reaction time experiments in which complex stimuli are used, one must take into account the asymmetry between the two hemispheres in their analysing capabilities. In other words, for a given material, there is one hemisphere which is highly competent and one which is less competent or incompetent in performing the analysis.

In the experiments in which large interhemispheric delays have been found, complex material has been sent to the competent and to the non-competent hemispheres, and the difference between reaction times in these two situations has been assumed to be the transmission time across the corpus callosum. This assumption is unjustified. When complex material is sent to the non-competent hemisphere, two possibilities arise: the first is that the stimulus is analysed completely by the non-competent hemisphere, until a decision about it is made; the second is that, at a certain level of elaboration, the non-competent hemisphere sends the information across the commissure to the other hemisphere which then completes the analysis and makes the required decision. In the first case, the so-called 'interhemispheric transmission time' represents essentially the difference in the rapidity with which the two hemispheres perform their analyses and has nothing to do with callosal transmission time. In the second case the 'transmission time' results from two factors: the real transmission time across the corpus callosum from the non-competent to the competent hemisphere, plus the time necessary for the competent hemisphere to analyse and decipher the message which has already been distorted by an inappropriate coding or processing by the non-competent hemisphere. It should be mentioned here that in such experiments a transfer of information cannot occur at the level of the primary visual cortical areas (where hemispheric differences in analysing stimuli are unlikely), because these areas are not connected with each other except along the vertical meridian (Berlucchi and Rizzolatti, 1968; Berlucchi et al., 1967; Hubel and Wiesel, 1967; Whitteridge, 1965; see also chapter 19).

The interpretation of the different delays found in simple and discriminative reaction times leads to the prediction that in certain conditions, 'transfer time' should covary with the absolute value of the reaction times. In simple reaction time experiments, since the 'transfer time' reflects the conduction velocity of callosal fibres, it should remain constant regardless of the absolute value of the responses. In contrast, in a discriminative reaction time experiment, an increase in the absolute reaction time due to a greater difficulty in discriminating the stimuli should produce an increase of the so-called 'transfer time', since now it would not be determined by the rigid properties of conduction velocity but rather would be a function of the relative rapidity with which the two hemispheres process visual information or of the capacity of the competent hemisphere to reconstruct and to recognise the message sent to it by the non-competent hemisphere.

Concerning the first prediction, the constancy of the delay between ipsilateral and contralateral responses to unstructured light stimuli in the simple reaction time paradigm, has a large experimental support. In spite of differences of stimulus intensity, background illumination, location on the retina and position of the hands, the magnitude of the advantage of the ipsilateral response has been found to be constant (see reference cited above). Figure 32.4 shows the validity of the second prediction. In this experiment we presented physiognomic material to 16 male subjects using two durations of stimuli: 100 ms and 20 ms. The stimuli used and the procedure employed was the same as in our previous studies (Rizzolatti *et al.*, 1971; Umiltà *et al.*, 1974). One can see that decreasing the stimulus duration (and thus making the task more difficult) did not greatly lengthen the reaction times to stimuli presented to the competent hemisphere (right in this case), whereas it had a dramatic effect when the stimuli were presented to the non-competent hemisphere. The mean difference between right and left visual fields with the 20 ms stimulus duration was approximately 150 ms and in two subjects the difference exceeded 200 ms. These differences are so large that any explanation in terms of simple transfer of visual information from one hemisphere to the other appears to be untenable.

In conclusion, the anatomical interpretation of the laterality effects in simple reaction time still remains valid, in spite of criticisms which have been raised against it in recent years. Furthermore, 2 ms as the measure of the time necessary for transmission across the corpus callosum appears, on the basis of available

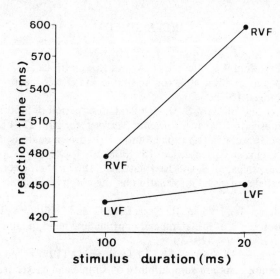

Figure 32.4. Means of median reaction times. RVF, right visual field; LVF, left visual field.
(After Rizzolatti and Buchtel, 1977)

evidence, to be the only acceptable one for reaction time experiments. It is worth mentioning that once one has a clear concept of which is the real callosal transfer time, one can attempt to solve the problems, already mentioned, of whether with complex material the non-competent hemisphere is able to analyse the stimuli by itself, or whether , on the contrary, a transfer of information to the competent hemisphere is necessary. If the first hypothesis is true, when the stimulus is sent to the non-competent hemisphere, the contralateral hand should be faster than the ipsilateral hand, since the analysis starts and finishes in this hemisphere. On the contrary, if the information must be transferred from the non-competent to the competent hemisphere, the ipsilateral hand, controlled by the competent hemisphere, will be faster than the contralateral one. In both cases, and regardless of hemispheric specialisation, the difference between the hands should be in the order of a few milliseconds—the time necessary to cross the corpus callosum.

ACKNOWLEDGEMENTS

I thank H. A. Buchtel for helpful discussion of the manuscript. Some of the work reported here was supported by a grant to the Istituto di Fisiologia Umana, University of Parma from C.N.R.

REFERENCES

Anzola, G. P., Bertoloni, G., Buchtel, H. A. and Rizzolatti, G. (1977). Spatial compatibility and anatomical factors in simple and choice reaction time. *Neuropsychologia*, **15**, 295–302

Arutyunova, A. S. and Blinkov, S. M. (1962). Latent period of motor reaction with hemianopsia (in Russian). *J. Higher Nervous Activity*, **12**, 432–36

Berlucchi, G. and Rizzolatti, G. (1968). Binocularly driven neurons in visual cortex of split-chiasm cats. *Science*, **159**, 308–10

Berlucchi, G., Gazzaniga, M. S. and Rizzolatti, G. (1967). Microelectrode analysis of transfer of visual information by the corpus callosum. *Arch. Ital. Biol.*, **105**, 583–96

Berlucchi, G., Heron, W., Hyman, R., Rizzolatti, G. and Umiltà, C. (1971). Simple reaction times of ipsilateral and contralateral hand to lateralized visual stimuli. *Brain*, **94**, 419–30

Berlucchi, G., Crea, F., Di Stefano, M. and Tassinari, G. (1977). The influence of spatial stimulus-response compatibility on simple and choice reaction time of ipsilateral and contralateral hand to lateralized light stimuli. *J. exp. Psychol.: Hum. Percept. Perform.*, **3**, 505–17

Brebner, J. (1973). S-R compatibility and changes in RT with practice. *Acta Psychol.*, **37**, 95–106

Brebner, J., Shephard, M. and Cairney, P. (1972). Spatial relationships and S-R compatibility. *Acta Psychol.*, **36**, 1-15

Broadbent, D. E. (1974). Division of function and integration of behavior. *The Neurosciences*, Third Study Program (F. O. Schmitt and F. G. Worden, eds.), MIT Press, Cambridge, Massachusetts, pp. 31-41

Filbey, R. A. and Gazzaniga, M. S. (1969). Splitting the brain with reaction time *Psychon. Sci.* **17**, 335-36

Fitts, P. M. and Seeger, C. M. (1953). S-R compatibility: spatial characteristics of stimulus and response codes. *J. Exp. Psychol.*, **46**, 199-210

Gazzaniga, M. S. (1971). Reply to McKeever and Huling. *Psychon. Sci*, **22**, 223-24

Hubel, D. H. and Wiesel, T. N. (1967). Cortical and callosal connections concerned with the vertical meridian of visual fields in the cat. *J. Neurophysiol.*, **30**, 1561-73

Jeeves, M. A. (1969). A comparison of interhemispheric transmission times in acallosals and normals. *Psychon. Sci.*, **16**, 245-46

Jeeves, M. A. (1972). Hemisphere differences in response rates to visual stimuli in children. *Psychon. Sci.*, **27**, 200-203

Lawrence, D. G. and Kuypers, H. G. J. M. (1968). The functional organization of the motor system in the monkey. *Brain*, **91**, 1-14

McKeever, W. F. and Gill, K. M. (1972). Interhemispheric transfer time for visual stimulus information varies as a function of the retinal locus of stimulation. *Psychon. Sci.*, **26**, 308-10

McKeever, W. F., Gill, K. M. and Van Deventer, A. D. (1975). Letter versus dot stimuli as tools for 'splitting the normal brain with reaction time'. *Q. Jl Exp. Psychol.*, **27**, 363-73

Moscovitch, M. and Catlin, J. (1970). Interhemispheric transmission of information: measurement in normal man. *Psychon. Sci.*, **18**, 211-13

Poffenberger, A. T. (1912). Reaction time to retinal stimulation with special reference to the time lost in conduction through nerve centers. *Archs Psychol.*, **23**, 1-73

Rizzolatti, G. and Buchtel, H. A. (1977). Hemispheric superiority in reaction time to faces: a sex difference. *Cortex*, **13**, 300-305

Rizzolatti, G., Umiltà, C. and Berlucchi, G. (1971). Opposite superiorities of the right and left cerebral hemispheres in discriminative reaction time to physiognomical and alphabetic material. *Brain*, **94**, 431-42

Tomasch, J. (1954). Size, distribution, and number of fibers in human corpus callosum. *Anat. Rec.*, **119**, 119-35

Tower, S. S. (1940). Pyramidal lesion in the monkey. *Brain*, **63**, 36-90

Travis, A. M. (1955). Neurological deficiences after ablation of the precentral motor area in *Macaca mulatta*. *Brain*, **78**, 155-73

Umiltà, C., Rizzolatti, G., Marzi, C. A., Zamboni, G., Franzini, C., Camarda, R. and Berlucchi, G. (1974). Hemispheric differences in the discrimination of line orientation. *Neuropsychologia*, **12**, 165-74

Wallace, R. J. (1971). S-R compatibility and the idea of a response code. *J. Exp. Psychol.*, **88**, 354-60

Whitteridge, D. (1965). Area 18 and the vertical meridian of the visual field. *Ciba Fdn Study Grps.*, **20**, 115-20

33
LEFT HEMIFIELD SUPERIORITY AND THE EXTRACTION OF PHYSIOGNOMIC INFORMATION

PAUL BERTELSON, HÉLÈNE VANHAELEN and JOSÉ MORAIS

INTRODUCTION

Data have accumulated in recent years which strongly suggest that the process of identifying human faces is critically dependent on functions for which the minor cerebral hemisphere is specialised. The notion is, in fact, supported by the now familiar pattern of neuropsychological evidence for hemispheric specialisation, which consists of (a) the existence of a specific pathological syndrome, (b) a correlation in brain-damaged patients between measures of the relevant capacity and side of injury, and (c) a perceptual asymmetry demonstrable in normal subjects. In the present case the syndrome is *prosopagnosia*, a rare condition involving the specific loss of the ability to recognise people from their faces, which is found mainly in patients with damage to the right hemisphere (Bodamer, 1947; Hecaen and Angelergues, 1962; Rondot and Tzavaras, 1969), although some lesion in a so-far unspecified region of the left hemisphere may also be necessary (Meadows, 1974).

When populations of non-prosopagnosic brain-damaged patients are submitted to tests involving recognition or comparisons of pictures of human faces, patients with right hemisphere lesions do more poorly (e.g. Benton and Van Allen, 1968; De Renzi *et al.*, 1968). The difference seems to be specific of a material picturing normally oriented human faces, since it is not found with pictures of other mono-oriented objects (Tzavaras *et al.*, 1970) nor with pictures of faces presented upside-down (Yin, 1970). Finally, faces presented in one visual hemifield of normal subjects are identified more accurately (Hilliard, 1973; Klein *et al.*, 1976; Marcel and Rajan, 1975) or faster (Geffen *et al.*, 1971; Rizzolati *et al.*, 1971) when presented in the left hemifield. This left side superiority is probably the reason behind the old finding (Wolff, 1933) that a composite picture made up by assembling two right halves of a face resembles the whole face more than one made up of two left halves (Gilbert and Bakan, 1973). There are however some conditions, not yet fully elucidated, under which the effect vanishes or gives way to right side superiority. One of these conditions is the use of names, another is familiarity with the pictures used in the test (Berlucchi *et al.*, 1976). We shall go back to that question later : understanding the apparent lability of left side superiority in face recognition was one of the motives of the present study.

Independently of data on lateralisation, the idea that the perception of the human face may involve specialised processes, sometimes called physiognomic, different from those involved in identifying other kinds of objects, has been entertained by many students of perception (e.g. Hochberg, 1972). The physiognomic mode of perception can however be applied to non-face stimuli, as when we see faces in clouds, Rorschach inkblots, etc., and can then lead to better recognition perfor- mance (Gibson, 1969). Consideration of the role played by the face in social inter- action as a source of both non-verbal communicative displays and of speech- accompanying signals on one hand, and as the main basis of individual recognition on the other, makes the emergence of specialised perceptual mechanisms plausible. There are also a number of remarkable features which appear to be specific of facial perception. One aspect, which has been well documented by Yin (1969), is the fact that recognition performance is affected by upside-down inversion in the case of faces much more than in the case of other mono-oriented objects such as houses or human figures. On the other hand, we can identify a person from his face across changes of viewing angle, of expression, of age, of health state and often in spite of the addition or elimination of paraphernalia such as moustache, beard, hair, glasses, etc. Physiognomic perception seems to imply the extraction of high order relational properties which are invariant across such changes.

The evidence regarding lateralisation undoubtedly fits in well with the notion of specialised processing facilities : some critical components of physiognomic perception would be based in the minor hemisphere. From that point of view, the sheer registration of lateral asymmetry is however unsatisfactory, and one is led to ask which are the critical operations, for which the right hemisphere is specialised, and which are essential to facial recognition (Teuber, 1972). An attractive propo- sition is that they consist of the extraction of those high order physiognomic in- variants we have just been considering.

If this assumption is correct, left hemifield superiority will only be detected reliably in a task which requires the extraction of properly physiognomic informa- tion. Now, this is not necessarily the case of any face-identification task. For instance, if the task is to decide if two simultaneously presented pictures are of the same person, but if one person is always represented by the same picture, so that the decision 'same' is made on the basis of two physically identical pictures, the extraction of physiognomic information is not necessary. In that situation, any aspect of the material can be valid for doing the task, so that the pictures can well be processed in a non-physiognomic mode. But if the decision 'same' must be made on the basis of two different pictures of a person, it becomes much less likely that low level routines be valid.

In the experiment to be described, subjects were asked to give speeded same- different reactions to successive pairs of photographs, the first member of each pair being presented at the fixation point and the second unpredictably in the left or right hemifield. In one condition, called 'physical identity' condition, a trial involved either two identical photographs or the photographs of two different people. In the other condition, called 'facial identity' condition, each trial involved two different photographs of the same person, taken from different viewing angles, or two photographs of two different persons. From the physiognomic invariant hypothesis, it was predicted that a larger left visual field superiority would be observed in condition 'facial identity'.

METHOD

Material and apparatus

The material consists of two photographs, one full-face and one three-quarter face, of 15 young men, aged ≈ 20 years. All models had dark hair, about the same haircut, were clean-shaven and wore no glasses. All were photographed wearing the same dark tee-shirt. Their expression was neutral. From each negative, two prints 24 mm × 35 mm were prepared with two opposite orientations.

The material was presented in an Electronic Developments 3-channel tachistoscope. In channel 1, a single small black cross, serving as fixation point, was presented in a central position. In channel 2, one photograph appeared in central position. In channel 3, a photograph was present either to the right or left of the centre. At the subject's eye, each face subtended a horizontal angle of about 1°50'. Those presented in lateral position extended from about 20' to about 2° 10'.

The subject started each trial by pressing a push button held in the left hand. He responded by operating with his right hand a vertical two-way joystick, located in a median position, which he had to move either away from or towards his body.

A digital timer (Advance Instruments TC-12) was used to measure the reaction time.

Procedure

The subject was instructed to fixate the fixation cross before starting the trial. Channel 2, with a photograph in the centre, was then lit for 300 ms (phase 1). One hundred millisec after its offset, channel 3 (with a photograph left or right of centre) came on for 100 ms (phase 2).

The subject was told to move the joystick in one direction if the second picture represented the same person as the first one, and in the other direction if it represented a different person. The two directions of movement were given opposite meanings for half the subjects (two males and two females) of each group. The timer was started at the beginning of phase 2 and stopped when the joystick was activated.

At the completion of each trial, the subject was told whether his response had been correct and, if 'yes', whether it had been fast or slow — 'fast' meaning faster than the mean of the previous session, for sessions 2–5, or the mean of a group of preliminary trials, on session 1.

Each subject participated in five sessions, a practice session of 120 trials and four experimental sessions of 180 trials each.

Eight subjects, four of either sex, were allocated to one of two groups. The subjects of one group worked under one of two conditions throughout.

In both conditions, the photograph appearing in phase 2, i.e. the one to which the reaction had to be given, was a three-quarter face, either left or right. In condition 'physical identity' the photograph appearing (in the centre) in phase 1 was also a three-quarter face one, in the same orientation. In group 'facial identity' the photograph appearing in phase 1 was full-face. In both groups a 'same' pair was presented on half the trials, a 'different' pair on the other half. From the preceding description, it follows that on 'same face' trials, the two successive photographs were identical in group 'physical identity' but differed by the angle of view in group 'facial identity'.

On experimental sessions 2–5 the order of presentation of the pictures was balanced in such a way that all faces appeared an equal number of times (6), in both phase 1 and phase 2, in each half-session.

Subjects

Sixteen students, all naive regarding the aim of the study, volunteered to participate. They were paid a fixed amount, plus a premium depending on both speed and accuracy.

RESULTS AND DISCUSSION

Mean correct reaction times per condition, side of presentation and judgement category appears in table 33.1, together with error percentages. Individual reaction times are given in figures 33.1 and 33.2

The main result is that a systematic difference in reaction time favouring the left hemifield appears in condition 'facial identity', not in condition 'physical identity'. Individual reaction times were submitted to a three-way analysis of variance, with hemifield and judgement category (same versus different) as within-subjects factors, and condition as between-subjects factor. It revealed a significant condition × hemifield interaction: $F(1;14) = 7.0; P < 0.025$. This outcome thus supports our main prediction: left hemifield superiority is at any rate weaker in condition 'physical identity'.

Since the finding of a significant interaction between systematic factors made the interpretation of main effects impossible, separate analyses were carried out on the data of the two groups of subjects. The effect of side of presentation is found significant in group 'facial identity', $F(1;7) = 18.4; P < 0.005$, not in group 'physical identity', $F(1;7) = 1.2$. In other words, left hemifield superiority is demonstrated in condition 'facial identity' only.

Table 33.1
Mean reaction times, (in ms) per group, hemifield and response category,
with percent errors (in parentheses)

Group	Response category	Hemifield		Difference left–right
		Left	Right	
Facial identity	Same	369 (5%)	375 (5%)	6
	Different	414 (8%)	437 (14%)	23
	Mean	391 (6.5%)	406 (9.5%)	14
Physical identity	Same	331 (4%)	330 (3%)	−1
	Different	370 (6%)	377 (8%)	7
	Mean	350 (5%)	353 (5.5%)	3

Left hemifield superiority occurs at the level of percent errors also. It can be seen in table 33.1 that the subjects of group 'facial identity' made more errors on right- than on left-side presentations. Seven subjects out of eight exhibited that pattern, the eighth showing no difference (7 out of 7 is significant at $P = 0.011$ by a unilateral sign-test). The effect of side of presentation on reaction time appears thus to reflect a genuine change in performance level, and is not obtained by trading off accuracy for speed. Presumably, had the subjects maintained the same accuracy level on right and left hemifield presentations, the difference at the level of reaction times would have been amplified.

So far, we have only considered mean data across the two judgement categories. It appears in the two figures that 'same' responses are systematically faster than 'different' responses. Variance analyses show that the difference is significant in both facial identity, $F (1;7) = 35.4; P < 0.005$, and physical identity, $F (1;7) = 80.7; P < 0.001$, groups. Shorter reaction times for choosing 'same' rather than 'different' responses are a constant feature of comparison tasks, and should thus come as no surprise. A more interesting feature of the data is the fact that in group 'facial identity', hemifield differences tend to be larger for 'different' responses than for 'same' responses: mean left field superiority is 23 ms for 'different' and only 6 ms for 'same' responses. The effect falls short of the 0.05 significance level in the variance analysis (hemifield × type of response interaction: $F (1;7) = 4.07; 0.05 < P < 0.10$). But the corresponding effect is observed at the level of percentage errors, which is larger for the right than for the left visual field in the case of 'different' responses, not for 'same' responses. Following the reasoning of the last paragraph, had the subjects adopted a strategy giving the same error rate for left and right visual fields on 'different' trials, the hemifield × judgement category interaction would presumably have been larger.

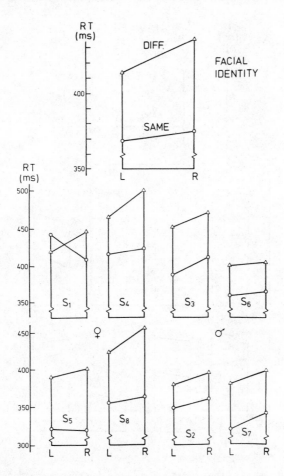

Figure 33.1. Group 'facial identity'. Mean correct reaction times as functions of hemifield (abscissa) and of type of judgement (parameter) for the group as a whole (above) and for each individual subject (below). Female subjects on the left and males on the right

Examination of figure 33.1 shows that there are rather large individual differences in pattern. One subject, S_1, is different from all others in that she exhibits right hemifield superiority for 'same' responses together with left hemifield superiority for 'different' responses. The data were examined for an effect of sex, since Rizzolati and Buchtel (1977) have reported data suggesting that women show lower laterality for faces than men. At the level of mean reaction time, only a small, non-significant, tendency is observed (mean left hemifield superiority = 15.5 ms for men, 10.5 for women). But the main difference is found at the level of the hemifield × type of judgement interaction. The four men give a mean left side superiority of 18 ms for 'different' response against 17 ms for 'same' responses. The corresponding figures for the women are 28 ms and −5 ms. Women appear thus to

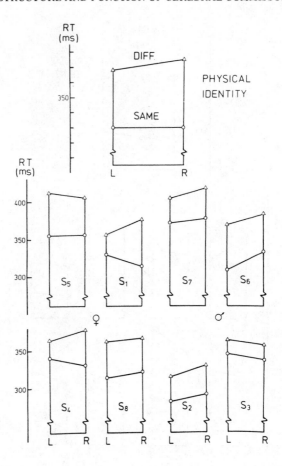

Figure 33.2. Group 'physical identity'. Mean correct reaction times as functions of hemifield (abscissa) and of type of judgement (parameter) for the group as a whole (above) and for each individual subject (below)

be responsible for the interaction observed at the level of mean reaction times. Even if we eliminate subject S_1, who exhibits the crossed interaction which has already been commented on, we find 30 ms and 5 ms for the three remaining female subjects. These observations can, of course, be considered as suggestive only and should be confirmed on a fresh sample of subjects before any interpretation is attempted.

CONCLUSION

The main prediction formulated in the introduction has been supported: left visual hemifield superiority was obtained in the task where the photographs to be compared were always physically different, and not when one of the possible situations was physical identity. The results are thus consistent with the notion that the operations which are performed better in the right hemisphere are concerned with the extraction of physiognomic invariants. Of course, only one of the changes considered in the introduction, change in viewing angle, has been manipulated. The study should obviously be extended to other cases such as change of expression, or as ageing. Such developments may help specify the critical cues and bring us beyond the very abstract 'physiognomic versus non-physiognomic' dichotomy, which is one of the most unsatisfactory aspects of the present attempt.

The observation that, in some subjects at least, lateralisation manifests itself mainly in decisions of difference may however constitute a difficulty for the conclusion. Given that the pictures involved in decisions of sameness were equivalent at the level of physiognomic invariants only, one would have expected left hemifield superiority for these decisions also.

There are two alternative interpretations for the absence of asymmetry on 'same' decisions. One is that the specialisation of the lateralised mechanism does not consist of the extraction of physiognomic invariants, but in a still more narrowly defined operation, is involved in 'different' decisions only. The other interpretation is that the present material did not make the extraction of physiognomic invariants really imperative. Some non-physiognomic cues might still have been valid bases of judgement, in spite of the change of viewing angle, and would have been used as such by some of the subjects. It is impossible to specify which these cues would be, but possible examples are details of haircut such as the presence of a flock or quiff on one side of the forehead. (It is here assumed that these non-physiognomic cues are used for decisions of sameness, but are not considered sufficient for decisions of difference. One may argue that, in this situation, the resistance of these cues to changes in viewing angle is only probabilistic, so that their presence in the second picture is a valid basis for deciding same, while their absence remains equivocal. In the 'physical identity' condition, on the contrary, absence and presence of a cue is equally informative, so that both 'different' and 'same' decisions can be made on the basis of low level visual data.)

While the first interpretation involves a qualification of the main conclusion, the second one keeps the conclusion and blames the material. It is of course impossible to choose between them on the basis of the present data. Further experiments, with more stringent obstacles to the use of non-physiognomic cues, are necessary before a decision can be reached. In the meantime, it is worth noting that Morais and Darwin (1974), in a task involving same–different reactions to lateralised CV syllables, observed right ear advantage for 'different' responses, not for 'same' responses, in spite of the fact that the two successive stimuli to be compared always differed in pitch, and were thus equivalent at a more abstract linguistic level only. A higher sensitivity of 'different' judgements to lateral specialisation might thus not be restricted to the present situation. (It must be noted however that in a same-different task with simultaneously presented schematic faces, Patterson and Bradshaw (1975) found right hemifield superiority for 'different' and left hemifield superiority for 'same' judgements—the opposite from the present interaction.)

After the present data had been gathered, a paper appeared whose results point to the same general conclusion (Moscovitch *et al.*, 1976). In same–different reactions to simultaneously presented 'identikit' pictures which were either identical or very different, no hemifield effect was obtained. But in another same–different task involving comparisons of photographs and caricatures, a clear left field superiority was obtained. This result clearly supports the notion that left hemifield superiority is connected with the extraction of physiognomic invariants. In the same study, it is shown also that left side superiority can be obtained in a 'physical identity' condition if delayed comparisons, imposing the retention of facial information, are used: with successive comparisons of either identical or different pictures, left hemifield superiority was observed with interstimuli intervals of 100 ms or more but not with shorter ones; it was also obtained whatever the interval where the first picture was pattern-masked. The results are in agreement with previous findings of Patterson and Bradshaw (1975). A possible interpretation is that faces are normally memorised in terms of physiognomic features.

With the idea that the lateralised physiognomic mechanism is best observed in tasks which involve either comparisons of different pictures of a same face, or comparisons of a picture to a memorised trace, we are in a position to understand several apparent difficulties in the literature. (The results showed by Rizzolatti, chapter 32 herein, reveal a third condition: asymmetry can be enhanced by shortening stimulus presentation. This manipulation may play a role similar to masking, by making low level visual cues unavailable for the decision.) Left side superiority has been found by authors who used a small constant set of pictures (Geffen *et al.*, 1971; Klein *et al.*, 1976; Moscovitch *et al.*, 1976; Rizzolatti *et al.*, 1971) because the presented picture had to be compared with a memorised face. Familiarity eliminated the effect (Berlucchi *et al.*, 1976) possibly because it made possible thè discovery of valid non-physiognomic cues.

Another difficulty which can now be explained is the result of Milner (1968) who found that right temporal lobe-excised patients were inferior to left ones in a task involving recognition of pictures of faces after a filled or unfilled 90 s interval, not if the recognition test was carried out immediately after presenting the target pictures. She concluded that the difficulty encountered by right temporal patients lies in retaining facial information, not in extracting it. On the other hand, Benton and van Allen (1968), De Renzi *et al.* (1968) and Tzavaras *et al.* (1970) all found right hemisphere patients inferior in tasks involving the matching of simultaneously presented pictures. But the tasks used by these authors involved the matching of different photographs of the same models, whereas in Milner's recognition task the target pictures were identical with those presented immediately before.

ACKNOWLEDGEMENTS

The present work has been partially subsidised by the Belgian 'Fonds de la Recherche fondamentale collective' under convention No. 2.4522.76. The illustrations were kindly supplied by Dr Tony Marcel of the MRC Applied Psychology Unit in Cambridge. Very useful suggestions were made by Dr Daniel Holender.

REFERENCES

Benton, A.L. and van Allen, M.W. (1968). Impairment in facial recognition in patients with cerebral disease. *Cortex*, **4**, 344-58

Berlucchi, G., Marzi, C. A., Rizzolatti, G. and Umiltà, C. (1976). Functional hemisphere asymmetries in normals : influence of sex and practice. Paper at 21st Int. Cong. Psychology, Paris

Bodamer, J. (1947). Die Prosop-Agnosie, *Archs Psychiat.*, **179**(6), 1

De Renzi, E., Faglioni, P. and Spinnler, H. (1968). The performance of patients with unilateral brain damage on face recognition tasks. *Cortex*, **4**, 17-34

Geffen, G., Bradshaw, J. L. and Wallace, G. (1971). Interhemispheric effects on reaction time to verbal and nonverbal visual stimuli. *J. exp. Psychol.*, **87**, 415-22

Gibson, E. J. (1969). *Principles of Perceptual Learning and Development*, Appleton-Century-Crofts, New York, pp. 105-107

Gilbert, C. A. and Bakan, P. (1973). Visual asymmetry in perception of faces. *Neuropsychologia*, **11**, 355-62

Hecaen, H. and Angelergues, R. (1962). Agnosia for faces (prosopagnosia). *Archs Neurol.*, **7**, 92-100

Hilliard, R. D. (1973). Hemispheric laterality effects on a facial recognition task in normal subjects. *Cortex*, **9**, 246-58

Hochberg, J. (1972). The representation of things and people. In *Art, Perception and Reality* (E. H. Gombrich, J. Hochberg and M. Black, eds.), Johns Hopkins University Press, Baltimore, pp. 47-96

Klein, D., Moscovitch, M. and Vigna, C. (1976). Attentional mechanisms and perceptual asymmetries in tachistoscopic recognition of words and faces. *Neuropsychologia*, **14**, 55-66

Marcel, T. and Rajan, P. (1975). Lateral specialisation for recognition of words and faces in good and poor readers. *Neuropsychology*, **13**, 489-97

Meadows, J. C. (1974). The anatomical basis of prosopagnosia. *J. Neurol. Neurosurg. Psychiatry* **37**, 489-501

Milner, B. (1968). Visual recognition and recall after right temporal-lobe excision in man. *Neuropsychologia*, **6**, 191-209

Morais, J. and Darwin, C. J. (1974). Ear differences for same–different reaction times to monaurally presented speech. *Brain Lang.*, **1**, 383-90

Moscovitch, M., Scullion, D. and Christie, D. (1976). Early vs late stages of processing and their relation to functional hemispheric asymmetries in face recognition. *J. exp. Psychol.: Hum. Perc. Perform.*, **2**, 401-16

Patterson, K. and Bradshaw, J. L. (1975). Differential hemispheric mediation of non-verbal visual stimuli. *J. exp. Psychol.: Hum. Perc. Perform.*, **1**, 246-52

Rizzolatti, G. and Buchtel, H. A. (1977). Hemispheric superiority in reaction time to faces : a sex difference. *Cortex*, **13**, 300-305

Rizzolatti, G., Umiltà, C. and Berlucchi, G. (1971). Opposite superiorities of the right and left cerebral hemispheres in discriminative reaction time to physiognomical and alphabetical material. *Brain*, **94**, 431–42

Rondot, P. and Tzavaras, A. (1969). La prosopagnosie après vingt années d'études cliniques et neuropsychologiques. *J. Psychol. Norm. Pathol.*, **9**, 133–65

Teuber, H. L. (1974). Why two brains? In *The Neurosciences*, 3rd Study Program (F. O. Schmitt and F. G. Worden, eds.) M.I.T. Press, Cambridge, Mass.

Tzavaras, A., Hecaen, H. and Le Bras, H. (1970). Le problème de la spécificité du déficit de la reconnaissance du visage humain lors des lésions hémisphériques unilatérales. *Neuropsychologia,* **8**, 403–16

Warrington, E. K. and James, M. (1967). An experimental investigation of facial recognition in patients with unilateral cerebral lesions. *Cortex*, **3**, 317–26

Wolff, W. (1933). The experimental study of forms of expression. *Char. Personal.*, **2** 168–76

Yin, R. K. (1969). Looking at upside-down faces. *J. exp. Psychol.*, **81**, 141–45

Yin, R. K. (1970). Face recognition by brain injured patients : a dissociable ability. *Neuropsychologia,* **8**, 395–402

34
CONSCIOUSNESS AFTER COMPLETE SURGICAL SECTION OF THE FORE - BRAIN COMMISSURES IN MAN

BRUNO PREILOWSKI

INTRODUCTION

For several years I have been concerned with a certain aspect of consciousness, i.e. the ability of self-reference by recognising self-attributions or photographs of one-self. In the following I shall present some results of attempts to test for this capacity in both hemispheres of 'split-brain' patients. In doing so, I shall include some observations made in preliminary tests with only one subject (NG), who has been described as one of the patients most representative of the disconnection syndrome (Sperry *et al.*, 1969). I think that these observations illustrate the difficulties in testing commissurotomy patients, which in turn tells something about the hemisphere functions in these patients.

In a first series of tests the standard procedure for investigating interhemispheric integration in 'split-brain' patients was used (Sperry *et al.*, 1969). Stimuli were projected for 0.1 s or less on to a rear-projection screen to the right and left of a centrally located red dot, on which the subject had to fixate with the dominant eye. The other eye was covered with an eye patch. Different colour slides of faces, including that of the patient and those of persons whom she knew quite well, were presented four times in a counterbalanced order, alternating right and left visual field presentations according to a Gellermann series (Gellermann, 1933). The patient was asked to indicate self-recognition by lifting the index finger of either hand, and later to describe what she had seen.

During the first sessions it was apparent that NG had difficulties in following the instructions; at times she would respond only to right visual field presenta-tions, but here to all stimuli. Also, several times, she asked the experimenter to repeat the instruction because she had forgotten what she was supposed to do. These difficulties were reduced as long as NG could be kept from giving a running commentary during testing, restricting verbal output to merely naming what she had seen. Under such conditions responses were made also to left visual field stimulation. However, responses to particular familiar faces were made at the same rate as those to her own face. None of these faces was correctly identified verbally. When asked to name what she had seen after left visual field stimulation, she either stated 'nothing' or 'a flash of light', and twice 'rocks' was given as the answer. With right visual field presentations familiar faces were described as 'a woman's face'. Her own picture, she thought, was that of a technical assistant, whose face actually was among the familiar faces presented in the same series.

The results pointed to two problems: because of the difficulties of the left hemisphere in recognising faces with brief visual exposures, reactions of this hemisphere no longer constituted a control for self-recognition. Secondly, on the basis of the finger signal, responses of correct self-recognition could not be distinguished from responses made merely on the basis of familiarity.

In previous unrelated tests of emotional arousal I had found that by showing a subject a picture of his own face rather dramatic skin resistance changes (GSRs) could be elicited, which were relatively resistant to habituation, in comparison with other visual stimuli.

I therefore repeated the above-mentioned experiment using the GSR and a heart-rate measure. A similar series of colour slides as before was presented six times to each visual field, with the same controls for order of stimuli and alternation of visual fields as in the previous experiment. This time, besides including faces of an unknown and a well-known person to control for effects of familiarity, slides of a surgical wound, of a red rose, and of scenery, as well as slides with red and orange colour filters, were interspersed in the series to control for general emotional arousal.

Besides NG, four female staff members (ages ranging from 25 to 41) were tested as controls. One of the controls suffered from rather severe cerebral palsy and her responses were analysed separately.

The GSR was recorded on an Offner polygraph together with the ECG, to determine heart rate, and breathing was recorded to control for artefacts. On the same record a signal from the projector indicated when a stimulus was presented. As a further control videotapes were made of the subjects' behaviour during testing.

Skin resistance changes were measured as a voltage drop between lead electrodes, which were taped to the palmar surface of the middle phalanges of middle and ring finger of the left hand. An a.c. measurement technique ($10 \mu A$, 3 Hz) was employed to avoid the influence of d.c. potential changes at the electrodes (Strong, 1970). The ECG was taken from the upper arms and left leg, to be able to determine heart rate from the R-wave to R-wave interval. Breathing was measured with an air-bellows strapped around the chest and a pressure transducer system.

The GSR was determined by measuring the largest deflection from the baseline within 10 s after stimulus onset. Since the average GSR to six preceding blank trials (slides with grey filters) was 300 Ω, only responses with values greater than 300 Ω were included in the analysis.

The results for the GSR measure are summarised in figure 34.1, which in the upper part shows the mean change in skin resistance for the three normal controls, for the control suffering from cerebral palsy, and for the 'split-brain' patient

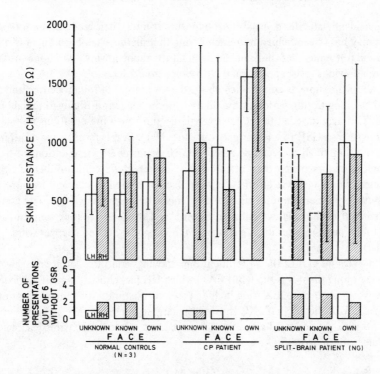

Figure 34.1. Average skin resistance changes to slides of faces presented to the left hemisphere (left column) and to the right hemisphere (right column) of three normal controls, a person suffering from cerebral palsy (CP) and a 'split-brain' patient (NG). In the lower part of the figure the number of presentations within six repetitions not followed by a GSR of at least 300 Ω is shown (data for normal controls are averaged)

(NG) in response to right and left visual field presentations of the face slides. While for each subject the largest single GSR was to her own photograph, because of the large variability of responses with repeated presentations the average responses only show a trend towards a differentiation between a familiar face and the subject's own face.

Results for presentations of the unknown and well-known face to the left hemisphere of NG are shown in bars with dotted outlines, since under these conditions only one response was observed to each slide. NG was unable to identify verbally any of the faces whether presented to the left or the right visual field. Videotape recordings showed an occasional frown or raising of the eyebrows with left visual field presentations of her own face, but she reported to have seen only flashes of light.

All of the controls stated that they had seen themselves. They also were able to give the name of the person belonging to the familiar face. However, from their reports it was apparent that they did not recognise the faces, including their own, every time. Although generally worse than the highly trained 'split-brain' patients in perceiving lateralised visual short-exposure stimuli, their recognition in this test may have been helped by remembering that pictures had been taken of them. NG did not remember that she had been photographed, which was done prior to the previous tests, approximately five months earlier.

All of the subjects complained about the monotony of the procedure and felt that the long testing period in the dimly lit room made it difficult to remain attentive. This may have led to the relatively large number of presentations not followed by a GSR (see lower part of figure 34.1). In this respect it is of interest to note that, in all subjects, responses to right hemisphere presentations of the subject's own face were least affected. Put a different way, the number of GSRs greater than 300 Ω was larger to the own face presented to the right hemisphere than to any other stimulus–visual field combination (see table 34.1). The non-facial control slides showed no significant GSRs after their first presentation. As far as the heart-rate results are concerned, no stimulus related changes were observed.

In a second part of the experiment line drawings and three-letter words were used. Among them was the word FAT, which NG had chosen as a self-attribute. The words DAY and SEX were included as control stimuli for general emotional arousal. With these stimuli NG showed the largest reaction to the self-attribute, both with right and left hemisphere presentations, while the controls reacted stronger to the word SEX.

Table 34.1
Total number of presentations followed by a GSR
greater than 300 Ω

Stimulus	Hemisphere	
	left	right
Unknown face	11	12
Well-known face	10	13
Own face	12	16

Note: There were 18 possible responses, including those from the 'split-brain' patient, the CP control and the mean number of responses from the three normal controls.

Two years later another experiment was run in which two 'split-brain' patients, NG and LB, were confronted with several different pictures of themselves, of faces of relatives, political personalities and unknown persons, as well as pictures of objects and pets, some of which belonged to the patients' households (for the description of the neurological status of these patients see Bogen and Vogel, 1975). For NG faces of babies and for LB pictures of semi-nudes were used as additional control stimuli for general emotional arousal.

The experiment was run in collaboration with Eran Zaidel, using his technique to achieve long-duration exposure of visual stimuli to only one hemisphere. This is accomplished through the use of a miniature collimator mounted on a contact lens, which is custom made for each subject and held to the eye by minimal suction. Through another lens system fixed above a working table anything visible on the table surface is projected through the collimator and the pupil. Covering one-half of the collimator opening prevents visual stimuli from reaching one hemi-retina without greatly restricting visual scanning with that eye. The other eye is covered with an eye patch (for details see Zaidel, 1973, 1975).

Four to nine black-and-white picture of various sizes were arranged on 20 cm × 25 cm large cards. On some cards the emotional stimuli, familiar objects and familiar faces, as well as the patients' own pictures, appeared together with other photographs of objects and faces. Two cards were prepared for each patient, containing four different pictures of them alone. There was a total of 16 cards shown twice to LB and 12 cards shown three times to NG in a counterbalanced order. Right and left hemispheres were tested on separate days, right hemisphere first. The patients had to look at the pictures on each card successively while the experimenter slowly pointed them out. They were then asked to point to a picture they liked best, to one they liked least, and to one that looked familiar. Occasionally, they were asked to name what they had pointed to.

GSR and basal skin resistance (BSR) were recorded from the middle and ring fingers of both hands separately with Beckman biopotential electrodes (diameter 11 mm) and a Beckman GSR/BSR coupler type 9842. A constant current of 10 μA and a time constant of 1s was used. Breathing was measured with a strain gauge around the chest and Beckman coupler 9853A. All signals were recorded on an Offner polygraph, on which the presentations of the stimuli were also marked. A protocol was kept by a technical assistant, and audiotape recordings were made during all four testing sessions. Again the amplitude of the GSR was measured, taking the largest deflection from the baseline during the presentation of each stimulus card, i.e. before pointing and speaking by the subject occurred.

Recordings from left and right hand of each subject showed some differences in the GSR, which were independent of electrode resistance and recording channel, and also did not appear to vary systematically with BSR differences between the hands. A detailed evaluation of lateral GSR differences, however, has not been done. Instead, only the record showing the largest overall GSRs was analysed, for NG in both sessions from the hand contralateral to the stimulated hemisphere, for LB both times from the right hand.

Figure 34.2 presents the average GSR reactions to the three groups of stimulus cards of main interest, i.e. those containing emotional and personal objects, familiar faces and faces of the patients themselves. As in the previous experiment the largest single responses were registered to their own face when presented to the right hemipshere. Even the averaged responses quite clearly indicate differences in reactions to their own face and to the other stimuli.

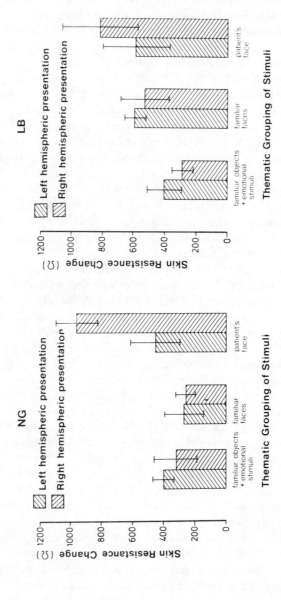

Figure 34.2. Average skin resistance changes to repeated presentations of pictures presented for prolonged periods to left and right hemispheres of two 'split-brain' patients (LB and NG)

When presented to the right visual field all pictures were verbally identified correctly. In the left visual field, on the other hand, NG was unable to describe correctly any stimulus except some of her own photographs, and this with some hesitation and uncertainty.

During right and left hemisphere testing NG showed quite different behaviours, with less verbal activity and more giggles and laughs during the right hemisphere session.

A similar, although much less marked, difference between both testing sessions was noticed in the verbal behaviour of LB, with more verbal comments during the left hemisphere session and mostly short, almost trite, answers during the right hemisphere testing. Nevertheless, in the latter session LB was able verbally to identify more of his own photographs than was NG, as well as the picture of his brother, his pet cat and dog, and his family's old car. Some of the verbal responses were preceded by left-hand tracing motions—a cross-cueing mechanism used quite often by LB during right hemisphere tests.

DISCUSSION

The demonstration of recognition of the patients' own face in pictures presented to both hemispheres means that still another aspect of consciousness has to be attributed to the 'mute, minor' hemisphere. As I described briefly at the beginning, this hemisphere also shows perceptions, it memorises, learns and directs actions, ranging from tactile explorations to conceptual categorisations, and to expressions of typically human emotions. And, all of this takes place outside of the awareness of the left hemisphere. Therefore, it is difficult to deny consciousness to the right half of the forebrain merely on the basis of a relative lack of speech.

Sperry even considers the right hemisphere to be a separate 'conscious system in its own right': 'The two disconnected hemispheres exhibit such independent properties and distinct mental capacities that we come to think of each hemisphere as having a separate mind of its own' (Sperry, 1976, p. 18). Sperry's conviction that both hemispheres are simultaneously and independently conscious is determined by his definition of consciousness as a 'functional property of the brain in action' (Sperry, 1966, p. 311). Furthermore, 'subjective awareness is conceived to be an emergent property of neural events generated at top levels in the brain hierarchy. The emergent (subjective) properties are conceived to have causal consequences in cerebral activity' (Sperry, 1976, p. 13).

If consciousness is defined not in terms of what it is, but rather in terms of particular aspects of observable behaviour, then in many situations the hemispheres of 'split-brain' patients do not appear to function completely independently. When cerebral cortical control is required bilateral functions show deficits in comparison with unilateral ability. This can be found in bilateral motor functions (for a review see Preilowski, 1975a), or bilateral stimulus conditions (e.g. Levy et al., 1972; Trevarthen, 1974).

A good example is the minor hemisphere dominance in a language-related task which involves the identification of tactually perceived letters and words: with vision excluded, various plastic letters were presented simultaneously to both hands, forming different words for each hand. These words then had to be pointed out when presented together with other words on lists printed in matching capital letters or written in script. Although no lateral differences were found during separate unilateral tests, with simultaneous presentation to both hands a right hemisphere dominance became apparent regardless of which hand was used in pointing or which transformation, e.g. from block letters to script, was required. It is especially important to note that the highly accurate retrieval of the left-hand stimuli in this test occurred together with a nearly total neglect of the right-hand stimuli.

In view of such data, the claims of a doubling of functional capacity following brain bisection (Gazzaniga, 1968; Gazzaniga and Young, 1967) appear questionable. Rather, in most complex behaviours, like behaviour involving decision processes, the 'split-brain' organism is still dependent upon a unified system. Deficits in complex bilateral tasks even point to a reduction in the effectiveness of this system due to a loss of part of its unifying structures.

As mentioned above, the reduction in efficiency is particularly apparent in tasks requiring simultaneous processing of stimuli and subsequent responses from both hemispheres. In testing the patients, I have however frequently noted—although not specifically investigated—that when a rapid or unpredictable change of stimulus input from one hemisphere to the other occurs, requiring a changeover of decision and action control between the hemispheres, the patients appear to have some problems. These problems do not appear as specific deficits but rather as a general obstacle during testing. The difficulties observed in giving finger signals of self-recognition, which finally led to the application of the GSR technique, may be an example of such a problem.

On the basis of extensive tests of visual behaviour and attentional mechanisms in the 'split-brain' patient, Trevarthen has convincingly demonstrated the importance of a unified subcortical control for active orientation. He differentiates these active selection processes from the 'relatively passive processes of immediate visual storage which may occur separately in two disconnected hemispheres, just as they may do for any two different areas of the visual field of the normal subject' (Trevarthen, 1974, p.250).

SUMMARY AND CONCLUSION

I have tried to show that, by using specific definitions of consciousness, a lot can be learned about it from the results of 'split-brain' research. The experiments of Sperry and his co-workers show that working within the confines of such definitions does not mean a restriction to trivial aspects of consciousness; I am however unable to say whether this approach can be extended to arrive at a final comprehensive and comprehensible description of the nature of consciousness itself, as Sperry has proposed for a long time (Sperry, 1952, 1966, 1968, 1969, 1970, 1976).

Summarising the present state of affairs, I would think that it has been conclusively shown that both hemispheres contribute to consciousness, if it is defined as the capacity to show higher order cognitive processes, typically human emotions and self-recognition. This consciousness is divided and doubled in the sense that these functions can take place in each hemisphere separately and independently, but not doubled in the sense of a duplication of functional capacity. Rather, the loss of direct hemispheric interconnections seems to affect the functional capacity negatively, although not to the extent that it would seriously alter general behaviour.

On the other hand, as long as we consider consciousness as wakefulness or attention separated from the rest of brain functions, the 'split-brain' individual possesses a unified consciousness. If we avoid this rather artificial distinction, then the individual possesses a doubled consciousness to the extent to which cerebral hemispheric and subcortical areas are seen as the organic substrate of functions included in our definition of consciousness.

Tying consciousness closely to the functions of the brain also implies that different lateralised inputs to each hemisphere would lead to a divergent development of functions in these hemispheres, as long as the critical neuro-anatomical substrate of these functions is found in both disconnected hemispheres and this substrate would possess functional plasticity, in the sense of allowing for learning to occur.

ACKNOWLEDGEMENTS

The experiments on self-recognition were conducted in 1971/72 and 1974 while the author was a postdoctoral fellow at the Psychobiology Laboratory of Professor R. W. Sperry at the California Institute of Technology. I am greatly indebted to Professor Sperry for his continued interest, encouragement and support. I also would like to thank Dr E. Zaidel for making the experiment with long duration lateralised stimulation possible. I am also grateful for technical assistance received by G. G. Gray, C. E. Johnson, P. Jonkhoff, L. MacBird and U.-A. Preilowski during the various experiments. Last but not least, I would like to thank Professors Bogen and Vogel for permission to examine their patients. (Financial support was provided through N.I.M.H. Grant MH 03372 to Professor Sperry and University of Konstanz Grant 38/73.)

REFERENCES

Bogen, J. E. and Vogel, P. J. (1975). Neurologic status in the long term following complete cerebral commissurotomy. In *Les syndromes de disconnexion calleuse chez l'homme* (F. Michel and B. Schott, eds.), Hôpital Neurologique, Lyon

Gazzaniga, M. S. (1968). Short-term memory and brain-bisected man. *Psychonomic Sci.* **12**, 161-2

Gazzaniga, M. S. and Young, E. D. (1967). Effects of commissurotomy on the processing of increased visual information. *Expl Brain Res., 3*, 368-71

Gellermann, L. W. (1933). Chance orders of alternating stimuli in visual discrimination experiments. *J. genet. Psychol., 42*, 206-208

Levy, J., Trevarthen, C. and Sperry, R. W. (1972). Perception of bilateral chimeric figures following hemispheric deconnection. *Brain, 95*, 61-78

Preilowski, B. (1975a). Bilateral motor interaction: perceptual-motor performance of partial and complete 'split-brain' patients. In *Cerebral Localization*, (K. J. Zülch, O. Creutzfeldt and G. C. Galbraith, eds.), Springer, Berlin

Preilowski, B. (1975b). Facial self-recognition after separate right and left hemisphere stimulation in two patients with complete cerebral commissurotomy. *Expl Brain Res., 23* (suppl.), 165

Sperry, R. W. (1952). Neurology and the mind-brain problem. *Am. Scient., 40*, 291-312

Sperry, R. W. (1966). Brain bisection and mechanisms of consciousness. In *Brain and Conscious Experience* (J. C. Eccles, ed.), Springer, New York

Sperry, R. W. (1968). Hemisphere deconnection and unity in conscious awareness. *Am. Psychol., 23*, 723-33

Sperry, R. W. (1969). A modified concept of consciousness. *Psychol. Rev., 76*, 532-36

Sperry, R. W. (1970). An objective approach to subjective experience: further explanation of a hypothesis. *Psychol. Rev., 77*, 585-90

Sperry, R. W. (1976). Changing concepts of consciousness and free will. *Pers. Biol. Med., 20*, 9-19.

Sperry, R. W., Gazzaniga, M. S. and Bogen, J. E. (1969). Interhemispheric relationships: the neocortical commissures; syndromes of hemisphere disconnection. In *Handbook of Clinical Neurology*, vol. IV (P. J. Vinken and G. W. Bruyn, eds.), North-Holland, Amsterdam

Strong, P. (1970). *Biophysical Measurements*, Tektronix Inc., Beaverton, Oregon

Trevarthen, C. (1974). Analysis of cerebral activities that generate and regulate consciousness in commissurotomy patients. In *Hemisphere Function in the Human Brain*, (S. J. Dimond and J. G. Beaumont, eds.), Elek, London

Zaidel, E. (1973). Linguistic competence and related functions in the right cerebral hemisphere of man following commissurotomy and hemispherectomy. Unpubl. doct. dissert., California Institute of Technology

Zaidel, E. (1975). A technique for presenting lateralized visual input with prolonged exposure. *Vision Res., 15*, 283-89

35

INTERHEMISPHERIC MODULATION OF LIGHT DIFFERENCE THRESHOLD IN THE PERIPHERY OF THE VISUAL FIELD

JOSEF ZIHL, DETLEV VON CRAMON,
ERNST PÖPPEL and WOLF SINGER

The distribution of light difference threshold throughout the visual field has been said to be mirrored rather exactly by the distribution of ganglion cells throughout the retina (e.g. Pöppel and Harvey, 1973). The close correlation between psychophysical results and anatomical data has suggested the hypothesis that light difference threshold is primarily determined by retinal mechanisms. Here we present evidence that light difference threshold can also be strongly influenced by non-retinal factors. Specifically we would like to suggest that light difference threshold at a given retinal location can be modulated by interhemispheric interactions which are most likely taking place at the subcortical level. A more extensive report of these observations has been published elsewhere (Singer *et al.*, 1977).

Light difference threshold was measured using the Tübinger perimeter (Sloan, 1971). The subject fixated a 30′ red fixation point presented in a centre of a homogeneously illuminated sphere (1 mL, low photopic range). Targets with either 27′ or 116′ visual angle and 500 ms duration were presented along the horizontal meridian at a defined eccentricity. One eye was covered by an opaque occluder. A psychophysical method of lower limits was used to determine the decremental light difference threshold; subsequent intensity levels differed by 0.1 log units.

When thresholds were measured in rapid succession at a given position, for instance at 30° eccentricity, a clear increase in threshold by as much as half a log unit is observed (figure 35.1). The main adaptation effect occurs within the first minutes of testing. If threshold measurements are discontinued it takes approximately 10 min until the original level of sensitivity is reached again.

The next experimental step was to decide whether the observed adaptation is a retinal or a non-retinal phenomenon. In order to answer this question it was tested whether adaptation would transfer between the two eyes. Adaptation was at first produced by successive threshold determination in the temporal visual

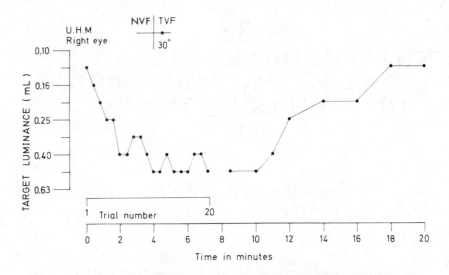

Figure 35.1. Change of sensitivity during successive determination of decrement threshold
at one position in the visual field. A stationary target with 116′ diameter was flashed
for 500 ms at an eccentricity of 30° along the horizontal meridian in the temporal visual
field (TVF) of the right eye. Abscissa: time in minutes starting with the beginning of
threshold measurements. Ordinate: target luminance, in mL, necessary to evoke a response.
Within the first 7 min, 20 thresholds were determined using approximately 150 target
presentations. The time course of *adaptation* indicates that after approximately 4 min a
stable sensitivity level is obtained. The recovery of decrement threshold was determined by
measurements at variable intervals after the adaptation series. As can be seen, it takes
approximately 10 min until the pre-adaptation sensitivity is reached again

field of the right eye. Then the right eye was occluded and it was tested whether
decrement threshold at the corresponding retinal point in the left eye was the same
as before (control measurement) or whether it had adapted as well. As can be
seen in figure 35.2, one gets an almost complete transfer of adaptation between the
two eyes. Thus the observed adaptation must be (at least in part) non-retinal.

Previously, Pöppel and Richards (1974) have suggested a mirror-symmetric
interaction between the two hemispheres at the mesencephalic level; this hypothesis
was derived from observations with brain-injured patients who showed a decrease
of light difference threshold at a mirror-symmetric position of a small cortical
scotoma in the visual field. On the basis of these observations the question was
asked whether light difference threshold and the course of adaptation can be
influenced by visual stimulation at a mirror-symmetric position in the contralateral
half-field. The result of such an experiment is shown in figure 35.3.

At first, adaptation was produced measuring successively threshold at 30°
eccentricity in the temporal visual field of the right eye. A stable level of adaptation
that is kept for a few minutes (figure 35.3, phases I and II) can be seen. Following
these measurements that led to an increase of light difference threshold by

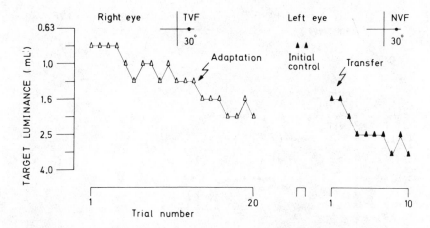

Figure 35.2. Binocular transfer of the adaptation effect. Abscissa: trial number of successive decrement threshold measurements. Ordinate: target luminance, in mL. Stimulus: 27', 500 ms. At first, decrement threshold was determined at 30° eccentricity along the horizontal meridian in the nasal visual field (NVF) of the left eye ('initial control'). It followed an adaptation series in the TVF of the right eye at 30° eccentricity ('adaptation'). Then decrement threshold was again measured in the NVF of the left eye, and an almost perfect interocular transfer of the adaptation was observed. Thus, the change in sensitivity observed during successive determination of decrement threshold must be non-retinal

approximately half a log unit, threshold was measured at 30° eccentricity in the nasal visual field of the right eye, i.e. at the mirror-symmetric position (Figure 35.3, phase III). Immediately after these mirror-symmetric measurements light difference threshold was again determined at 30° eccentricity in the temporal visual field (figure 35.3, phase IV). The mirror-symmetric measurement has produced a rather dramatic effect. As can be seen, threshold is immediately reset to its original pre-adaptation level, or even lower, i.e. adaptation is immediately cancelled. Such a resetting does not occur when thresholds are determined during phase III at areas non-symmetric to the previously tested location (cf. Singer et al., 1977).

Presumably the presentation produced by successive measurements at one position in the visual field is cancelled on the basis of disinhibiting or facilitating mechanisms that operate in a mirror-symmetric interhemispheric fashion. The resetting of threshold cannot be explained by a spontaneous recovery; the two-minute break between phases I and II, that corresponds roughly in time to phase III, does not indicate a change of adaptation; thus the resetting must be due to the interhemispheric interaction.

Several observations suggest that subcortical centres play an essential role in processing visual information in the human visual system (e.g. Perenin and Jeannerod, 1975; Pöppel et al., 1973; Richards, 1973; Weiskrantz et al., 1974), specifically in that they may participate in the programming of saccadic eye movements (Frost and Pöppel, 1976). It is therefore of interest to find out whether the resetting of

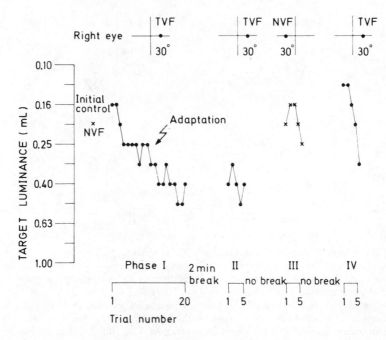

Figure 35.3. Resetting of the adaptation effect measuring of decrement threshold at a mirror-symmetric position in the contralateral visual hemifield. Abscissa: trial number of successive decrement threshold measurements. Ordinate: target luminance, in mL. Stimulus: 27′, 500 ms. At first a control measurement was obtained in the NVF of the right eye at 30° eccentricity. Then, central adaptation was provoked through 20 successive measurements of decrement threshold at 30° eccentricity in the TVF of the right eye. As can be seen, the adaptation effect was still present after a break of 2 min. It followed five measurements of decrement threshold at 30° eccentricity of the NVF at the mirror-symmetric position of the adaptation locus. Apparently as a consequence of these measurements, decrement threshold at 30° eccentricity of the TVF is reset immediately by approximately half a log unit to its pre-adaptation level, possibly even lower

light difference threshold is due to interhemispheric interactions at the cortical or at the subcortical level. In order to investigate this question, experiments with patients who had suffered lesions of the central visual pathways were performed. In figure 35.4 the result of such an experiment in one patient is demonstrated. At first adaptation was produced by successive measurements of light different threshold at 30° eccentricity. As this patient had his hemianopsia on the right side, adaptation was obtained in the left hemi-field. As can be seen, a clear adaptation lasting at least several minutes was obtained. Then (figure 35.4, phase III) a point in the 'blind' area of the visual field was stimulated (30°, nasal visual field); the patient was unable to 'see' these targets. As a result of this target presentation in the 'blind' visual field, light difference threshold was reset immediately to its pre-adaptation level as in the normal subjects. It has therefore to be concluded that the

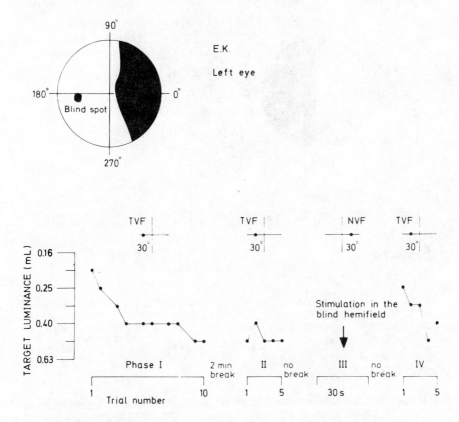

Figure 35.4. Resetting of the adaptation effect by stimulation of the blind area as determined by perimetry. Top: visual field of a patient who suffered a lesion of the central visual pathways; a hemianopsia is seen on the right side of the visual field sparing a strip of vision along the vertical meridian. Bottom: successive measurements of decrement threshold at 30° eccentricity in the TVF of the left eye indicate a clear adaptation effect which is still present after a break of 2 min. After phases I and II of the experiment the mirror-symmetric locus of the visual field within the hemianopic area (30°, NVF) was stimulated; the patient detected none of the targets. Although the patient did not 'see' the targets, this manipulation resulted in an immediate resetting of decrement threshold at 30° eccentricity of the TVF. Thus, resetting most likely involves non-cortical pathways.

interhemispheric interaction takes place at the subcortical level because the more central visual centres have been destroyed.

A control experiment with a patient who had suffered a compression of the left optic tract indicates no interhemispheric modulation of light difference threshold (figure 35.5). As can be seen, a similar adaptation as in the other patient, lasting at least for a few minutes, is obtained. The mirror-symmetric stimulation, however, does not result in a resetting of light difference threshold. This is strong evidence that the observed adaptation is a central phenomenon and not the result

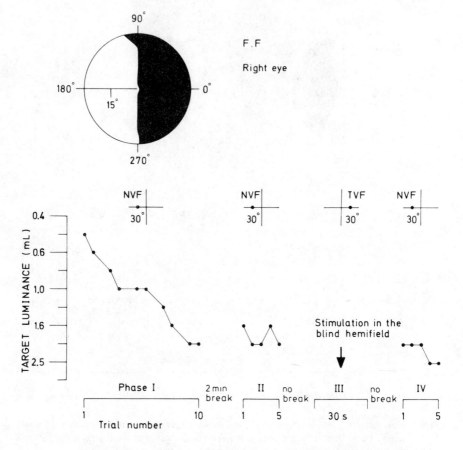

Figure 35.5. Failure of resetting the adaptation effect in a patient who suffered a pre-geniculate lesion. Top: visual field of the right eye of a patient with a compression of the left optic tract showing a hemianopsia on the right side. Bottom: phases I and II show the adaptation effect. In phase II the mirror-symmetric locus (TVF, 30°) was stimulated, but this stimulation did not result in a resetting of decrement threshold (phase IV)

of a change in retinal sensitivity, and it can also not be accounted for by stray-light effects.

The data presented here suggest that light difference threshold can be influenced by non-retinal factors. It appears to be likely that this modulation of threshold is partly due to neuronal activity at the midbrain level. The presence of resetting in patients with 'cortical blindness' leaves no doubt that non-cortical areas in the human brain are engaged in visual information processing; these experiments can thus be viewed as independent control experiments for the initial reports on residual vision (Pöppel et al., 1973).

The interhemispheric interaction presumably taking place at the midbrain level appears to be related to effects described by Sprague (1966). His observations on the cat visual system suggested a facilitory action of each visual cortex on its ipsilateral superior colliculus and an inhibitory interaction between the two colliculi. Our observations can add to this that the interhemispheric interaction at the midbrain level in the human visual system is organised with a clear retinotopy, i.e. in a mirror-symmetric fashion.

ACKNOWLEDGEMENT

This work was supported by Deutsche Forschungsgemeinschaft.

REFERENCES

Frost, D. and Pöppel, E. (1976). Different programming modes of human saccadic eye movements as a function of stimulus eccentricity: indications of a functional subdivision of the visual field. *Biol. Cybernetics,* **23**, 39-48

Perenin, M. T. and Jeannerod, M. (1975). Residual vision in cortically blind hemifields. *Neuropsychologia,* **13**, 1-7

Pöppel, E. and Harvey, L. H., Jr. (1973). Light difference threshold and subjective brightness in the periphery of the visual field. *Psychol. Forschung,* **36**, 145-61

Pöppel, E. and Richards, W. (1974). Light sensitivity in cortical scotoma contralateral to small islands of blindness. *Expl. Brain Res.,* **21**, 125-30

Pöppel, E., Held, R. and Frost, D. (1973). Residual visual function after brain wounds involving the central visual pathways in man. *Nature (Lond.),* **243**, 295-96

Richards, W. (1973). Visual processing in scotomata. *Expl Brain Res.,* **17**, 333-47

Singer, W., Zihl, J. and Pöppel, E. (1977). Subcortical control of visual threshold in humans: evidence for modality specific and retinotopically organized mechanisms of selective attention. *Expl Brain Res.,* **29**, 173-90

Sloan, L. L. (1971). The Tübinger perimeter of Harms and Aulhorn. *Archs Ophthal.,* **86**, 612-22

Sprague, J. M. (1966). Interaction of cortex and superior colliculus in mediation of visually guided behavior in the cat. *Science,* **153**, 1544-47

Weiskrantz, L., Warrington, E. K., Sanders, M. D. and Marshall, J. (1974). Visual capacity in the hemianopic field following a restricted occipital ablation. *Brain,* **97**, 709-28

36

A REVIEW OF BEHAVIOURAL STUDIES OF AGENESIS OF THE CORPUS CALLOSUM

A. D. MILNER and M. A. JEEVES

INTRODUCTION

Psychological investigations of the consequences of surgical section of the cerebral commissures over the past 15 years have yielded some dramatic and thought-provoking findings (Sperry, 1968a). It is in the light of those studies, carried out predominantly with the patients of Bogen and Vogel (1962), that a renewed interest in the unusual neurological condition of congenital absence of the corpus callosum has been kindled. These patients present an intriguing picture which is in most respects very different from that typical of surgical 'split-brain' patients. Studies of the latter during the 1960s established a clear and internally consistent 'disconnection syndrome' which led Sperry (1968c) to the conclusion that 'these patients behave in many ways as if they have two independent streams of conscious awareness, one in each hemisphere, each of which is cut off from and out of contact with the mental experiences of the other'. But the same author, following a series of comparable tests carried out upon a congenitally acallosal subject (Saul and Sperry, 1968), found 'not one of the numerous symptoms of cerebral disconnection exhibited by the surgical cases under exactly the same testing conditions (Sperry, 1968b, p. 311).

In the present review, then, we shall take as our template the relatively securely based findings from studies of commissurotomy patients and examine the results of experimental studies of complete agenesis concerned with the interhemispheric integration of sensory input through the modalities of sight, touch and hearing. Studies of bimanual co-ordination and skilled performance will form a separate section, and will be followed by a discussion of possible mechanisms of neural and behavioural compensation which may help to account for the lack of behavioural deficits on many tasks.

THE ACALLOSAL BRAIN

The corpus callosum originates in the commissural part of the primitive lamina terminalis, and its growth seems to be correlated with the maturation of particular

428

cortical areas (e.g. Hewitt, 1962). Depending on the embryological stage at which a developmental arrest occurs, there may be partial or complete agenesis of the corpus callosum, associated with the presence or absence of other commissures. Complete agenesis of the corpus callosum seems more often than not to be accompanied by an intact anterior commissure, and is not necessarily associated with absence of the hippocampal commissure (Loeser and Alvord, 1968). After reviewing some developmental and clinical aspects of agenesis of the corpus callosum and presenting their own study of 12 autopsied cases these authors conclude that 'agenesis of the corpus callosum is one manifestation of dysgenesis of the telencephalic midline structures and that the concomitants of this malformation are explicable if their embryogenesis is considered'. They concur with the widely expressed view that 'agenesis of the corpus callosum is itself asymptomatic but is frequently associated with other malformations which appear to play the dominant role in the production of symptoms'.

By 1965, 210 cases of agenesis of the corpus callosum had been reported, including that of Harcourt-Webster and Rack (1965). Of these, 138 were diagnosed at necropsy and 72 by pneumoencephalography. Of the 210, 25 were said to be neurologically asymptomatic during life and the defect was an incidental finding on necropsy; of these 25, 17 were cases of total agenesis.

Bossy (1970), in an extremely detailed study, reports a further case of pure agenesis—a man who died at age 66. He found that the brain fell well within the normal range of weight and volume and that microscopic study of the cortex did not show any marked differences from normal. However, the anterior commissure was slightly increased in size and included a group of callosal fibres. A hippocampal commissure was found just above the anterior commissure and the volume of the other commissures was slightly increased. An enlarged anterior commissure in agenesis has occasionally been reported by others (e.g. Geschwind, 1974).

More recently, in contrast to Bossy (1970), Shoumura et al. (1975) have reported that the microstructure of 'OBg' (a narrow zone of Brodmann's area 18 at the boundary with area 17) differed from normal in two brains completely lacking the corpus callosum. They found that layer III of OBg contained a slightly reduced number of smaller pyramidal cells than normal, and that the characteristic large pyramidal cells were scarcely detectable whilst other layers of OBg were not definitely changed. They suggested that the large layer III pyramids of OBg might normally send or receive callosal fibres, as indeed seems to be the case in the monkey (Glickstein and Whitteridge, 1974). The inference would seem to be that these particular callosal connections had not been rerouted, e.g. through the anterior commissure.

That 'pure' cases of agenesis exist is important in that it comes as a corrective to the widely expressed view that 'agenesis . . . occurs as a frequent malformation . . . very often associated with other malformations . . . of the brain . . . ' (Myers, 1962). None the less, it goes without saying that no behavioural studies of acallosals are complete without the inclusion of appropriate control subjects. These would ideally have neurological symptoms matching the acallosals (e.g. epilepsy, hydrocephaly) and would normally need to be matched on subnormal IQ. A full discussion of associated brain anomalies may be found in the recent review of Ettlinger (1977). Clearly it would be absurd to suppose that any acallosal brain could be entirely normal except for its lack of a corpus callosum.

A distinction must be drawn, however, between on the one hand associated cerebral pathology, and on the other an aberrant brain organisation which has developed in response to the lack of a corpus callosum. It may well be that the occasionally enlarged anterior commissure (Bossy, 1970; Geschwind, 1974) is one feature of such an aberrant organisation, whilst others may be an elaboration of ipsilateral pathways and/or an increased development of subcortical pathways. We shall return to these questions in the discussion.

VISUAL PERCEPTION

Information from each hemiretina travels via the classical geniculostriate pathway to the cerebral hemisphere ipsilateral to it. The fact that in this way the two halves of visual space are primarily represented in opposite hemispheres causes no trouble for the normal brain. Efficient cross-connections through the splenium of the corpus callosum (and to a lesser extent the anterior commissure) exist which permit interhemispheric integration between all known cortical areas concerned with visual processing, starting with the primary projection area, V1 (or area 17) (Berlucchi, 1972; Zeki, 1970) and extending into the temporal lobe (Zeki, 1973). Complete split-brain surgery, in which the corpus callosum, anterior commissure and hippocampal commissure are sectioned, excludes such cross-communication. Clearly, therefore, aspects of visual processing which depend primarily upon cortical mechanisms must be divided following such surgery, and several instances of 'disconnection' in vision have been well documented (Gazzaniga et al., 1965; Levy et al., 1972).

In the majority of tests for 'disconnection' between the two visual half-fields, tachistoscopic presentation is employed, normally with stimulus durations in the region of 100 ms. By this means the experimenter is able to project stimuli separately to left or right of the *fovea centralis* (provided, of course, that the subject maintains fixed gaze) and hence separately to either hemisphere.

Unlike the 'split-brain' patients, subjects with total agenesis of the corpus callosum have been found able both to read words and to name drawn objects, when these stimuli were presented in the left half (or the right half) of the visual field (Dunne, 1977; Ettlinger et al., 1972, 1974; Gazzaniga, 1970, ch. 8; Lehman and Lampe, 1970; Persson, 1970; Sperry, 1968b). The patient of Solursh et al. (1965) was reported to have a unilateral inability to name drawings, in this case in the right half-field. This finding is difficult to interpret, since the opposite asymmetry was reported for identifying letters.

Ettlinger et al. (1974) found that although their patients with agenesis were able to read words and to name pictures shown to either visual half-field, they did so slightly less well on the left than on the right. Such asymmetries are well known in normal subjects and were found to a similar extent in the partial-acallosal and non-acallosal control groups tested by these investigators. Reversed, but still small-scale, asymmetries in the efficiency of reading alphabetical material have been reported by Sperry (1970b) for his patient SK, and by Reynolds and Jeeves (1978) for their patient KC. In a more recent study, a 10-year-old acallosal girl made significantly more errors in naming pictures of common objects presented to the right visual field (Jeeves and Geffen, in preparation). (This girl's performance on a dichotic listening test favoured the left ear. If, then, language were lateralised in her right hemisphere, this would help to explain the left-field advantage on the picture naming task.)

Again, unlike the operated patients, acallosal subjects are generally able to cross-match correctly verbal or non-verbal visual stimuli presented in opposite visual half-fields (Ettlinger et al., 1972, 1974; Saul and Sperry, 1968). Similarly, Ettlinger et al. (1972) found their patients able to judge alignment or misalignment between horizontal lines presented to the two half-fields: a related (but probably easier) task was failed by a commissurotomised patient (case 2 of Gazzaniga et al., 1965).

There are, however, two contrary reports. Although Ettlinger et al. (1972) found their acallosal subjects able to cross-match colours, saturations and patterns, they reported an apparent deficit in the matching of dot density. (The stimuli involved fields of dots varying in dot size as well as density, to compensate for brightness differences, and accuracy scores were analysed relative to 'up–down' matching scores.) The two patients with complete agenesis tested both performed at a lower level than any of the control subjects (2 partial-acallosal, 4 non-acallosal). Secondly, Mackay (1976) and Dunne (1977) found that their acallosal subject (KC of Reynolds and Jeeves, 1974), like split-brain patients, failed to detect the join when shown bilateral 'chimaeric' faces (Levy et al., 1972) tachistoscopically. Largely confirmatory findings are reported by Jeeves (see chapter 37 herein) in his studies of three more acallosals on this task. There would seem to be a failure to detect a difference between the constituent half-faces which form a chimaeric face (the join falling along the vertical midline of the visual field). There is evidence that the immediate 2° or so of visual angle at either side of the midline are crucial for a normal subject's capacity for spotting the mismatch in such conditions (Milner and Dunne, 1977). At the same time, however, the cross-matching ability of acallosals appears to be good in the same visual-field region in the work of Ettlinger et al. (1972, 1974) whose stimuli fell within 2° at either side of the midline. One possible way of resolving this discrepancy is to postulate that the perception of symmetry in a single pattern is a different process from that of judging a mirror-image match between two separate stimuli. This proposal (Corballis and Beale, 1976) would seem to merit further investigation.

Perhaps not surprisingly, acallosal subjects never fail to see the incompleteness of partial pictures or words cut off at the visual midline (Dunne, 1977; Trevarthen, 1974b), and so never experience total perceptual completion, as split-brain subjects sometimes do (Trevarthen, 1974a, 1974b).

Complex tasks requiring visual cross-integration are possible in some cases of agenesis: Sperry (1968b) found his patient able to read correctly and without hesitation single words spanning both sides of the vertical midline. This was so even when the stress of the first half of the word differed according to the nature of the second half (e.g. al-ign and al-ly). (Sperry, 1970a, reports further than even when the size and thickness of the letters constituting such a word were reduced almost to the acuity threshold, she was able to perform as well with divided input as with unified input to either half-field alone.) This patient was also able to add or multiply two numerals presented to opposite visual half-fields (Sperry, 1968b).

Judgements of simultaneity and temporal succession have been investigated by Ettlinger et al. (1974). Acallosal patients were not especially inaccurate in such a task even though they were required to compare the temporal occurrence of visual stimuli presented to opposite half-fields. No such test has been described using commissurotomised patients. Presumably the acallosal brain has learned to make compensatory adjustment for any additional time taken for signals to cross via an extracallosal route.

Such compensation must also be a prerequisite for the intact perception of apparent ('phi') movement found by Ettlinger et al. (1972). They reported that apparent movement was described by two out of three of their acallosal patients, and by three out of four non-acallosal controls, under circumstances where the inducing sources of light lay on opposite sides of the fixation point. However, Bridgeman and Smith (1945) found intact phi movement across the midline amongst three out of four patients with complete section of the corpus callosum, under conditions where 'considerable care was taken to see that the subject's head was held stationary and the eye fixated constantly on the fixation point'. Bridgeman and Smith argued that the phenomenon could be mediated by either (a) the anterior commissure, (b) possible remnants of the callosum, or (c) midbrain visual centres. It is not known at present whether phi movement can be seen across the midline by the commissurotomy patients of Bogen and Vogel. If it can, then alternative (c) would seem most likely to account for the findings in all of these cases.

Tests for the ability to judge stereoscopic depth have produced conflicting results. Early studies, both on the callosal-sectioned cases of van Wagenen (van Wagenen and Herren, 1940) by Bridgeman and Smith (1945), and on Bogen and Vogel's first reported case by Gazzaniga et al. (1962), failed to reveal deficit. Although Jeeves (1965) reported that the 9-year-old acallosal boy he studied had difficulty in judging distance and that his stereoscopic vision was defective as tested on a co-ordinascope, his adult acallosal subject showed no abnormalities under the same test conditions. Similarly, Ettlinger et al. (1974) observed accurate depth judgements in their acallosal subjects. More recently, however, Mitchell and Blakemore (1970) did find an apparent impairment in a commissure-sectioned subject under conditions of midline stereopsis, but not with more peripheral stimuli. Only in the former case does the retinal information carrying the cue of binocular disparity fall on opposite sides of the vertical meridian: hence only under such circumstances would the perception of binocular fusion and stimulus depth require callosal participation. Ettlinger and co-workers, like the earlier workers, used central presentation, and steady fixation was required of their subjects; however, tachistoscopic exposures were not used. Rogers and Mackay (1977) have tested the clinically asymptomatic acallosal patient KC using conditions similar to those of Mitchell and Blakemore, and have found a similar deficit: i.e., significantly poorer central than peripheral performance. This result has now been replicated on a different acallosal subject (see chapter 37 herein).

A possible interpretation of the discrepancies between these tachistoscopic studies, as against those of Bridgeman and Smith, Gazzaniga and co-workers, Jeeves (1965), and Ettlinger and co-workers, could be that the former involved 'coarse stereopsis' whilst the others were operating mainly in the zone of 'fine' stereopsis (Bishop and Henry, 1971). This distinction is based primarily on degree of binocular disparity, with fine stereopsis operating at low disparities in conjunction with binocular fusion, and coarse stereopsis at higher disparities where double images tend to result. If this distinction does apply to the present experiments, the findings are consistent with Bishop and Henry's suggestion that fine stereopsis at the midline may be mediated by the slight nasotemporal overlap known to exist in the retinogeniculate projections in animals (Stone et al., 1973), and presumably intact in acallosals. Coarse midline stereopsis, on the other hand, would require some form of interhemispheric integration.

Finally, the interocular transfer of a movement after-effect (MAE) generated monocularly has been studied in acallosals. The subjects first viewed a rotating random pattern through one eye, and then indicated the duration of after-effect experienced when only the other eye was open (and viewing a grey card). The three acallosal patients tests reported interocular MAEs significantly shorter than a control group of 18 normal subjects, with two of them reporting none at all (Dixon and Jeeves, 1970). More recently, Reynolds and Jeeves (1977a) have found the interocular MAE to be absent in the acallosal patient KC, not only using Dixon and Jeeves' method, but also when the after-effect was tested with the second eye viewing the stationary random pattern (a technique much more effective in revealing both monocular and interocular MAEs). They used six control subjects of similar age and IQ to the patient, including the patient's sister; all six showed an interocular MAE using the random pattern as test field. The most recent report of lack of interocular transfer comes from a study by Jeeves (chapter 37 herein) using the Archimedes Spiral and with the stationary spiral as the test surface.

Barr (1977) has carried out further studies on KC, in which an effort was made to exclude knowledge of which eye was being stimulated in adaptation and test phases, by use of polarising filters. The intention was by this means to reduce expectancy effects.

Like Reynolds and Jeeves, she reports the absence of interocular MAE, but also exceptionally short monocular MAEs in KC in both of the testing conditions used.

In addition, mental-age-matched controls showed low average interocular MAEs, with two of the six showing none at all in one test condition. (This did not occur in any of a group of university students tested.) It is difficult to make a firm conclusion on these studies. On the one hand, it could be argued that KC may fall within the range of 'normal' interocular MAEs for her age and IQ, given a reduced overall tendency to experience MAEs, which is typical of brain-damaged populations (Holland, 1965). But on the other hand, the consistency with which acallosals have been found to report reduced or absent interocular MAEs is remarkable and ultimately demands explanation (chapter 37 herein).

TACTUAL PERCEPTION

As in vision, the best-known features of the disconnection syndrome in touch are also absent in agenesis. Thus, acallosal patients are able to name objects and shapes held out of sight in the left hand (Ettlinger et al., 1972; Gazzaniga, 1970; Persson, 1970; Reynolds and Jeeves, 1977b; Solursh et al., 1965; Sperry, 1968b). They are also able to match them correctly with objects perceived through the right hand (Ettlinger et al., 1974; Lehman and Lampe, 1970; Sperry, 1968b). Stimulus dimensions used by investigators include length (Lehman and Lampe, 1970), roughness (Ettlinger et al., 1974) and phase of to-and-fro sinusoidal movement (Ettlinger et al., 1974).

With some reservations, a similar picture appears in regard to the intermanual transfer of tactual training. Thus, Ettlinger et al. (1972) report that two out of three acallosal patients tested did show transfer of shape-discrimination training (as did six out of seven of their control patients). On the other hand, such transfer was reported to be absent following commissurotomy in case 1 of the Vogel series (Gazzaniga et al., 1963). Again, Goldstein and Joynt (1969) were unable to demonstrate transfer of training where repeated trials of a form-sorting task and of a form-board task were given to the two hands of one of van Wagenen's callosum-sectioned patients some 28 years postoperatively.

However, the picture is not uniformly so clear. Transfer of stylus maze training was found impaired relative to control patients (though not absent) among acallosals by Lehman and Lampe (1970) and by Jeeves (chapter 37 herein) and among a group of van Wagenen's commissurotomy patients (Smith, 1951, 1952), but was stated to be intact in the first of the Vogel series (Gazzaniga et al., 1962) and was clearly so in the acallosal girl KC (Reynolds and Jeeves, 1977b). Whilst good transfer might be plausibly explained as the result of ipsilateral projection of information regarding 'shoulder movement and trunk adjustments' (Gazzaniga et al., 1962), such an account should apply just as well to those studies where impairment was reported. One way to reconcile the reports would be to argue that the patient of Gazzaniga and co-workers might have revealed some degree of impaired transfer, if his performance had been compared with appropriate controls, but to accept that in acallosals the results vary from subject to subject.

Acallosals have also been tested for intermanual transfer of timed tactual form-board learning, with variable results (Jeeves, 1965; Reynolds and Jeeves, 1977b; Russell and Reitan, 1955; Solursh et al., 1965). There are evidently no comparable data for surgical patients. It seems that a reduction in transfer tends to occur in agenesis, but strong conclusions are hazardous, since performance on either hand is invariably slow, and the degree of transfer even in controls is often low.

Thus it seems that acallosal patients show positive, though often subnormal, intermanual transfer of tactual discrimination learning (whilst commissurotomised patients show none), but that both types of patient tend to show reduced though finite transfer of tactual maze learning.

Given his patient's abilities in visual and tactual cross-matching, it is perhaps not surprising that Sperry (1968b) found her able to recover, with either hand, objects, drawings of which had been shown tachistoscopically to a single visual half-field. When two different drawings were presented simultaneously, one to each half-field, either hand would be used in selecting the corresponding objects tactually, without preference. This capacity is, of course, completely absent in split-brain patients (Sperry, 1968c).

This patient was also able to perform cross-localisation of stimulated points on one limb, without the aid of vision, upon the contralateral limb, as had earlier been reported by Jeeves (1965) for his first case. This latter finding has been replicated in a recent study of the same subject (chapter 37 herein). An impairment in cross-localisation was first noted as characteristic of commissurotomised patients by Gazzaniga et al. (1962). More recent studies, however, have uncovered deficits in acallosal patients too (Dennis, 1976; Ettlinger et al., 1972; Gazzaniga, 1970; Reynolds and Jeeves, 1977b). Several explanations for these disagreements are possible. There could be differences of test procedure between some studies. Perhaps also there could be individual differences between cases of agenesis in the extent to which compensatory mechanisms have come into play. Since the patients of Ettlinger and co-workers, Dennis, and Reynolds and Jeeves all performed at levels of 75–80% correct, clearly their deficit is not absolute, as seems to be the case following commissurotomy (there are no published figures). If compensation can occur to that degree, it is conceivable that in some cases it could occur almost totally.

Despite these deficits, Ettlinger et al. (1974) have shown that the accuracy of locating one hand (passively positioned in space) by means of the other, in the blindfold agenesis subjects, is as good as that of control patients. A comparable test was administered by Gazzaniga et al. (1963) to their first split-brain patient, and he was 'unable to reach accurately'. However, no indication of the degree of inaccuracy is given, and quite high average error scores were obtained even by the control patients of Ettlinger and co-workers (3.73 cm for partial-agenesis patients, 2.77 cm for non-agenesis patients).

AUDITORY PERCEPTION

Apparently normal test performance has been reported in studies of dichotic listening in agenesis. It has been found that the slight asymmetry of recall of verbal material presented under dichotic conditions (i.e. different words presented simultaneously to the two ears, through headphones) which is characteristic of normal subjects, is also present in acallosal subjects (Bryden and Zurif, 1970; Ettlinger *et al.*, 1972, 1974; Reynolds, 1975). Commissure section, on the other hand, results in a marked inability to recall from the left ear under these conditions (Milner *et al.*, 1968; Sparks and Geschwind, 1968; Springer and Gazzaniga, 1975). This latter finding suggests that during such competitive auditory stimulation, in normal individuals input from the left ear to the left ('talking') hemisphere can only be achieved via right hemisphere and corpus callosum. Clearly some other mechanism must be at work to produce a similar end-product in callosal agenesis.

As in visual half-field studies using verbal stimulation, the gross asymmetry in favour of the left hemisphere which is found following commissurotomy is absent; however, it would be wrong to infer a diminished cerebral asymmetry from a diminished behavioural asymmetry. In the case of auditory tasks two major alternatives are available: increased commissural exchange at a subcortical level and increased exploitation of ipsilateral projection pathways.

SKILLED PERFORMANCE

Hand preferences for carrying out unimanual skilled actions have been mentioned in several reports on callosal agenesis. Sperry (1968b) described his subject as being, unlike all the surgical patients that had been studied, 'left-handed and somewhat ambidextrous', and claimed this to be 'a finding that is common among patients with agenesis'. In point of fact, only one published case has been assessed in detailed fashion for hand preference (Smith, 1945; Smith and Akelaitis, 1942). This patient was strongly right-handed. In most of the other behavioural reports on patients with agenesis, the authors have simply stated (often probably on the basis of a cursory examination) the patient's apparent hand preference. (The principal exception is the study by Ettlinger *et al.*, 1972). Fifteen have been described as right-handed, four as mixed, and three as left-handed. (Among partial agenesis cases, eleven are reported as right-handed, one as mixed-handed, and one as left-handed.) In the absence of further detailed evidence of the type collected by Smith, it would seem unwise to claim that there is other than an ordinary cross-section of handedness (Annett, 1967) amongst acallosals.

Skill in performing certain 'visuospatial' tasks (copying perspective line drawings and assembling block designs), normally the province of the preferred hand, has been reported as favouring the non-preferred (left) hand following commissurotomy

(Gazzaniga *et al.*, 1965) This reversal of manual superiority has not been found to be present in agenesis (Ettlinger *et al.*, 1972). However, even following commissurotomy the asymmetry appears to disappear in time (presumably through the development of ipsilateral motor control).

None the less a general impairment, irrespective of hand used, in visuospatial aptitudes has been reported. This ranges from rather low-level visuomotor skills, such as threading beads and plugging pegs into holes (Jeeves, 1965; Reynolds and Jeeves, 1977b; Sperry *et al.*, 1969) to non-verbal reasoning and spatial aspects of mathematics and geography (Sperry, 1970a). Whilst none of these are obviously 'disconnection' symptoms, it should be noted that many visuospatial difficulties are also found in the surgical cases (Bogen *et al.*, 1972; Sperry *et al.*, 1969). Moreover, Zaidel and Sperry (1977) have recently found abnormally slowed performance in split-brain subjects on a series of standardised motor co-ordination tasks, many involving visuomotor co-ordination.

It is possible that the difficulties of acallosals in motor co-ordination are related to the observation by Dennis (1976) of a high rate of unintended 'associated movements' during contralateral manual activity in her acallosal subjects. (Ettlinger *et al*, 1972, failed to uncover any evidence of such synkinesia in their cases of complete agenesis, but they did not use such a sensitive measure as Dennis).

A further possibility is that skilled performance suffers from the lengthening of simple reaction time which has been observed in acallosals. This was first reported by Jeeves (1965), who pointed out that manual reaction times were especially high when 'crossed', i.e. when the visual stimulus fell in the half-field contralateral to the responding hand. A difficulty in the interpretation of the results of that pilot study arises, however, from the fact that within the test session, either hand could be called upon to respond, on a random basis; if the stimulus was on the left, the right hand was required to respond, and vice versa. These conditions would maximise the 'incompatibility' between stimulus and response (Broadbent and Gregory, 1965) and so exaggerate the reaction times obtained for reasons not directly related to callosal transmission. (Conversely, ipsilateral combinations in control sessions would be maximally compatible.) Not surprisingly, therefore, the results of Jeeves' later work on the same two patients (Jeeves, 1969), in which this problem was circumvented, indicate less dramatic (though none the less statistically significantly greater than normal) differences between contralateral and ipsilateral reaction times (differences of 17.00 and 61.33, as opposed to 350 and 183 ms, respectively). (The comparable difference scores for normal groups of adults (Jeeves, 1969) and 9–11-year-old children (Jeeves, 1972) average 1.58 and 1.33 ms, respectively). Confirmatory data have been obtained on a third acallosal patient (Reynolds and Jeeves, 1974), whose difference score averages out at 12.93 ms—again significantly greater than the normal mean.

Other investigators have not reported such clear-cut results. Persson (1970) (two patients with partial agenesis tested) and Ettlinger *et al.* (1972) (three total acallosal patients, three partial) did not even find a clear retardation of crossed relative to uncrossed reactions; and Kinsbourne and Fisher (1971) (one total patient) report that their differences (12.4 and 13.1 ms in their two experiments) failed to reach statistical significance. However, these three studies have in common the fact that relatively small numbers of relevant reaction time observations were made on each subject (80 by Persson, 100 by Ettlinger and co-workers, and 100 and 60 by Kinsbourne and Fisher). In contrast, 600 observations were recorded on each of Jeeves' acallosal and normal subjects, except for the adult acallosal (Jeeves 1969, 1972; Reynolds and Jeeves, 1974). It would seem that the high variance found in the reaction time scores of neurological patients, together with the need for prolonged practice, demand large numbers of responses in order for the impairment to appear clearly.

In all three of these recent papers the procedure required simultaneous responding with the two hands; however, use of the more conventional single-handed procedure appears to produce an even clearer retardation of crossed responding (Reynolds and Jeeves, 1974), as indeed it does with normal subjects (Jeeves, 1969).

There seems unfortunately to have been no fully comparable study of commissurotomised patients. Smith (1947a, 1947b) did test a group of Van Wagenen's patients, and found that on average crossed reaction times increased to the same extent as the result of surgery as did uncrossed. However, this study suffers both from the 'compatibility' objections referred to above and from insufficient data (80 trials preoperatively, 80 trials postoperatively). Gazzaniga *et al.* (1965) reported that crossed visual reactions were not possible at all in their case 1 in early postoperative tests. However, 24 months after surgery he could use either hand to locate a visual target in either half-field; at this time uncrossed responses remained superior to crossed, 'in speed, accuracy and general coordination'. Case 2 is described in the same report as showing 'no difference between ipsilateral and contralateral combinations in reaction time to a simple flash of light in either half-field'. No further details are given.

Although a degree of 'disconnection' seems apparent in callosal agenesis when simple reaction time is investigated, such is not clearly the case in two tests where manual response is required in imitation of crossed stimulation. First, when a drawing of a hand held in a particular posture or finger-configuration was shown only to one-half of vision (or when one hand was moulded in such a way), Sperry (1968b) found his patient able to reproduce it correctly by use of the contralateral hand. Such had not been found possible for the commissurotomised patients.

In the second task, first used by Gazzaniga *et al.* (1962), the patient is required to reproduce, by tapping with one hand, a sequence of taps of a particular rhythm or number received by the other hand. Gazzaniga and co-workers reported an inability in the first of the Vogel series of patients even to correctly reproduce between 1 and 4 taps. Solursh *et al.* (1965) report that their acallosal patient, whilst making 90% errors with numbers of taps exceeding 8, did so 'using either the left or right *or the same* hand'. It would appear therefore that the patient was not selectively deficient in contralateral reproduction. Kretschmer (1968) reports an impairment in the crossed reproduction of rhythms in his patient with total agenesis; however, he seems to have omitted to confirm that ipsilateral reproduction was possible in this patient. It therefore seems premature to conclude that callosal agenesis *per se* impairs performance on this crossed tapping task: such a conclusion must await further and more refined investigation. Until then, it seems reasonable to suppose that it does not.

POSSIBLE MECHANISMS OF COMPENSATION

Cross-cueing

The development in commissurotomised patients of subtle behavioural strategies by means of which the cerebral hemispheres can interact in an indirect fashion, has been described by Sperry (1968c) and by Gazzaniga (1970). Acallosal patients would have a lifetime in which to acquire such 'cross-cueing' habits, and thus would be expected to have them even more deeply ingrained in their everyday behaviour than the surgical patients (Sperry, 1968b). But, of course, this does not imply that they actually engage in more cross-cueing than the latter. In fact, one would expect that if any neurological compensation has occurred at all over their lifetime, then there would be less need for, and therefore less, cross-cueing. It is known that neurological compensation occurs following split-brain surgery even in adulthood: Gazzaniga (1970) documents the growth of ipsilateral motor control of the extremities. It therefore would seem a little difficult to maintain that acallosals 'appear integrated across the split' merely 'because the patients are enormously clever at developing behavioural strategies to deal with their physical incapacities' (Gazzaniga, 1970, p. 136).

There is also considerable direct empirical evidence against such a view: performance on the cross-localisation test, in which Gazzaniga (1970) states that cross-cueing is eliminated, is generally around 75% correct in agenesis, far better than could be expected on the basis of guessing. Furthermore, several tests of visual and tactual cross-matching are performed at a high level.

None the less, behavioural strategies must play some part in the test performances which have been the subject of this review. Sperry (1970a) has pointed to the need, in the absence of the corpus callosum, for continuous oculomotor scanning of the visual world, in order for both hemispheres to keep fully informed. It is possible that in some individuals this kind of activity becomes ingrained and difficult to suppress. If this is so, it should be borne in mind when considering apparently successful cross-integration in visual experiments where fixed gaze is crucial (i.e. tachistoscopic work). Furthermore, failure of steady fixation might provide an explanation of the 'positive' result that monocular movement aftereffects are of shorter duration in agenesis.

It would be possible to test empirically (by electromyographic or photographic recording) whether such increased scanning does characterise the perceptual behaviour of acallosal patients. In the meantime it is possible to use the 'positive' finding of impaired dot-field matching (Ettlinger *et al.*, 1972), and failure to 'see the join' in chimaeric faces (Dunne, 1977; Mackay, 1976; see also chapter 37 herein) as internal evidence for satisfactory fixation in tachistoscopic testing of at least some acallosal subjects.

Bilateralisation of language

An additional hypothesis which has been advanced to supplement a behavioural-strategy account of the findings in agenesis is that language capacity develops in both hemispheres (Gazzaniga , 1970; Gazzaniga *et al.*, 1962; Sperry, 1968b). This would help explain the ability to make appropriate verbal response to lateralised visual or tactual inputs on either side, and for the ability to recall left-ear words in dichotic listening tasks. However, it would not permit explanation of the above-mentioned relative success in cross-localisation, nor of the evident success in visual and tactual matching. Nor would bilateral language capacity account for the observation that words spanning the visual midline were correctly and promptly read aloud.

There have been two (published) direct investigations of speech-capacity localisation in agenesis. By means of intracarotid injection of sodium amytal, it was found in one instance that the capacity was unilateral (B. Milner, referred to by Gazzaniga, 1970, p. 138), and in the other (a left-hander) bilateral (Saul and Gott, 1973). Unfortunately nothing further of a behavioural nature has been reported on these patients, though it may be that the second one is the much-studied patient SK of Saul and Sperry (1968) (see Sperry, 1974). For the present it would appear appropriate to assume normal lateralisation of language in agenesis, just as the evidence summarised earlier is consistent with an assumption of a normal inci-dence of hand-preference. The findings which bilateral language could help to explain can all be accounted for in terms of other forms of compensation, which in any case have to be inferred on the basis of other findings.

Visual cross-connections

Given the numerous examples of intact visual cross-integration in agenesis (e.g. tachistoscopic matching; phi phenomenon; crossed visual reaction, though retarded) it would seem necessary to postulate compensatory specialisation of extracallosal commissures. Two main proposals have been made for such cross-communication: increased usage of the anterior commissure (Doty and Negrão, 1973; Ettlinger *et al.*, 1974) and of the commissures of the midbrain visual system (Ettlinger *et al.*, 1972; Jeeves, 1965; Sperry, 1968b, 1970a).

The 'onset' and 'place' information required to permit crossed judgements of temporal order and the experience of apparent movement could perhaps be carried by the latter system, even without supernormal development (Ettlinger and Blakemore, 1969, p. 38). But where more complex patterns are concerned, it seemed until recently that only the anterior commissure could be considered as a possible channel. However, Trevarthen and Sperry (1973) have found that even in the patients of Vogel (with presumed complete section of all neocortical commissures), cross-integration of simple patterns can occur, providing the stimuli are moving or changing, and are presented in the periphery of vision. It is now conceivable that this (presumed) midbrain system could develop sufficiently in callosal agenesis to account for the tachistoscopic findings; and it is possible that increased ocular scanning might assist in bringing the system into play. A definitive decision between the anterior and midbrain commissures must await a careful comparison between acallosals who do and do not possess an anterior commissure. (Diagnosis in this respect has not generally been possible with traditional radiological techniques.) In either case, the commissural development must be considerable if there is to be essentially perfect preservation of acuity for alphanumeric material carried by it (Sperry 1970a). And yet if the findings of Ettlinger *et al.* (1972) are borne out in other patients, it would seem that the system cannot operate efficiently within certain visual dimensions.

Furthermore, it would seem from the tests of Mackay (1976), Dunne (1977) and Jeeves (chapter 37 herein) that compensation has failed to occur in respect to the perception of asymmetry about the midline. According to the observations of Julesz (1971, 1975) it would seem that the normal subject's perception of symmetry or asymmetry in a random dot pattern generally depends upon a central band of the pattern; it matters little whether the outer portions are or are not symmetrically disposed. The work of Milner and Dunne (1977) indicates that a similar conclusion applies to the perception of asymmetry in tachistoscopically presented facial photographs; the absence of a central 5° panel of the photograph usually prevents normal subjects from distinguishing chimaeric from 'normal' faces.

The callosal cross-connections of the primary (retinotopic) visual projection areas (V1, V2, V3) seem to be limited to the portions of those areas devoted to the 2-3° of the visual field adjacent to the vertical midline (Fisken *et al.*, 1975; Hubel and Wiesel, 1967; Zeki, 1969). It would seem possible then that the normal homotopic cross-connections of these areas have failed to achieve compensation. If so, the observed impairment in midline stereopsis (Rogers and Mackay, 1977) also gains a ready explanation (Berlucchi, 1972). Such an explanation would certainly find support from the study of Shoumura *et al.* (1975) of 'callosal' OBg in human callosal agenesis. They reported that the characteristic large pyramidal cells normally present in layer III of OBg were scarcely detectable in the two acallosal brains they studied. A similar observation was made following callosal section or contralateral occipital ablation in macaques (Glickstein and Whitteridge, 1974). In monkeys, OBg is clearly to be identified with visual area V2, and it is area V2 where binocularly driven visual cells are to be found which are tuned for stereoscopic disparity (Hubel and Wiesel, 1970). Perhaps, on the other hand, fibres from (relatively) non-retinotopic visual regions in prestriate and temporal cortex which pass through the splenium of the corpus callosum in the normal brain (Zeki, 1970, 1973) might be redirected through the anterior commissure in total callosal agenesis. This could permit cross-matching of stimulus features independent of precise spatial location on the retina.

A further failure of compensation occurs in the neural mechanisms underlying the performance of spatial problems and visuomotor co-ordination tasks. Sperry (1970a) has suggested the possibility that this could be the result of a bilateral development of language, which might be said to use up 'processing capacity' which in a normal individual would be dedicated to spatial functions. However, this explanation is not compelling, since 'split-brain' patients also perform poorly on spatial and dexterity tasks (Sperry et al., 1969; Zaidel and Sperry, 1977). Presumably some high level co-operation between the hemispheres must be necessary, which cannot be carried out efficiently by means of extracallosal structures.

Impaired visuomotor skill has been attributed to slow crossed reaction times (Jeeves, 1965); since it is now known that the surgical cases are also impaired, the plausibility of this account is enhanced.

Ipsilateral pathways

A different explanation of visuomotor loss would be to postulate a heavy development of ipsilateral motor control in agenesis, which would not be so readily available following commissurotomy in adulthood. This might result in less precise motor control, and could explain the reported tendency for synkinetic movements to occur (Dennis, 1976). It might also be the mechanism by which 'crossed' manual reactions to light are made in agenesis (Kinsbourne and Fisher, 1971) (although an alternative mechanism would exist in one or other of the proposed routes for visual cross-integration). If so, it might be expected that in the bimanual response task of Jeeves (1969) and Reynolds and Jeeves (1974), a single hemisphere (depending on the side of visual input) controls both hands, whilst in non-acallosal controls, one would expect that the crossed efferent routes would be used, so that different motor processing centres would control the two hands in this situation. In this way, it might be expected that the response times of the two hands would correlate more closely with each other in the acallosal than in the normal. If, on the other hand, responses were organised independently in the two hemispheres (by virtue of visual information crossover in the midbrain for the contralateral combinations), there might be (if anything) even less correlation of times than in the controls. Such a re-analysis of the data is in progress.

For tactual cross-communication, the most likely explanation is an increased development of ipsilateral somatosensory pathways (Ettlinger et al, 1974; Sperry, 1968b) perhaps through lack of callosal suppression during early brain development (Dennis, 1976). The limits of this development are indicated by the results of cross-localisation tests; the punctate mapping of the body surface characteristic of the crossed (lemniscal) system can evidently still not be achieved ipsilaterally.

Dennis (1976) reports an impairment even in unimanual localisation ability in her acallosal subjects (using a model hand), a control condition which had been omitted by other workers. She therefore argues that 'congenital acallosals develop a reliance on uncrossed sensory and motor systems'; implicitly at the expense of the crossed tracts. None the less the system is able to mediate matching along a number of tactual dimensions and transfer of simple tactual learning. The contralateral reproduction of finger configurations could be handled by the crossed sensory pathway in conjunction with ipsilateral motor control of the fingers.

Two broad alternative accounts of the ability to recall words from the left ear in dichotic listening are possible: bilateral language capacity and freer direct access of auditory information from the left ear to the language-dedicated areas of the ipsilateral cortex. The former seems unlikely as a general explanation, since one of the two known direct tests goes against it. Furthermore it has been argued above to be superfluous in accounting for the ability to respond verbally to information presented to left hand or visual half-field. (It is also notable that the distribution of handedness in agenesis is consistent with a normal incidence of left-hemisphere 'dominance'.) On the other hand, the ipsilateral auditory pathway appears to operate effectively in monaural presentation conditions (Milner *et al.*, 1968) and perhaps even in dichotic conditions after practice (Sparks and Geschwind, 1968), following commissure section; it could therefore reasonably be assumed to provide the compensatory pathway in agenesis (Ettlinger *et al.*, 1974).

GENERAL CONCLUSIONS

The main demonstration of the investigations reviewed here is the remarkable ability of the human brain to compensate (neurally and/or behaviourally) for the congenital absence of the major commissure linking the left and right cerebral hemispheres. It has been securely established by the study of the surgical cases that this huge forebrain commissure is normally active in a variety of cognitive, perceptual and motor processes. Yet there is only minimal loss of efficiency in such processes in individuals lacking this pathway. Near-intact behaviour is ensured in these patients by virtue of the immature brain's capacity to reprogramme its development subsequent to an earlier developmental error, making use both of alternative neural structures and of behavioural skills which modify its own inputs.

Evidence (both structural and behavioural) nevertheless suggests that there are limits to the amount of compensation, of whatever kind, that can occur. In particular, it seems that an absent corpus callosum cannot be compensated for where cross-mapping of fine-grain sensory information, in vision or in touch, is necessary. For these, callosal communication seems to be indispensable. In addition, there seem to be clear constraints upon the rate at which skilled movements can be co-ordinated, and upon spatial intelligence; evidently these cannot be wholly overcome by compensatory processes.

ACKNOWLEDGEMENT

The authors owe a debt of gratitude to Professor G. Ettlinger, for critical and constructive comments on an early draft of this chapter.

REFERENCES

Annett, M. (1967). The binomial distribution of right, mixed and left handedness. *Q. Jl exp. Psychol.*, **19**, 327-33

Barr, J. E. (1977). An investigation of the interocular transfer of the movement aftereffect in an acallosal subject. *M.A. dissert.*, University of St Andrews

Berlucchi, G. (1972). Anatomical and physiological aspects of visual functions of corpus callosum. *Brain Res.*, **37**, 371-92

Bishop, P. O. and Henry, G. H. (1971). Spatial vision. *A. Rev. Psychol.*, **22**, 119-60

Bogen, J. E. and Vogel, P. J. (1962). Cerebral commissurotomy in man. Preliminary case report. *Bull. Los Angeles neurol. Soc.*, **27**, 169-72

Bogen, J. E., De Zure, R., Tenhouten, W. D. and Marsh, J. F. (1972). The other side of the brain. IV, The A/P ratio. *Bull. Los Angeles neurol. Soc.*, **37**, 49-61

Bossy, J. G. (1970). Morphological study of a case of complete, isolated, and asymptomatic agenesis of the corpus callosum. *Archs. Anat. Histol. Embryol.*, **53**, 289-340

Bridgeman, C. S. and Smith, K. U. (1945). Bilateral neural integration in visual perception after section of the corpus callosum. *J. comp. Neurol.*, **83**, 57-68

Broadbent, D. E. and Gregory, M. (1965). On the interaction of S-R compatibility with other variables affecting reaction time. *Br. J. Psychol.*, **56**, 61-67

Bryden, M. P. and Zurif, E. B. (1970). Dichotic listening performance in a case of agenesis of the corpus callosum. *Neuropsychologia*, **8**, 371-77

Corballis, M. C. and Beale, I. L. (1976). *The Psychology of Left and Right*, Erlbaum, Hillsdale, New Jersey

Dennis, M. (1976). Impaired sensory and motor differentiation with corpus callosum agenesis: a lack of callosal inhibition during ontogeny? *Neuropsychologia*, **14**, 455-69

Dixon, N. F. and Jeeves, M. A. (1970). The interhemispheric transfer of movement aftereffects: a comparison between acallosal and normal subjects. *Psychon. Sci.*, **20**, 201-203

Doty, R. W. and Negrão, N. (1973). Forebrain commissures and vision. In *Handbook of Sensory Physiology*, Vol. VII/3 B (R. Jung, ed.), Springer-Verlag, Berlin

Dunne, J. J. (1977). The role of the corpus callosum in midline perception. *M.A. dissert.*, University of St. Andrews

Ettlinger, G. (1977). Agenesis of the corpus callosum. In *Handbook of Clinical*

Neurology, vol. 30, part 1; ch. 12 (P. J. Vinken and G. W. Bruyn, eds.), North-Holland, Amsterdam

Ettlinger, G. and Blakemore, C. B. (1969). The behavioural effects of commissure section. *Contributions to Clinical Neuropsychology,* ch.2 (A. L. Benton, ed.), Aldine, Chicago

Ettlinger, G., Blakemore, C. B., Milner, A. D. and Wilson, J. (1972). Agenesis of the corpus callosum: a behavioural investigation. *Brain,* **95**, 327–46

Ettlinger, G., Blakemore, C. B., Milner, A. D. and Wilson, J. (1974). Agenesis of the corpus callosum: a further behavioural investigation. *Brain,* **97**, 225–34

Ferriss, G. S. and Dorsen, M. M. (1975). Agenesis of the corpus callosum. 1. Neuropsychological studies. *Cortex,* **11**, 95–122

Fisken, R. A., Garey, L. J. and Powell, T. P. S. (1975). The intrinsic, association and commissural connections of area 17 of the visual cortex. *Phil. Trans. R. Soc. Lond. B.,* **272**, 487–536

Gazzaniga, M. S. (1970). *The Bisected Brain,* Appleton-Century-Crofts, New York

Gazzaniga, M. S., Bogen, J. E. and Sperry, R. W. (1962). Some functional effects of sectioning the cerebral commissures in man. *Proc. natn. Acad. Sci. U.S.A.,* **48**, 1765–69

Gazzaniga, M. S., Bogen, J. E. and Sperry, R. W. (1963). Laterality effects in somesthesis following cerebral commissurotomy in man. *Neuropsychologia,* **1**, 209–15

Gazzaniga, M. S., Bogen, J. E. and Sperry, R. W. (1965). Observations on visual perception after disconnexion of the cerebral hemispheres in man. *Brain,* **88**, 221–36

Geschwind, N. (1974). Late changes in the nervous system: an overview. In *Plasticity and Recovery of Function in the Central Nervous System* (D. G., Stein, J. J. Rosen, and N. Butters, eds), Academic Press, New York

Glickstein, M. and Whitteridge, D. (1974). Degeneration of layer III pyramidal cells in area 18 following destruction of callosal input. *Anat. Rec.,* **178** 362–63

Goldstein, M. N. and Joynt, R. J. (1969). Long-term follow-up of a callosum-sectioned patient. *Archs. Neurol.,* **20**, 96–102

Harcourt-Webster, J. N. and Rack, J. H. (1965). Agenesis of the corpus callosum. *Postgrad. Med. J.,* **41**, 73–79

Hewitt, W. (1962). The development of the human corpus callosum. *J. Anat.,* **96**, 355–58

Holland, H. C. (1965). *The Spiral Aftereffect,* Pergamon, London

Hubel, D. H. and Wiesel, T. N. (1967). Cortical and callosal connections concerned with the vertical meridian of visual fields in the cat. *J. Neurophysiol.,* **30**, 1561–73

Hubel, D. H. and Wiesel, T. N. (1970). Cells sensitive to binocular depth in area 18 of the macaque monkey cortex. *Nature (Lond.),* **225**, 41–42

Jeeves, M. A. (1965). Psychological studies of three cases of congenital agenesis of the corpus callosum. In *Functions of the Corpus Callosum,* vol. 20, CIBA Foundation Study Groups, Churchill, London pp 73–94

Jeeves, M. A. (1969). A comparison of interhemispheric transmission times in acallosals and normals. *Psychon. Sci.,* **16**, 245–46

Jeeves, M. A. (1972). Hemisphere differences in response rates to visual stimuli in children. *Psychon. Sci.,* **27**, 201–203

Julesz, B. (1971). *Foundations of Cyclopean Perception*, University of Chicago Press, Chicago

Julesz, B. (1975). Experiments on the visual perception of texture. *Scient. Am.*, **234** (4), 34–43

Kinsbourne, M. and Fisher, M. (1971). Latency of uncrossed and of crossed reaction in callosal agenesis. *Neuropsychologia*, **9**, 471–73

Kretschmer, H. (1968). Zur Klinik des Balkensyndroms. *Arch. Psychiat. Z. Ges.| Neurol.*, **211**, 250–65

Lehman, H. J. and Lampe, H. (1970). Observations on the interhemispheric transmission of information in 9 patients with corpus callosum defect. *Eur. Neurol.* **4**, 129–47

Levy, J., Trevarthen, C. and Sperry, R. W. (1972). Perception of bilateral chimeric figures following hemispheric deconnexion. *Brain*, **95**, 61–78

Loeser, J. D. and Alvord, E. C., Jr. (1968). Agenesis of the corpus callosum. *Brain*, **91**, 553–70

Mackay, B. (1976). An investigation into two perceptual impairments with agenesis of the corpus callosum: depth perception and the completion of one visual half-field for a chimeric stimulus. *M.A. dissert.*, University of St Andrews

Milner, A. D. and Dunne, J. J. (1977). Lateralised perception of bilateral chimaeric faces by normal subjects. *Nature (Lond.)*, **268**, 175–76

Milner, B., Taylor, L. and Sperry, R. W. (1968). Lateralized suppression of dichotically-presented digits after commissural section in man. *Science*, **161**, 184–86

Mitchell, D. E. and Blakemore, C. (1970). Binocular depth perception and the corpus callosum. *Vision Res.*, **10**, 49–54

Myers, R. E. (1962). Discussion, Second Session. In *Interhemispheric Relations and Cerebral Dominance* (V. B. Mountcastle, ed), Johns Hopkins Press, Baltimore

Persson, V. G. (1970). Untersuchungen bei drei fällen mit angeborenem Balkenmangel. *Psychiat. Neurol. Med. Psychol.*, **22**, 448–55

Reynolds, D. McQ. (1975). Hemisphere differences and interhemispheric relations with special reference to the functions of the corpus callosum. *Ph.D. thesis*, University of St Andrews

Reynolds, D. McQ. and Jeeves, M. A. (1974). Further studies of crossed and uncrossed pathway responding in callosal agenesis—reply to Kinsbourne & Fisher. *Neuropsychologia*, **12**, 287–90

Reynolds, D. McQ. and Jeeves, M. A. (1977a). The interocular transfer of movement aftereffects in a case of agenesis of the corpus callosum. *Neuropsychologia*, *in preparation*

Reynolds, D. McQ. and Jeeves, M. A. (1977b). Further studies of tactile perception and motor coordination in agenesis of the corpus callosum. *Cortex*, **13**, 257–72

Reynolds, D. McQ. and Jeeves, M. A. (1978). A study of hemisphere lateralization in the visual perception of alphabetical stimuli in a case of agenesis of the corpus callosum. *Neuropsychologia, in press*

Rogers, B. J. and Mackay, B. (1977), *in preparation*

Russell, J. R. and Reitan, R. M. (1955). Psychological abnormalities in agenesis of the corpus callosum. *J. nerv. ment. Dis.*, **121**, 205–14

Saul, R. E. and Gott, P. S. (1973). Compensatory mechanisms in agenesis of the corpus callosum. *Neurology,* **23**, 443

Saul, R. E. and Sperry, R. W. (1968). Absence of commissurotomy symptoms with agenesis of the corpus callosum. *Neurology,* **18**, 307

Shoumura, K., Ando, T. and Kato, K. (1975). Structural organization of 'callosal' OBg in human corpus callosum agenesis. *Brain Res.,* **93**, 241–52

Smith, K. U. (1945). The role of the commissural systems of the cerebral cortex in the determination of handedness, eyedness and footedness in man. *J. gen. Psychol.,* **32**, 39–79

Smith, K. U. (1947a). The functions of the intercortical neurones in sensorimotor coordination and thinking in man. *Science,* **105**, 234–35

Smith, K. U. (1947b). Bilateral integrative action of the cerebral cortex in man in verbal association and sensory motor coordination. *J. exp. Psychol.,* **37**, 367–76

Smith, K. U. (1951). Learning and the associative pathways of the human cerebral cortex. *Science,* **114**, 117–20

Smith, K. U. (1952). Experimental analysis of the associative mechanism of the human brain in learning functions. *J. comp. physiol. Psychol.,* **45**, 66–72

Smith, K. U. and Akelaitis, A. J. (1942). Studies on the corpus callosum I. Laterality in behavior and bilateral motor organization in man before and after section of the corpus callosum. *Archs Neurol. Psychiat.,* **47**, 519–43

Solursh, L. P., Margulies, A. I., Ashem, B. and Stasiak, E. A. (1965). The relationship of agenesis of the corpus callosum to perception and learning. *J. nerv. ment. Dis.,* **141**, 180–89

Sparks, R. and Geschwind, N. (1968). Dichotic listening in man after section of neocortical commissures. *Cortex,* **4**, 3–16

Sperry, R. W. (1968a). Mental unity following surgical disconnection of the cerebral hemispheres. *Harvey Lect.,* **62**, 293–323

Sperry, R. W. (1968b). Plasticity of neural maturation. *Devl Biol. Suppl.,* **2**, 306–27

Sperry, R. W. (1968c). Hemisphere deconnection and unity in conscious awareness. *Am. Psychol.,* **23**, 723–33

Sperry, R. W. (1970a). Perception in the absence of the neocortical commissures. In *Perception and its Disorders,* vol. 48, Res. Publ. Assoc. Nerv. Ment. Dis., Williams & Wilkins, Baltimore, pp. 123–38

Sperry, R. W. (1970b). Cerebral dominance in perception. In *Early Experience and Visual Information Processing in Perceptual and Reading Disorders* (F. A. Young and D. B. Lindsley, eds.), Natl. Acad. Science, Washington

Sperry, R. W. (1974). Lateral specialization in the surgically separated hemispheres. In *The Neurosciences,* Third Study Program (F. O. Schmitt and F. G. Worden, eds.) MIT Press, Cambridge, Massachusetts

Sperry, R. W., Gazzaniga, M. S. and Bogen, J. E. (1969). Interhemispheric relationships: the neocortical commissures: syndromes of hemisphere disconnection. In *Handbook of Clinical Neurology,* vol. 4, ch. 14 (P. J. Vinken and G. W. Bruyn, eds.), North-Holland, Amsterdam

Springer, S. P. and Gazzaniga, M. S. (1975). Dichotic testing of partial and complete split brain subjects. *Neuropsychologia,* **13**, 341–46

Stone, J., Leicester, J. and Sherman, S. M. (1973). The naso-temporal division of the monkey's retina. *J. comp. Neurol.,* **150**, 333–48

Trevarthen, C. B. (1974a). Analysis of cerebral activities that generate and regulate consciousness in commissurotomy patients. In *Hemisphere Function in the Human*

Brain, ch. 9 (S. J. Dimond and J. G. Beaumont, eds.), Elek, London

Trevarthen, C. B. (1974b). Functional relations of the disconnected hemispheres with the brain stem and with each other: monkey and man. In *Hemispheric Disconnection and Cerebral Function* (M. Kinsbourne and W. L. Smith, eds.), Thomas, Springfield, Illinois

Trevarthen, C. and Sperry, R. W. (1973). Perceptual unity of the ambient visual field in human commissurotomy patients. *Brain,* **96,** 547–70

Van Wagenen, W. P. and Herren, R. Y. (1940). Surgical division of commissural pathways in corpus callosum: relation to spread of epileptic attack. *Archs Neurol. Psychiat.,* **44,** 740–59

Zaidel, D. and Sperry, R. W. (1977). Some long-term motor effects of cerebral commissurotomy in man. *Neuropsychologia,* **15,** 193–204

Zeki, S. M. (1969). Representation of central visual fields in prestriate cortex of monkey. *Brain Res.,* **14,** 271–91

Zeki, S. M. (1970). Interhemispheric connections of prestriate cortex in monkey. *Brain Res.,* **19,** 63–75

Zeki, S. M. (1973). Comparison of the cortical degeneration in the visual regions of the temporal lobe of the monkey following section of the anterior commissure and the splenium. *J. comp. Neurol.,* **148,** 167–76

37

SOME LIMITS TO INTERHEMISPHERIC INTEGRATION IN CASES OF CALLOSAL AGENESIS AND PARTIAL COMMISSUROTOMY

M. A. JEEVES

INTRODUCTION

Complete section of the corpus callosum and anterior commissure, at a single operation, produces a set of specific and enduring behavioural symptoms that may be directly correlated with loss of the forebrain commissures (Sperry 1974). By contrast, congenital absence of the corpus callosum is notable for the lack of 'disconnection syndromes' (Ettlinger et al., 1972, 1974; Jeeves, 1965; Jeeves and Rajalakshmi, 1964; Saul and Sperry, 1968 see also chapter 36 herein). This striking contrast has been variously explained; Sperry (1968) and Gazzaniga (1970) hypothesised the development of language and speech mechanisms in both hemispheres; Jeeves (1965, 1969), impressed by the reduced efficiency evident on some cross-integration tasks in acallosals, suggested the use of alternative mid-brain pathways and emphasised the potentially high capacity of the human brain to use small, intact remnants of the commissures to compensate for and conceal disconnection deficits; Gazzaniga (1970) stressed the possibility of increased usage of ipsilateral projections. Such explanations, in terms of neural and/or behavioural compensations, raise more general issues concerning neural plasticity and recovery of function in the central nervous system (Stein et al., 1974).

In this chapter we present evidence from two continuing studies of the fore-brain commissures which, in their differing ways, address themselves to these issues. The first is a 15-year longitudinal follow-up of two acallosal patients, the second is a preliminary report of three cases of partial commissurotomy.

The longitudinal study of the three acallosals has been supplemented by testing on two visual perceptual tasks previously given to surgical-split patients, namely, chimaeric faces and midline stereopsis. The findings on these tasks indicate that there are limits to the extent of neural compensation possible in the absence of the corpus callosum.

PROCEDURE

The tests reported here were conducted during a four-month visit to Australia, the prime object of which was to re-examine two acallosal patients first studied 15 years ago (Jeeves and Rajalakshmi, 1964; Jeeves, 1965). At the same time the opportunity arose to study three patients who had undergone brain surgery for the removal of colloid cysts or tumours involving a transcallosal approach. Most of the testing methods were similar to those we or others, notably Sperry and his colleagues, have developed for detecting impairments in interhemispheric cross-integration. The particular tests used for any individual case were chosen in order to detect changes in compensation which may have occurred over a number of years (in the case of acallosals), to follow up leads given in recent work in related areas of brain research (e.g. concerning the midline visual system) or because of specific deficits likely to be present in the light of known anatomical connections through the corpus callosum (in the case of the partial commissurotomy patients).

Testing of all five patients is still in progress. The aim of the present chapter is to focus upon the limits of the compensation evident in callosal agenesis. The existence of such limits should be seen against the background of a trend which has developed to minimise deficits in such cases. The results reported below serve as a reminder that specific behavioural deficits can occur in callosal agenesis and that circumscribed disconnection symptoms result from partial sectioning of the corpus callosum. Since the testing is continuing and data on control groups is in some cases incomplete, due caution is exercised in interpreting the findings.

METHODS AND TASKS USED

Bimanual co-ordination

(a) Stringing beads

A box containing wooden beads is placed in front of the patient who is told that on the command 'GO' he is to thread as many of them as he can on to a string until told to stop. The string is a lace with a knot in one end and a metal clip on the other to facilitate putting the string through the holes. The time allowed is 2 min. Subjects normally chose to hold the string in the preferred hand.

(b) Winding a string

A length of string is attached at one end to a pencil and the patient is asked to wind the string round the pencil as quickly as possible on the word 'GO'.

Tactile learning

(a) Three-hole formboard

The three cutout forms are a circle, a triangle and a square. The patient slides his hand under a curtain stretched to prevent his looking at the board and is allowed to feel the edges of the board and the location of the forms. On the word 'GO' he fits the forms into the board as quickly as possible. Normally, after five such trials with the preferred hand, the untrained hand is tested for transfer. Each trial is timed.

(b) Pencil maze

A metal 10 choice-point pencil maze (Corkin 1965) (Lafayette Instrument Company) is placed behind the screen. The subject's hand is guided to the start hole and the finish hole and the extremities of the maze are felt. He is instructed to get from the start to the finish as quickly as possible. The time for each trial is recorded. Depending on the patient's motivation he is encouraged to complete 20 such trials with the preferred hand. The average intertrial interval was 15 sec. This is followed by several timed trials with the non-preferred hand. This is a difficult task and if it seemed likely to upset the patient testing was discontinued.

Cross-matching of cutaneous localisation

The subject's hands were placed under the screen palms upwards. It was explained that the tip of one of their fingers would be lightly touched and that they should then indicate which finger was touched by touching that finger with the thumb of the same hand. In the contralateral testing condition it was explained that they should indicate in the same manner but on the non-stimulated hand. Within each batch of 20 trials each finger was touched five times in a pseudo-random order. The order of testing was (1) ipsilateral right hand (RR), (2) ipsilateral left hand (LL), (3) contralateral right hand (RL) (i.e. touch right indicate with left), (4) contralateral left (LR).

Verbal identification of tactual stimuli

(a) Common objects

The patient placed each hand in turn beneath the screen and was asked to name a series of familiar objects placed in his hands (e.g. ball, ring, key, eraser).

(b) Digits

A set of nine digits approximately 2 × 1½ inches in size was placed in either hand and the patient was required to identify them.

Chimaeric faces

A set of 36 colour slides previously used in testing an acallosal in St Andrews (see below and Milner and Dunne, 1977) were presented tachistoscopically. Before each exposure of 125 ms the patient fixated a red dot on a white screen at a distance of 200 cm. The pictures from ear to ear ranged in width from 44 to 54 cm on the screen. Of the 36 slides, 12 were normal whole faces and 24 were chimaeric faces. They were presented in a predetermined randomised order. The first time through the patient was required to point with his right hand to the photograph laid out horizontally in front of him corresponding to the picture just flashed to the screen. The complete set of slides was then projected once again and the patient pointed with his left hand. At the completion of all 72 presentations he was asked if he had noticed anything unusual about any of the slides.

Midline stereopis

Slits of light were projected either side of a fixation point (a light-emitting diode) to produce crossed or uncrossed disparity at the midline. Movement of the slits could also produce peripheral fusion 3.5° out from foveal fixation, again crossed or uncrossed for divergent and convergent disparities. The data reported on the St Andrews acallosal were gathered using a 100 ms exposure. The Australian data were gathered on a modified apparatus using very brief exposures produced by photographic flash bulbs with filters fitted to reduce the level of illumination and avoid persistent after images. In the event, these very brief exposures increased the difficulty of the test significantly. The patient on each exposure had to report whether the slit appeared to be in front of or behind the fixation point. Twenty trials, 10 in front and 10 behind, were run in a pseudo-random order.

I. LONGITUDINAL STUDIES OF CALLOSAL AGENESIS

Results

Case A

Since a detailed account of this patient is given elsewhere (Jeeves, 1965) only a brief summary is presented here. PH was born in June 1954 and, when aged 6, referred for neurological examination because of an enlarged head. Further examination, including ventriculography, presented a picture which led to the conclusion that 'the appearances are those of agenesis of the corpus callosum, probably total'.

Psychological investigations carried out between October and December 1960 indicated a W.I.S.C. IQ of 75. On specific tasks requiring bimanual co-ordination he was markedly slower than matched controls; he showed no transfer on tactual learning of a three-hole formboard. Two years later, following the reports by Geschwind (1962), Geschwind and Kaplan (1962) and Gazzaniga et al. (1962), the patient's ability to cross-localise tactile stimulation to the fingers was tested and he showed no deficit. His handwriting was poor and with his non-preferred hand very poor indeed.

Between February and June 1977 this patient was re-examined. He has grown into a strong and physically healthy young man and is married. He co-operated enthusiastically in all the tasks given to him and conversed fluently and intelligently about a wide range of contemporary issues. He claimed to be a keen reader but showed considerable difficulty when asked to read a prose passage aloud. A selection of the tasks given to him 15 years ago was administered, the choice being determined by the availability of suitable materials.

Handwriting. It is interesting to compare his handwriting now (figure 37.1), at the age of 22 years, with a specimen collected when he was 9 years old and published in earlier reports (Jeeves, 1965). The outstanding feature continues to be the very marked discrepancy between writing with his preferred (right hand) and non-preferred hand.

Bimanual co-ordination. As a test of bimanual co-ordination he was given the bead-threading task and whilst appearing to perform well, in fact, when compared with three normal controls of different ages it was evident that he showed a deficit (table 37.1).

Tactile transfer: (a) Pencil maze learning. Because of his great enthusiasm for the testing procedures I decided to give him the task of learning a difficult pencil maze without vision. He had previously shown no difficulty on transferring the learning of a three-hole formboard from the preferred to the non-preferred hand. On the pencil maze he not only showed no transfer on the first attempt with the non-preferred hand but continued, when switched back and forth from the preferred to the non-preferred hand, to behave as if his left hand literally did not know what his right-hand had been doing. (See table 37.2 and especially the times for trials 21–24 on this task.)

Tactile transfer: (b) Cross-localisation of touch. When tested for cross-localisation of light touch to the fingertips he showed 100% correct both ipsilaterally and contralaterally, repeating the picture obtained 12 years earlier.

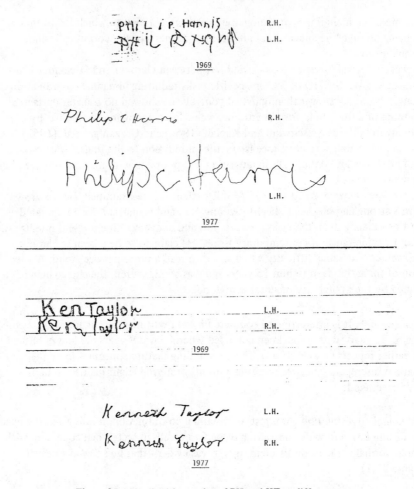

Figure 37.1 Handwriting styles of PH and KT at different ages

Cerebral asymmetries. Preliminary testing by Dr G. Geffen on a dichotic listening task showed a slight asymmetry, with a right ear advantage; in fact, a normal appearance for right-handers. (A detailed account of the study of this acallosal and a number of new cases is in preparation by Jeeves and Geffen.)

Chimaeric faces. He showed no asymmetry of responding either with the right hand or the left hand; a result neither in line with the reports on commissurotomy patients nor on other acallosals tested (see below and Milner and Dunne, 1977). In response to the question of whether he had noticed anything unusual about any of the slides, he replied that 'some seemed to be made up of twó photos'. When asked how many were of that kind he replied 'two or three'. Further questioning revealed

Table 37.1
Tests of bimanual co-ordination under speed stress

Subject	Number of beads threaded in 2 min	Winding string on to a stick (s)
PH (age 22)	21	not given
KT (age 19)	15	8
Controls	36 ($N = 3$)	5 ($N = 3$)
PH (age $6\frac{1}{2}$)	15	60
Controls (taken from Jeeves, 1965)	21 ($N = 8$)	43 ($N = 6$)
KT (age $5\frac{1}{2}$)	10	132
Controls (taken from Jeeves, 1965)	23 ($N = 6$)	74 ($N = 6$)

Note: The raw data gathered in 1960–64 are not comparable with those gathered in 1977. The beads were of different sizes and the lengths of string for the winding tasks were different.

that 'two or three' literally meant 'two or three' and not an indeterminate small number. One explanation of the lack of asymmetry would be that, as Sperry has suggested for language and speech, so in such a case, the perception of faces is bilaterally represented. Against there being bilateral representation for other functions, such as language, is the evidence of the normal slight right ear advantage from the dichotic listening tests.

Case B

The second case (KT) was born in December 1958 and first presented in June 1961 following an epileptic episode. Plain X-rays and pneumoencephalography revealed that this was a case of agenesis of the corpus callosum with some evidence of right atrophy, more posterior than anterior and more right than left. Routine psychological investigations in 1963 showed a sturdy boy of about average intelligence. A more detailed psychometric assessment in June 1964 indicated on the Binet test (form L) an IQ of 88. The results of testing on the W.I.S.C. showed a full scale IQ of 80.

Bimanual co-ordination. When he was tested on tasks of bimanual co-ordination in 1964 (for details see Jeeves, 1965) he was markedly slower than matched controls. When he was seen again between February and June 1977, testing on two of the tasks used 13 years previously indicated that the deficits observed in 1964 were still evident (see table 37.1).

Table 37.2

Transfer of learning of a pencil maze

Subject	Left hand (preferred hand) mean time, trials 1–5	mean time, trials 21–25	Right hand trial 26	Left hand trial 27	Right hand trial 28	Left hand trial 29	Right hand trial 30	Left hand trial 31
KT	2' 59"	46"	2' 40"	61"	36"	29"	1' 19"	22"

Subject	Right hand (preferred hand) mean time, trials 1–5	mean time, trials 16–20	Left hand trial 21	Right hand trial 22	Left hand trial 23	Right hand trial 24	Left hand trial 25
PH	1' 57"	33"	2' 17"	32"	2' 7"	33"	3' 2"

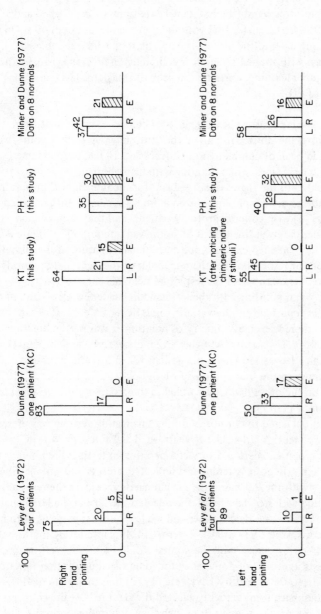

Figure 37.2 Summary of results: percentage choices favouring left (L) or right (R) half of chimaeric faces, and errors (E)

Tactile transfer. When he was tested on the complex pencil maze given to PH he performed to some extent in a similar manner. Whilst the last four trials of testing with his preferred hand (the left hand) gave times of 28, 22, 36 and 28 s his time on the first transfer trial with the right hand was 2 min 40 s. On the next trial, switching back to the preferred hand, he took 61 s (see table 37.2). The following trial with the right hand was completed in 36 s, suggesting either transfer or very rapid learning. Certainly the lack of transfer is less convincing than in the case of PH.

Chimaeric faces. During testing with the slides of chimaeric faces, heat from the projector caused the shutter to jam on the 20th slide. Up to that point five of the pictures had been of complete normal faces and 14 had been chimaeric faces. Of the chimaeric faces, when pointing with his right hand he pointed to 9 in the left visual field, 3 in the right visual field and for the remaining 2 he was in error on both half-faces. This pattern of responding is similar to that reported by Levy *et al.* (1972) with commissurotomy patients and that shown by an acallosal (KC) recently given this task at St Andrews (Dunne, 1977) (figure 37.2). Once the 20th slide remained exposed, and the chimaeric nature of the stimuli was known, his pattern of responding for the remainder of the right hand pointing still showed a slight tendency to select the left visual field, his choices being LVF 7, RVF 5, errors 4. When pointing with the left hand he made few errors and in many instances correctly reported both halves, the totals being LVF 22, RVF 18; once again, in so far as there was an asymmetry of pointing, it was in the direction observed with split-brain patients. As figue 37.2 indicates, the patient KC (Dunne 1977; Reynolds and Jeeves 1974) and the patient KT in this study present a pattern of responding similar to the four commissurotomy patients of Levy *et al.* (1972). The patient PH, on the other hand, performed as the group of normal subjects of Milner and Dunne (1977).

   A further acallosal came to our notice during this testing and she was presented with the chimaeric faces. A girl aged $10\frac{1}{2}$ years, she has a full scale W.I.S.C. of 84 and appears well groomed, alert and very co-operative on testing. Preliminary testing on Dr G. Geffen's dichotic listening test indicated a left ear advantage. She writes and throws with the left hand. On the chimaeric faces test she responded as follows: pointing with her right hand, she selected the face in the left visual field 8 times, the right visual field 5 times and made 11 errors; pointing with her left hand, the results were LVF 2, RVF 7, errors 14. It is interesting that if one considers the correct responses only, she points with her preferred left hand in a way which suggests a reversal of dominance for some visual perception functions. This finding is akin to the report by Levy *et al* (1972) that their patient (PD), a left-handed commissurotomy patient, selected the right half of the chimaeric stimulus twice as frequently as the left, though they only report pointing with the right hand. Their other results, however, led them to conclude that no switch of the minor hemisphere visual perception functions had occurred, a conclusion which we should endorse (Jeeves and Geffen, in preparation) in the light of additional visual testing on this girl.

Midline stereopsis. One further test of visual perception was undertaken with KT
in order to follow up a preliminary study of midline stereopsis in an acallosal
carried out recently in St Andrews (Mackay, 1976). Given 20 trials in a pseudo-
random order he performed at chance level, making 11 correct judgements out of
20 presentations. When the same task was given but with the test slit more than
$2\frac{1}{2}°$ from the vertical meridian KT scored 15 out of 20 correct. Using the same
apparatus on a colleague he gained 9/10 correct with the midline condition and
when tested by the colleague, the present writer scored 10/10 correct. It was
certainly a difficult judgement to make, which may partly have accounted for KT's
less than perfect performance under the second condition when the stimulus was
more than $2\frac{1}{2}°$ from the vertical meridian. Data on this condition for controls are
not yet available.

Transfer of the after-effect of seen movement. Since PH had been tested some
years earlier on his ability to show interocular transfer of a movement after-
effect (Dixon and Jeeves, 1970), KT was given the same task. The stimulus was
a rotating black and white spiral, viewed at a distance of 1 m and rotating at 36 rpm
for 20 s. The results for KT are shown in table 37.3, where the interocular transfer
(IOT) is expressed as a percentage of the mean monocular after-effect. He was
quite categorical in reporting no after-effect under the transfer condition. This
finding is in line with our earlier results (Dixon and Jeeves, 1970) and more
recent findings with an acallosal in St Andrews (Reynolds and Jeeves, in prepara-
tin; Barr, 1977).

Recently the St Andrews acallosal (KC) has taken part in further testing,
this time using polarised light in an effort to overcome any effects due to the
patient knowing which eye has been stimulated (Barr, 1977). The results are
ambiguous and are summarised in table 37.3. Under condition A, a photographic
transparency of a high contour disc bearing a radial random dot pattern was
projected on to a silvered screen 2.4 m from the subject and subtending a visual
angle of $9.74°$. The illumination of the patttern could be varied by means of a
dimmer control, and experiments were always carried out beside the window and
during daylight hours to maintain a relatively constant background illumination. The
disc rotated at 20 rpm for 25 s. The patient viewed the screen through eyepieces
set in a rubber mask. The orientations of the polaroid filters in the two halves
of the eyepiece differed by $90°$. A polaroid lens was also positioned in front of
the projector and could be swiftly and accurately rotated through a $90°$ orientation
change. This arrangement gave maximum occlusion to either eye at choice.

In condition B the only difference was the introduction of another projector
with polaroid filter so as to give polarised, unpatterned, homogeneous light over
the same area of the screen as that filled during stimulation by the patterned disc.
Appropriate orientations of the polaroid filters in front of each projector directed
the patterned stimulus to one eye, and the homogeneous field to the other eye,
the coincident central spots facilitating fixation and convergence in the rivalrous
situation. In both conditions A and B a sufficiently low level of illumination was

Table 37.3

Results of studies of the interocular transfer of after-effect of seen movement with acallosals, normals and mental matches under a variety of stimulating and viewing conditions

Reference	Subject	Percentage IOT	Nature of stimulus	Nature of test field
Dixon and Jeeves	PH Normals (N=18)	4 13	Rotating black and white disc	Sheet of matt grey paper
Reynolds and Jeeves (1978)	KC Normals (N=20) Mental match (N=5)	0 32 60	Rotating black and white disc	Matt grey surface
Reynolds and Jeeves (1978)	KC Normals (N=20) Mental match (N=5)	0 64 75	Rotating black and white disc	Stationary black and white disc

Study	Subject		Rotating black and white spiral	Stationary spiral
This study	KT	0	Rotating black and white spiral	Stationary spiral
	Normal (N=1)	40		
Barr, 1977 (condition A)	KC	0	Rotating black and white disc using polarised light	Stationary disc
	Normals (N=6)	35		
	Mental match (N=5)	19		
Barr, 1977 (condition B)	KC	47	Rotating black and white disc using polarised light	Stationary test pattern illuminated with polarised, unpatterned, homogeneous light of matched brightness to stimulating field
	Normals (N=6)	46		
	Mental match (N=5)	52		

used in an effort to ensure that no pattern was being leaked.

The patient KC reported shorter MAE's than the normal and mental match controls. Her monocular MAE's were outside the range of scores for the normal subjects. Under condition A she gave 0% in the transfer test, whereas under condition B she gave the same percentage as the controls. However her *actual* MAE's were markedly lower than the controls throughout all the experiments, a finding that calls for comment and, if possible, explanation.

II. THE EFFECTS OF PARTIAL SECTIONING OF THE CORPUS CALLOSUM

Case A

SF was born in August 1968. At the age of five years an intraventricular tumour was removed and at operation the corpus callosum was transected in the midline. There was a dramatic improvement and the boy remained well for 16 months. He was readmitted on 18 September, 1975 and an air encephalogram demonstrated a mass in the right lateral ventricle. A second transcallosal exploration was performed on 29 September, 1975; this time the corpus callosum was approached by a right frontal craniotomy, and sectioned posterior to the genu but anterior to the previous exploration. The surgeon did not specify the precise extent of these two callosal sections, but evidently they must have involved the whole of the body of the corpus callosum, with preservation of the genu and the rostrum. Posteriorly the section certainly did not reach the splenium, which was not visualised. When reviewed on 20 April, 1977, prior to the psychological testing reported below, he presented as a happy and co-operative child, speaking fair English (his parents were of Italian origin) and without any obvious speech defect. His general intellectual retardation is considered to represent the effects of generalised tuberose sclerosis as well as the damage inflicted by his two intraventricular astrocytomas.

Case B

WF was admitted at age 14 and investigations revealed what appeared to be a midline tumour of the septum pellucidum. Following an earlier attempt to perform a ventriculocisternal shunt, a further operation was performed during which the body of the corpus callosum was incised, posterior to the genu, which was preserved. The surgeon reports that the length of incision was probably less than 3 cm. The pillars of the fornix were also dissected and a tumour was stripped away from the tela choroidea. Histological evidence confirmed the removal of a colloid cyst. Five years after the operation she is very well and has no neurological symptoms and is attending a tertiary educational institution.

Case C

GO was admitted at age 64 and investigations revealed a mass, of 2 cm diameter, occupying the anterior third ventricle. At operation the corpus callosum was exposed in a distance of almost 3 cm and was incised. It was also necessary to incise white matter (probably the thinned out fornix) to expose the posterior surface of the cyst. There was no damage to neurological structures other than the corpus callosum and a portion of the right fornix. Though suffering subsequently from intermittent depression he seemed physically well when the studies reported here were carried out and he co-operated well in all testing.

Each of the patients was given such of the tests listed above as time and circumstances would permit. In two cases (WF and SF) it was possible to arrange for them to visit a psychological laboratory, whereas in the third case (GO) testing was limited to one session at a hospital; hence the variation in testing between patients. In a subsequent and fuller report (Jeeves, Geffen and Simpson, in preparation) it is intended to include the same testing on all patients together with more adequate data from control groups.

Results

Individual scores for the patients and the control data available at present are summarised in table 37.4. The results of the testing so far completed reveal nothing of the usual 'disconnection syndrome' except on those tasks which call for the interhemispheric transfer of tactile stimulation (cross-localisation of light touch), for tactual learning (formboard and pencil maze) and for bimanual co-ordination (stringing beads). As table 37.4 shows, on each of these one or other of the partial commissurotomy patients showed a deficit.

The results of tests on touch localisation are particularly worthy of comment. On ipsilateral testing all three patients performed as do normals. All showed deficits on cross-localisation, in two cases (WF and GO) the deficit being more marked when the left hand was touched and the right hand had to respond, than in the opposite direction; the third (SF) showed a greater deficit the other way round. The two patients (W.F. and S.F.) who were able to attend for further testing both showed an improvement of cross-localisation on second testing and, in one case (S.F.), a further improvement still on third testing. The success rates at each testing are shown in table 37.5. In the case of WF, I noticed that at second testing she was, on some trials, labelling the finger touched as 'forefinger', 'little finger', etc., and thus utilising the kind of cross-cueing previously reported by Gazzaniga (1970). SF used a different form of cross-cueing, in that on some of the trials he first touched the stimulated finger with the ipsilateral thumb before indicating the finger touched with the contralateral thumb. Such cross-cueing presumably enabled

Table 37.4

Results of tests on partial commissurotomy patients

		Case A (SF) age 8½	Case B (WF) age 20	Case C (GO) age 68	Controls
Touch localisation (percentage success)	RR	100	100	100	100
	LL	100	100	100	100
	RL	30	75	90	100
	LR	50	35	70	100
String beads (number strung in 2 min)		4	21	13	36
Three-hole form-board (5 trials with preferred hand followed by 5 trials with non-preferred hand)		Not given	Not given	No savings on transfer	

Pencil maze	Not given	Clear savings on transfer of learning after 15 trials with right hand. Trials 1–5 mean 2'4" trials 11–15 mean 59 s; transfer trial 1–46s; transfer trial 2–64 s	No savings on transfer after 6 trials
Naming familiar object by touch (each hand tested in turn)	All correct	All correct	All correct
Naming digits by touch (each hand tested in turn)	All correct	All correct	All correct
Chimaeric faces	Saw chimaeric character of slides at once. Correctly reported both halves of faces	Aware of chimaeric nature of stimuli. Pointed to 'half which seemed dominant' LVF REV ERRORS 17% 46% 37%	Not given

Table 37.5
Changes in contralateral touch localisation performance
on repeated testing of two partial commissurotomy
patients

		RL	LR
Case A	1st testing	30	50
(SF)	2nd testing	40	55
	3rd testing	75	65
Case B	1st testing	75	35
(WF)	2nd testing	96	40

alternative and intact intra- or interhemispheric pathways to provide information
about which finger had been touched, thus raising performance levels.

The better performances under the 'stimulated right hand, test left hand'
condition as compared with 'stimulated left hand, test right hand' condition, of both
WF and GO may be due to the former condition producing afferent sensory input
to the language hemisphere and thus facilitating the verbal coding referred to
above.

The two patients (WF and SF) when shown the chaemeric faces immediately
noticed that there were two different faces joined at the vertical meridian. They
were, none the less, asked to continue the test and point to the faces they had
seen. SF pointed correctly to both faces combined in a chimaeric slide and gave no
evidence of asymmetry of pointing, whereas WF chose to point to the face she
felt 'was the dominant half'. In her case there was evidence of asymmetry in her
pointing. Of the 24 chimaeric slides presented she pointed correctly to 4 in the
left visual field, 11 in the right visual field and made errors on the remaining 9.
This asymmetry is in the opposite direction to that reported with total commissurotomy patients.

We may conclude from these preliminary findings that partial sectioning of
the body of the corpus callosum along a length of approximately 3 cm produces
deficits only on tactile and somatosensory tasks: a result we should expect from
anatomical considerations (Jones and Powell, 1969a, 1969b) and from the results
of animal studies (e.g. Myers, 1962, in Mountcastle, pp. 117–129).

Earlier reports of partial commissurotomy include those of Gazzaniga et al.
(1975), Gordon et al. (1971), and Zaidel and Sperry (1974). Gordon et al (1971)
reported that hardly any of the symptoms which follow the surgical separation of
the anterior commissure and the corpus callosum were present in two cases in whom
the splenium of the callosum was spared. In one of their cases (DM), the anterior
commissure was cut together with the anterior 5 cm of the corpus callosum; in
the other (NF), the same operation was performed and the section was said to
include all of the genu and body of the callosum as well as the anterior part of the
splenium.

Zaidel and Sperry (1974), studying eight total commissurotomies, used standardised memory tests involving visual reproduction, temporal sequential relations, verbal and logical retention, free picture recall, and related memory factors and reported consistent marked impairment in short term money. The two patients with only partial section of the commissures also obtained subnormal scores on the majority of tests. They comment that this similarity in memory impairment between total and partial commissurotomies contrasts with the marked differences between partials and totals in basic disconnection symptoms (Gordon et al., 1971). The partials scored higher on non-verbal, presumed right hemisphere, tests but lower on some of the verbal left hemisphere tests. They comment that 'the frontal two-thirds of the callosum thus seems to be implicated as being involved in mnestic functions even for highly verbal semantically complex material such as prose passages'.

Gazzaniga and co-workers report on four patients, two with sectioning of the corpus callosum and anterior commissure, one with sectioning of the corpus callosum except for the sparing of a few splenium fibres and one with the anterior commissure and anterior one-third of the corpus callosum sectioned. They conclude that the deficits they discover are 'consistent with the theory that fibers of specific portions of the commissural system transfer particular kinds of information, and that 'While interhemispheric transfer of some *primary* sensory information has been shown to be dependent on the integrity of specific portions of the commissural system, the more *secondary* forms of processed information seem to transfer readily across any available pathway'. Amongst the *secondary* forms they appear to include linguistically encoded material which they regard as more easily transferable. If they are correct, it would certainly be consistent with one of our patient's (WF) use of verbal encoding to cross-cue during later testing sessions of touch cross-localisation. Certainly our findings here are consistent with their views of specificity within the commissural system, pointing as they do to the body of callosum, perhaps more posteriorly than anteriorly, being involved in the cross-integration of tactile and somatosensory information.

DISCUSSION

When comparing the performances of surgically sectioned split-brain patients with congenital agenesis patients, it has become customary to do as I have done in the introduction of this paper, namely, to emphasise the absence of the 'disconnection syndrome' in callosal agenesis. Whilst this is understandable there is a danger that in so doing we may fail to give due weight to the remaining deficits exhibited by the acallosals and thus fail to differentiate between those tasks on which compensation of some kind, neural or behavioural, has occurred and those where it has not. By looking more closely at these two kinds of performance, the compensatable and the non-compensatable, we may get further clues concerning the limits of plasticity of the central nervous system (Stein et al., 1974).

Gazzaniga (1970) speculated that in callosal agenesis extremely sophisticated cross-cueing strategies may develop which serve to compensate for deficits observed in commissurotomy patients. He believes that one implication of this is that neonate commissurotomy in animals should produce hemisphere disconnection which is not compensated for by adulthood, presumably on the grounds that animals lack the ability to devise sophisticated cross-cueing strategies. He cites in support of his view the, at that time unpublished, study by Yamaguchi and Myers (1972) using monkeys. We found (Jeeves 1972; Jeeves and Wilson, 1969) that on a test of tactile learning the effect of total sectioning of the corpus callosum in kittens was to produce the same effects as sectioning in adulthood, but that where there was sparing of either the anterior one-third or posterior one-third of the callosum normal transfer occurred when testing was carried out in adulthood. More recently, Sechzer et al (1977) have reported that neonatal sectioning of the corpus callosum in kittens produced a syndrome bearing striking similarities to the minimum brain dysfunction (MBD) syndrome observed in children. This observation is certainly an interesting one, since some at least of the MBD symptoms are observed in some acallosal children.

The 15-year follow-up of the two acallosal boys reported above suggests that there is no further compensation beyond that which was evident at five years old. Some aspects of the evidence, moreover, are not easily accommodated by the views of neural compensation in callosal agenesis advocated by Sperry and Gazzaniga. Thus, if there was the bilateral development of speech and language suggested by these authors we may ask why do both patients still exhibit a marked deficit when writing with the non-preferred as compared with the preferred hand (see figure 37.1 above)? Why, moreover, does the patient tested on dichotic listening exhibit the degree of asymmetry found in normals—a finding in line with the earlier studies of Bryden and Zurif (1970), Ettlinger et al., (1972, 1974) and Reynolds (1975)?

The unchanged deficit on tasks of bimanual co-ordination and of the more difficult task of the intermanual transfer of tactile learning, taken together with the finding of Ettlinger et al. (1972) of a deficit of matching dot patterns, suggest that alternative pathways, whether interhemispheric or intrahemispheric, can compensate for the absence of the corpus callosum either when only easy tasks are presented or when there is no time constraint on performance. Such alternative pathways may not, however, be able to handle the information transmission called for by complex tasks or when there is a speed stress on performance. If this is a correct interpretation, then, presumably, on a task such as that used by Ettlinger et al. (1972), one should be able to increase systematically the difficulty of the dot pattern discrimination and find that whereas on simple versions of the task acallosals did not differ from normals yet when the task difficulty increased the acallosals' performance should systematically fall below that of normals. A similar approach could be taken to the intermanual transfer of pencil maze learning, progressing from simple mazes to complex mazes.

The other tasks on which there seemed to be little or no compensation were

those involving the integration of the visual information falling 2-3° either side
of the vertical meridian. Thus, the acallosals in general failed to notice the join
of the two halves of the chimaeric faces (this paper; Milner and Dunne, 1977)
and showed deficits on midline steropsis akin to that reported by Mitchell and
Blakemore (1970) on a surgically sectioned patient. Support for the view that
the deficits on these two tasks may be enduring ones attributable to structural
changes in the brains of acallosals comes from the study of Shoumura *et al*.
(1975). They reported that in the brains of two acallosals layer III of OBg contained a slightly reduced number of smaller pyramidal cells than normal, and that
the characteristic large pyramidal cells were scarcely detectable. Since other studies
have shown that, in monkeys (Cragg, 1969; Karol and Pandya, 1971; Myers, 1962;
Zeki, 1970, 1971), OBg is a specialised zone of the cortex which sends and receives
callosal fibres, and since Glickstein and Whitteridge (1974) found that OBg large
pyramids of macaque monkeys were shrunk and reduced in number following
sectioning of the corpus callosum, this is further circumstantial evidence that our
acallosals' deficits on these visual tasks are attributable to these specific structural
changes affecting the integration of visual information close to the vertical meridian.

The other visual task on which the evidence is less clear is the continuing deficit
in the interocular transfer of a movement after-effect (Barr, 1977; Dixon and Jeeves,
1970; Reynolds and Jeeves, 1977). That interocular transfer is *either* absent *or*
greatly reduced now seems clear but how this is to be explained remains a puzzle.
The shortened monocular movement after-effects of the acallosals could be explained as resulting from the kind of continuous oculomotor scanning suggested
by Sperry (1970) reducing fixation of the stimulating target, a condition known
to reduce the length of the movement after-effect (Holland, 1965; Pickersgill and
Jeeves, 1964). In view of the associated absence of midline stereopsis in these
patients the question arises of whether the stimulation falling on that part of the
retina 2-3° either side of the vertical meridian has a major role to play in the interocular transfer of the movement after-effect. One way to test this could be to study
normals for whom the monocular stimulation is absent from the strip 2-3° either
side of the vertical meridian and testing for interocular transfer.

An alternative possibility would be that suggested by Dixon and Jeeves (1970)
of a storage function for some of the callosal cells. This possibility has, as we
noted above, since been put forward in another context by Zaidel and Sperry
(1974), where they wrote 'Taken collectively the results support the conclusion
that the interhemispheric commissures are important to memory especially in
the initial grasping and sorting for storage of perceived information and at late
stages in the retrieval and read-out of contralateral or bilateral engrams'. If 'the
bilateral engrams' laid down in both hemispheres by monocular stimulation need
to be stored and available in the callosum for the transfer effect but not when
the stimulated eye is tested, this may account for the absence of transfer in the
callosal agenesis patients. Such an *ad hoc* explanation does not, however, on the
face of it, seem very plausible. More compelling is the possibility that reduced
transfer of MAEs is linked to the observed deficit in stereopsis, since several

studies have shown that stereoblind subjects are less likely to transfer the MAE than normals (Mitchell *et al*, 1975; Wade, 1976; Ware and Mitchell, 1974).

Two recent reports (Dennis, 1976; Zaidel and Sperry, 1977) have helped to resolve issues which were outstanding at the time of the 1972 and 1974 studies reported by Ettlinger and his colleagues. Dennis has produced evidence from a study of two cases of callosal agenesis, one complete and one partial, which she believes supports the view that the intermanual deficits reportedly shown by some acallosals on a test of fingertouch localisation (Ettlinger *et al*., 1972; Gazzaniga, 1970; Reynolds and Jeeves, 1978) arise because of a deficit in intra-manual localisation. However, she discovered intramanual deficits only when testing against a model hand and like us found no difficulty with intramanual localisation when testing on the patient's own hand. The evidence presented here from the studies of four further acallosal patients points to a deficit in intermanual localisation being evident even when intramanual performance is at the 100% correct level (table 37.6). Dennis' other results certainly support the contention that the intermanual transfer on discriminative tasks shown by her two patients may be most parsimoniously attributed to the increased functional use of ipsilateral sensory and motor connections.

However, the evidence presented above could suggest that such ipsilateral systems may be of limited capacity. Thus, whilst they may cope with simple dis-criminative matching tasks and hence, in some cases, with the learning of a form-board, they seem insufficient to handle tasks of the complexity of difficult pen-cil mazes. Dennis limited her task difficulty to that of formboards.

Table 37.6
Cross-localisation of touch by four acallosal patients

Subjects	Percentage correct responses			
	RR	LL	RL	LR
JW (age $10\frac{1}{2}$) (in preparation)	100	100	65	70
KC (age 13) (Reynolds and Jeeves, 1977a)	100	100	85	65
KT (age 19) (this study)	100	100	90	90
PH (age 22) (this study)	100	100	100	100

Zaidel and Sperry (1977) have now shown that in commissurotomy patients, as in the case of the acallosals (Jeeves 1965; Reynolds and Jeeves, 1978; this study), whilst qualitative performance on tasks involving complex intermanual co-ordination appears essentially unimpaired, nevertheless on most tests the scores for speed were consistently below normal and also inferior to those reported for patients with various unilateral brain lesions. Such reduced efficiency may be due to the limited capacity of alternative interhemispheric pathways to carry information normally carried by the intact corpus callosum, and it may in part be due to delays in interhemispheric transmission times reported in a number of earlier studies (Dixon and Jeeves, 1970; Jeeves, 1965; Reynolds and Jeeves, 1974).

Further confirmatory evidence comes from the report of Saul and Gott (1973) who found that two young adult patients with radiologically verified total agenesis performed subnormally on the blind intermanual transfer of tactile formboard learning and related tests in which 'spatial information has to be continually related to sequential motor activity'. This latter phrase is an apt description of part of what is involved in pencil maze learning on which some of our patients have shown marked deficits. It may also be due in part, as Dennis (1976) suggests, to the congenital acallosals' inability to suppress ipsilateral systems. She points out that the acquisition of normal sensory and motor competence involves a suppression of the information contained in uncrossed pathways. Thus, when the corpus callosum is missing throughout ontogeny, the behavioural expression of uncrossed sensory and motor systems persists into adulthood and the corpus callosum is not present to provide the inhibition necessary for the development of precise motor control. That such inhibitory action of callosal cells in the neurons of the motor system exists has been documented for both evoked and spontaneous activity (Asanmura and Okamoto, 1959).

The report by Zaidel and Sperry (1977) referred to earlier shows that some years after total commissurotomy, deficits remain on tasks of intermanual co-ordination done under speed stress. It is precisely on tasks of this kind that we found deficits in the absence of other typical 'disconnection' symptoms. The impairment on the task of tactual cross-localisation evident in all three partial commissurotomised patients is present though the splenium has not been divided. That the middle and posterior callosal regions are implicated in cross-localisation was evident from the results that Dennis obtained with her partial acallosal case (JE). The evidence from our three patients, however, does not support her further contention that the splenium is the callosal region essential for cross-localisation and distal motor control. Rather, our evidence argues for the posterior portion of the body of the callosum being crucially involved in cross-localisation of touch. On the evidence so far available from these three cases there is nothing to support Geschwind's suggestion (Geschwind, 1974) that more severe syndromes are seen as a result of the sudden onset of the callosal lesions produced in previously largely normal brains, or that the syndrome is more severe in the adults (68 and 20 years old) than in the boy (8 years old).

In view of the differences, some slight, some more substantial, found between the performances of different patients, whether acallosals or partial commissuro-tomies, within this study and as between the results of this and earlier studies, it is well to remember that 'differences in the effects of lesions' may be attributable 'to what one might describe as host variation' (Geschwind, 1974, p. 501). As Geschwind points out: 'Despite the tremendous interest in individual differences dating back for nearly a century there has been comparatively little attention paid to variations in the nervous system that might account for different responses to lesion.' A thought echoed by Marshall (1973) in his review of problems and paradoxes of hemispheric specialisation, when he wrote: 'The search for generality in the study of brain-mechanisms is no doubt laudable—but it seems more than likely that a theory of individual differences is a necessary prerequisite for success in this enterprise.'

REFERENCES

Asanmura, H. and Okamoto, K. (1959). Unitary study on evoked activity of callosal neurons and its effect on pyramidal tract cell activity on cat. *Jap. J. Physiol.*, **9**, 437-83

Barr, J. (1977). *MA thesis*, University of St Andrews

Bryden, M. P. and Zurif, E. B. (1970). Dichotic listening performance in a case of agenesis of the corpus callosum. *Neuropsychologia*, **8**, 371-77

Corkin, S. (1965). Tactually-guided maze learning in man: effects of unilateral cortical excisions and bilateral hippocampal lesions. *Neuropsychologia*, **3**, 339-51

Cragg, B. G. (1969). The topography of the afferent projections in the circumstriate visual cortex of the monkey studied by the Nauta method. *Vision Res.*, **9**, 733-47

Dennis, M. (1976). Impaired sensory and motor differentiation with corpus callosum agenesis: a lack of callosal inhibition during ontogency? *Neuropsychologia*, **14**, 455-69

Dixon, N. F. and Jeeves, M. A. (1970). The interhemispheric transfer of movement aftereffects: a comparison between acallosal and normal subjects. *Psychon. Sci.*, **20**, 201-203

Dunne, J. J. (1977). *MA thesis*, University of St Andrews

Ettlinger, G., Blakemore, C. B., Milner, A. D. and Wilson, J. (1972). Agenesis of the corpus callosum: a behavioural investigation. *Brain*, **95**, 327-46

Ettlinger, G., Blakemore, C. B., Milner, A. D. and Wilson, J. (1974). Agenesis of the corpus callosum: a further behavioural investigation. *Brain*, **97**, 225-34

Gazzaniga, M. S. (1970). *The Bisected Brain*, Appleton-Century-Crofts, New York

Gazzaniga, M. S., Bogen, J.E. and Sperry, R. W. (1962). Some functional effects of sectioning the cerebral commissures in man. *Proc. natn Acad. Sci.*, *U.S.A*, **48**, 1765-69

Gazzaniga, M. S., Risse, G. L., Springer, S. P., Clark, E. and Wilson, D. H. (1975). Psychologic and neurologic consequences of partial and complete cerebral commissurotomy. *Neurology*, **25**, 10-15

Geschwind, N. (1962). Disconnection of the cerebral hemispheres in man. Paper read at 7th Ann. VA Conf., Cincinatti

Geschwind, N. (1974). Late changes in the nervous system: an overview. In *Plasticity and Recovery of Function in the Central Nervous System* (D. G. Stein,

J. J. Rosen, and N. Butters, eds.), Academic Press, New York

Geschwind, N. and Kaplan, E. (1962). A human cerebral deconnection syndrome. *Neurology*, **12**, 675

Glickstein, M. and Whitteridge, D. (1974). Degeneration of layer III pyramidal cells in area 18 following destruction of callosal input. *Anat. Rec.*, **178**, 362-63

Gordon, H. W., Bogen, J. E. and Sperry, R. W. (1971). Absence of deconnexion syndrome in two patients with partial section of the neocommissures. *Brain*, **94**, 327-36

Holland, H. C. (1965). *The Spiral Aftereffect*, Pergamon Press, London

Jeeves, M. A. (1965). Psychological studies of three cases of congenital agenesis of the corpus callosum. In *Functions of the Corpus Callosum* (E. G. Ettlinger, ed.), Churchill, London, pp. 77-94

Jeeves, M. A. (1969). A comparison of hemispheric transmission time in acallosals and normals. *Psychon. Sci.*, **16**, 245-46

Jeeves, M. A. (1972). Further psychological studies of the effects of agenesis of the corpus callosum in man and neonatal sectioning of the corpus callosum in animals. In *Cerebral Interhemispheric Relations* (J. Cernacek and F. Podivinsky, eds.). Publishing House of the Slovak Academy of Sciences, Bratislava

Jeeves, M. A. and Rajalakshmi, R. (1964). Psychological studies of a case of congenital agenesis of the corpus callosum. *Neuropsychologia*, **2**, 247-52

Jeeves, M. A. and Wilson, A. F. (1969). Tactile transfer and neonatal callosal section in the cat. *Psychon. Sci.*, **16**, 235-37

Jones, E. G. and Powell, T. P. S. (1969a). Connexions of the somatic sensory cortex of the rhesus monkey, I—Ipsilateral cortical connexions. *Brain*, **92**, 477-502

Jones, E. G. and Powell, T. P. S. (1969b). Connexions of the somatic sensory cortex of the rhesus monkey, II—Contralateral cortical connexions. Brain, **92**, 717-730

Karol, E. A. and Pandya D. N. (1971). The distribution of the corpus callosum in the rhesus monkey. *Brain*, **94**, 471-86

Levy, J., Trevarthen, C., and Sperry, R. W. (1972). Perception of bilateral chimeric figures following hemispheric deconnexion. *Brain*, **95**, 61-78

Mackay, B. (1976). *MA thesis*, University of St Andrews

Marshall, J. C. (1973). Some problems and paradoxes associated with recent accounts of hemispheric specialization. *Neuropsychologia*, **11**, 463-70

Milner, A. D. and Dunne, J. J. (1977). Lateralised perception of bilateral chimaeric faces by normal subjects. *Nature (Lond.)*, **268**, 175-76

Mitchell, D. E. and Blakemore, C. (1970). Binocular depth perception and the corpus callosum. *Vision Res.*, **10**, 49-54

Mitchell, D. E., Reardon, J. and Muir, D. W. (1975). Interocular transfer of the motion aftereffect in normal and stereoblind observers. *Expl. Brain Res.*, 22, 163-73

Myers, R. E. (1962). Transmission of visual information within and between the hemispheres: a behavioural study. In *Interhemispheric Relations and Cerebral Dominance* (V. B. Mountcastle, ed.), Johns Hopkins Press, Baltimore

Pickersgill, M. J. and Jeeves, M. A. (1964). The origin of the aftereffect of movement. *Q. Jl exp. Psychol.*, **16**, 90-103

Reynolds, D. M. (1975). *PhD thesis*, University of St Andrews

Reynolds, D. M. and Jeeves, M. A. (1974). Further studies of crossed and uncrossed pathway responding in callosal agenesis—reply to Kinsbourne and Fisher. *Neuropsychologia,* **12**, 287-90

Reynolds, D. M. and Jeeves, M. A. (1977). Further studies of tactile perception and motor coordination in agenesis of the corpus callosum. *Cortex,* **xiii**, 257

Reynolds, D. M. and Jeeves, M. A. (1978). The interocular transfer of movement aftereffects in a case of agenesis of the corpus callosum. *Neuropsychologia, in press*

Saul, R. E. and Gott, P. S. (1973). Compensatory mechanisms in agenesis of the corpus callosum. *Neurology,* **23**, 443

Saul, R. and Sperry, R. W. (1968). Absence of commissurotomy symptoms with agenesis of the corpus callosum. *Neurology,* **18**, 307

Sechzer, J. A., Folstein, S. E., Geiger, E. H. and Morris, D. F. (1977). Effects of neonatal hemispheric disconnection in kittens. In *Lateralization in the Nervous System* (S. Harnad, R. W. Doty, L. Goldstein, J. Jaynes and G. Krauthamer, eds.), Academic Press, New York

Shoumura, K., Ando, T. and Kato, K. (1975). Structural organization of 'callosal' OBg in human corpus callosum agenesis. *Brain Res.,* **93**, 241-52

Sperry, R. W. (1968). Mental unity following surgical disconnection of the cerebral hemispheres. *Harvey Lect.,* **62**, 293-323, New York, Academic Press

Sperry, R. W. (1970). Perception in the absence of the neocortical commissures. In *Perception and its Disorders: ARNMD*, Williams and Wilkins, Baltimore, pp. 123-38

Sperry, R. W. (1974). Lateral specialization in the surgically separated hemispheres. In *The Neurosciences,* Third Study Program (F. O. Schmitt and E. G. Worden, eds.), MIT Press, Cambridge, Mass., pp. 5-19

Stein, D. G., Rosen, J. J. and Butters, N. (1974). *Plasticity and Recovery of Function in the Central Nervous System,* Academic Press, New York

Wade, N. J. (1976). On interocular transfer of the movement aftereffect in individuals with or without normal binocular vision. *Perception,* **5**, 113-18

Ware, C. and Mitchell, D. E. (1974). On interocular transfer of various visual aftereffects in normal and stereoblind observers. *Vision Res.,* **18**, 731-34

Yamaguchi, S. and Myers, R. E. (1972). Age effects of forebrain commissure section and interocular transfer. *Expl Brain. Res.,* **15**, 225-33

Zaidel, D. and Sperry, R. W. (1974). Memory impairment after commissurotomy in man. *Brain,* **97**, 263-72

Zaidel, D. and Sperry, R. W. (1977). Some long-term motor effects of cerebral commissurotomy in man. *Neuropsychologia,* **15**, 193-204

Zeki, S. M. (1971). Cortical projections from two prestriate areas in the monkey. *Brain Res.,* **34**, 19-35

Zeki, S. M. (1970). Interhemispheric connections of prestriate cortex in monkey. *Brain Res.,* **19**, 63-75

38
ON THE ROLE OF CEREBRAL COMMISSURES IN ANIMALS

L. WEISKRANTZ

The cerebral commissures consist of fibres interconnecting symmetrically placed regions in the two hemispheres. What functional role might they have? Of course, one could ignore the fact that the connections are interhemispheric and argue that they are simply like any other connection, intra- or interhemispheric. But if that were the case, we would expect that cutting the commissures would interfere with various behavioural capacities in much the same way that intrahemispheric lesions do. But this evidently is not the case in animals. What is interfered with is interhemispheric communication, e.g. the access that one hemisphere has to the results of experience imposed on the other hemisphere via inputs exclusively directed to it.

There would be no need for such a quantitatively impressive communication system (in the cat it has been estimated that there are 700 000 fibres per mm^2 cross-section of the corpus callosum; Myers, 1959) if there were nothing to communicate, i.e. if each of two hemispheres did not have information or functions unique to it. Therefore, *a priori* one is led to assume that indeed the two hemispheres in animals *are* specialised, even though it is commonly assumed that hemispheric specialisation or dominance does not occur in animals other than man. Putting the assumption in this form draws attention to the important need to distinguish between specialisation and dominance. That the two hemispheres are specialised in animals cannot be disputed, if only because each has a stronger relationship to inputs from and outputs to the contralateral parts of the body (and to the contralateral visual field) than it does to the ipsilateral parts. Were each hemisphere to receive equally strong projections from both sides of the body then no doubt there would be much less need for a corpus callosum.

The question of dominance, however, arises from evidence that suggests that there is an *asymmetry* of specialisation, i.e. that lesions to one hemisphere are more destructive of a particular capacity than lesions to the other hemisphere. In man the evidence for such asymmetry is overwhelming. Evidence for asymmetrical specialisation in infrahuman animals is said to be weak or non-existent. But where there is asymmetrical specialisation, then no doubt the corpus callosum is an even more essential communication pathway than is required merely for symmetrical specialisation (because in the latter case adjustments of peripheral parts of the body are normally taking place more or less continuously so that both hemispheres are engaged in the same task, e.g. both visual hemifields are stimulated by the same display as the eyes scan it).

The evidence for asymmetrical specialisation in man derives mainly from the fact that in the large majority of persons damage to the left hemisphere is much more likely to interfere with linguistic function than is damage to the right hemisphere, at least beyond a certain young age. Language is, by its very nature, an abstract system that is not related to the left or the right half of the body, and a second *a priori* assumption might be that it would be much less efficient for the nervous system to duplicate all the machinery in both hemispheres than it would be to have just one piece of machinery, but with access open to it through the corpus callosum. At any rate, that broadly speaking is how it appears to be organised in man.

In this case, it might be that a similar argument might be put for other functions that are not logically related to the left side or the right side of the body or of each eye, whether in man or an infrahuman mammal. For example, animals live in a semantically rich world, a world that is both categorised and has acquired meaning independently of any unique relation to external or body space. They also live in a world of temporal sequences of events about which the same could be said. Might it not be redundant for the animal brain also to duplicate the processing machinery for such properties in both hemispheres? It seems worth considering the possibility that there is asymmetry of specialisation in the animal as well as the human brain.

Some years ago, James Dewson, Alan Cowey and I decided that the perception of auditory sequences might serve as a candidate for the study of such a possible asymmetry in the monkey. Aside from anything else, perception of auditory sequences must be a necessary condition for the comprehension of speech, and while the monkey might not comprehend speech (although for all we know it may!) it might at least possess an evolutionary prerequisite for further development of speech comprehension. And so we taught the monkeys, in effect, to play a two-key piano, except that one key always produced a tone and the other always produced white noise. The animal's task was to listen to a pair of sounds presented randomly to it (noise and tone in any of the four possible combinations) and then to reproduce the sequence by pressing the keys in the correct order, for which it obtained a food reward. The animals learned the task. We then varied the duration of each member of the auditory pair and also the interval between the members systematically, so that temporal limits of performance could be measured. Then the animals were given *unilateral* lesions of auditory association cortex in the superior temporal gyrus, sparing primary auditory cortex (or control lesions).

The result was that even a unilateral lesion was sufficient to produce an enduring deficit in the task (Dewson *et al.*, 1970). The deficit was primarily expressed in the narrowing of the range of temporal parameters within which the animal could perform successfully. But there was no suggestion that damage to the left hemisphere was any more detrimental than damage to the right hemisphere over the group as a whole. Since that time, Cowey and I have mainly pursued the question of the nature of the deficit itself, e.g. whether it might be an auditory short-term memory impairment (Cowey and Weiskrantz, 1976). But Dewson, who returned to Stanford University, developed the task along a very interesting and rather different line. What he did, in effect, was to convert the task (actually in a somewhat simpler form) to a non-spatial form. In our original situation, the animal had to press one key on the left and another on the right in the correct order. It is possible that when he listened to a particular sequence, he could transform it into and remember it as a left–right response pattern. Dewson required the animal to press one of two keys, but the spatial location of the key was made irrelevant. Instead, for a particular sound it had to press a red key and for another sound a green key, but the actual location of red and green varied randomly from trial to trial. There was no obvious way in which the animal could remember the sounds according to a left–right spatial code. When Dewson and colleagues made the same unilateral lesion in the superior temporal gyrus, they reported that only left hemisphere and not right hemisphere lesions interfered with performance on his task (Dewson, 1977; Dewson *et al.*, 1975).

This dramatic finding obviously requires replication and elaboration, but it at least indicates that the possibility of asymmetrical hemispheric specialisation in the monkey is one worth pursuing. There are a number of other approaches to the problem that might well be worth considering. Deficits in man that lead us to conclude that there is asymmetrical specialisation commonly involve cognitive *systems* or categories, not just isolated discrimination tasks. Left hemisphere deficits of language are an obvious example, and many of the linguistic errors that left hemisphere tumour cases show, it has been claimed, are semantic errors (Coughlan and Warrington, 1978). Non-verbal visual disorders of the agnosia type are also possible to view as semantic disorders, i.e. disorders of meaning within a hierarchical structure.

This is not to say that all unilateral deficits in man are of this type — there are reports of left hemisphere motor sequencing deficits (Kimura, 1977), left hemisphere acoustic short-term memory deficits (Warrington and Shallice, 1969), various perceptual disorders associated with right hemisphere lesions, etc., but one wonders whether a human subject with a lesion in one or the other hemisphere would ever be impaired on the typical task on which animals have been shown to be impaired (typically only with bilateral lesions), e.g. visual discrimination tasks (inferotemporal cortex lesions) or delayed response tasks (frontal cortex lesions). Indeed, one is inclined to doubt whether human subjects would be impaired even with bilateral lesions!

Until animal subjects are tested on a much richer range of tasks, particularly those that force the subject to reveal its cognitive structuring of its world, I am reluctant to accept the universal negative conclusion that dominance does not occur in animals. The universal negative is not only impossible to prove, but Dewson's work, if it holds up, disconfirms it. I am also reluctant to assume that there is a sharp discontinuity in hemispheric organisation between man and all other animals, and that the richness and profusion of commissural pathways and connections in animals has evolved merely to allow the two halves of the body or of space to be joined.

REFERENCES

Coughlan, A. K. and Warrington, E. K. (1978) Word-comprehension and word-retrieval in patients with localized cerebral lesions. *Brain,* **101**, 163–85

Cowey, A. and Weiskrantz, L (1976). Auditory sequence discrimination in *Macaca mulatta*: the role of the superior temporal cortex. *Neuropsychologia*, **14**, 1–10

Dewson, J. H. (1977). Preliminary evidence of hemispheric asymmetry of auditory function in monkeys. In *Lateralization in the Nervous System* (S. Harnad, R. W. Doty, L. Goldstein, J. Jaynes and G. Krauthamer, eds.). Academic Press, New York and London, pp. 63–71

Dewson, J. H., Cowey, A. and Weiskrantz, L. (1970). Disruptions of auditory sequence discrimination by unilateral and bilateral cortical ablations of superior temporal gyrus in the monkey. *Expl Neurol.*, **28**, 529–48

Dewson, J. H., Burlingame, A., Kizer, K., Dewson, S., Kenney, P. and Pribram, K. H. (1975). Hemispheric asymmetry of auditory function in monkeys. *J. Acoust. Soc. Am.*, **58**, S66

Kimura, D (1977). Acquisition of a motor skill after left hemisphere damage. *Brain*, **100**, 527–42

Myers, R. E. (1959). Localization of function in the corpus callosum. *Archs Neurol.*, **1**, 74–77

Warrington, E. K. and Shallice, T. (1969). The selective impairment of auditory verbal short-term memory. *Brain*, **92**, 885–96

39
ANATOMICAL ASPECTS OF THE AGENESIS OF THE CORPUS CALLOSUM IN MAN

S. Z. STEFANKO and V. W. D. SCHENK

The corpus callosum is the largest and phylogenetically one of the oldest of the commissures, yet its function is an enigma. In primitive mammals (edentata) it is formed by a thin membrane. In phylogenesis the corpus callosum becomes larger and larger. It is proportional to the growing size of the telencephalon and to the number of cerebral convolutions. Congenital absence of the corpus callosum in man is a rare occurrence. However, we have had the opportunity to observe 24 cases of agenesis of this commissure. The main purpose of this chapter is to demonstrate some typical variations of this pathological condition.

There are many classifications of the types of aplasias or hypoplasias of the corpus callosum. The system that we used is that proposed by Rogalski (1924).

(1) total agenesis of the corpus callosum
    (a) without any other significant dysplasias of the brain
    (b) with other developmental abnormalities
(2) partial agenesis of the corpus callosum
(3) 'secondary' hypoplasia or aplasia of the corpus callosum (coexistent with the tumours in the vicinity of the callosum).

CASE REPORTS

Case A (no. 278-77); 36-year-old man.
Clinical diagnosis: Imbecility.
Cause of death: Cystopyelonephritis, uraemia.

The most important abnormality in the brain was the total agenesis of the corpus callosum. The gyri of the medial parts of the hemispheres showed an abnormal picture. The cingulate gyrus was imperfectly formed and in its place radially oriented convolutions were present.

The two columns of the fornix (columnae fornicis) were separated throughout their length (figure 39.1). Between them protruded the membranous roof (lamina

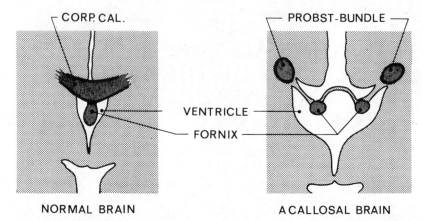

NORMAL BRAIN   A CALLOSAL BRAIN

Figure 39.1   Coronal sections of normal and acallosal brains at the level of the foramen of Monro

chorioidea epithelialis) of the enlarged third ventricle. The lateral ventricles showed an abnormal oblique position, and were considerably dilated. There was no septum pellucidum. This structure was represented by the two laminae running obliquely between the fornix and the unusual prominent rounded bundles of fibres running longitudinally above the fornix. Each bundle took its origin from the white matter of frontal pole, passed through the medial part of the roof of the lateral ventricle and merged with the white matter enclosing the posterior horn. The basal ganglia, truncus and cerebellum showed no abnormalities. Microscopically the cytoarchitecture of the cortex was not disturbed.

This case is typical for total agenesis of the corpus callosum without any significant dysplasias of the brain. In the normal brain the two leaves of the septum pellucidum are vertical, and they attach the fornices to the corpus callosum in the midline. In the acallosal brain the course at the septa is directed sharply laterally. The schematic drawing (figure 39.1) of coronal sections of normal and acallosal brains, at the level of the foramen of Monro, illustrates this situation. The course of the septa pellucida is directed laterally in the acallosal brain. The septa are attached to the longitudinal Probst bundles. The massive longitudinal bundle lying above the fornix and running fronto-occipital in the medial wall of each hemisphere is called the 'Balkenlängsbündel' of Probst, or 'Fasciculus callosus longitudinalis'. The anatomy and the function of this bundle is still unclear.

According to Vogt (1905) the callosal longitudinal bundle is always present in the acallosal brains. However, it can be absent when the agenesis of the corpus callosum is associated with other severe abnormalities of the forebrain. (We have found this bundle indeed in all cases of our series of callosal agenesis.) The observations of King (1936) are of special interest. He found a longitudinal bundle in a strain of mice with a congenital absence of the callosum. According to him the longitudinal bundle is thought to be composed of fibres from the cells of origin of the corpus callosum. Due to genetic factors, these fibres run in a well-defined course in the ipsilateral hemisphere. They are derived from the medial, dorsal and lateral cortex, and run in the anteroposterior direction. Connections with different parts of the olfactory system have been described. Rakic and Yakovlev (1972) believed that agenesis of the corpus callosum is not a failure of the fibres to grow, but is instead a misdirection of their growth (see figure 39.2).

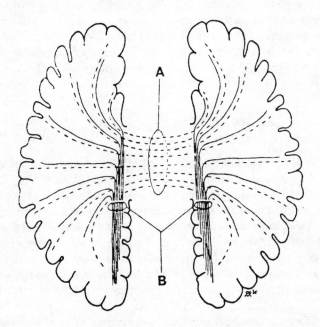

Figure 39.2   Failure of commissuration without agenesis of callosal fibres. The commissural fibres of corpus callosum (A) in a normal brain are shown by dashed lines. The abnormal longitudinal bundles ('Balkenlängsbündels' of Probst) (B) consist of normal callosal fibres which failed to cross in 'agenesis' of corpus callosum (solid lines) (After Rakic and Yakovlev, 1972)

We believe that support for the interpretation that the Probst bundle as an aberrant corpus callosum comes from observations of cases with a subtotal callosal aplasia. We have chosen two cases from our series:

(1) A 9-year-old boy (no. 208-77)
    Clinical diagnosis: Idiocy and epilepsy.

The autopsy of the brain showed a microcephaly. A most important finding was the absence of the body and splenium of the corpus callosum, with hypertrophy of the anterior commissure and of the massa intermedia. In the cingulate gyrus the abnormal, radially orientated convolutions were present (corresponding with a 'foetal' arrangement of the medial gyri). In the coronal section of the frontal lobe the corpus callosum and a short septum were visible. The septum was normally attached to the septal peduncle.

In a section through the anterior commissure the picture was different. A prominent bundle of myelinated fibres (under the cingulum) was visible, derived anatomically from the callosum at the frontal pole. An oblique lamina corresponding with the laterally displaced lamina septi connected the bundle with the laterally displaced fornix, which is analogous with the acallosal brain. These longitudinal bundles reached their largest diameter as they extended caudally.

As the development of the corpus callosum during ontogeny is rostrocaudal, then we believe this case of partial 'agenesis' is an example of arrested normal development. During the later foetal period, subsequent growth of the callosal fibres was misdirected. In this particular case the cause of the interference with normal development cannot be identified. This, however, need not always be the case.

The next case of our series shows the causal development of the Probst bundle more clearly.

(2) A 3-year-old girl (no. 156-76);
    Clinical diagnosis: Imbecility and epilepsy.

An agenesis of the posterior part of the callosum was found. The acallosal part of the brain originated at the location of a lipoma (5 mm in diameter).

Anatomical examination showed a hypoplastic and atrophic corpus callosum with the fornix attached normally to the callosum. There was an asymmetry of the basal ganglia and of the internal capsules. The third ventricle was dilated and showed an abnormal configuration. Under the right cingulum the lipoma was visible. The interhemispheric connections of the corpus callosum were disrupted posterior to the lipoma. The anatomical disruption of the callosal body was accompanied by degenerative processes of the myelin, which strongly suggests that the interruption of the callosal fibres was a secondary feature and was due to the presence of the tumour. Thereafter the fibres continued caudally, and both anatomically and histologically corresponded with the bundles of Probst. No signs of degeneration on the periphery of these bundles was seen. We believe that in this case the congenital lipoma hindered the interhemispheric development of the corpus callosum during the late foetal period and led to the heterotopia, closely related to the bundle of Probst.

In conclusion, we agree with Yakovlev, that the so-called longitudinal bundle of Probst is a heterotopic corpus callosum. Furthermore, in the majority of cases of so-called acallosal brains in which the Probst bundle is found, we believe that it is due to the failure of commissuration of the callosal fibres, and not because a 'true' agenesis has taken place.

REFERENCES

King, L. S. (1936). Hereditary defects of the corpus callosum. *J. comp. Neurol.,* **64,** 337-63

Probst, M. (1901). Über den Bau des Vollständigen Balkenlosen Groszhirns sowie über Heterotopie der grauen Substanz. *Archs Psychiat.,* **34,** 709-86

Rakic, P. and Yakovlev, P. I. (1968). Development of the corpus callosum and the cavum septi in man. *J. comp. Neurol.*, **132**, 45–72

Rogalski, J. (1924). *Wrodony Brak Spoidla Wielkiego*, Krakow.

Stefanko, S. (1960). A case of congenital agenesis of the corpus callosum. *Patologia Polska*, **11**, 275–84

Vogt, H. (1905). Über Balkenmangel im Menschlichen Gehirn. *J. Psychol. Neurol., Lpz.*, **5**, 1–17

AUTHOR INDEX

SUBJECT INDEX